ADDICTION AND CHANGE

Addiction and Change

*How Addictions Develop
and Addicted People Recover*

Carlo C. DiClemente

THE GUILFORD PRESS
New York   London

© 2003 The Guilford Press
A Division of Guilford Publications, Inc.
72 Spring Street, New York, NY 10012
www.guilford.com

Printed in the United States of America

This book is printed on acid-free paper.

Last digit is print number: 9 8 7 6 5 4 3 2 1

Library of Congress Cataloging-in-Publication Data

DiClemente, Carlo C.
   Addiction and change: how addictions develop and addicted people
recover / Carlo C. DiClemente
          p. cm. — (Guilford substance abuse series)
Includes bibliographical references and index.
      ISBN 1-57230-057-4 (alk. paper)
   1. Addicts—Rehabilitation. 2. Substance abuse—Treatment. I. Title.
II. Series.
RC564.D535 2003
616.86′03—dc21   2002015477

To
Albert and Rose
Lyn
Cara and Anna

About the Author

Carlo C. DiClemente, PhD, is Professor and Chair of the Department of Psychology at the University of Maryland, Baltimore County. He received his MA in Psychology at the New School for Social Research and his PhD in Psychology at the University of Rhode Island. Dr. DiClemente is the codeveloper with Dr. James Prochaska of the Transtheoretical Model (TTM) of behavior change. He is the author of numerous scientific articles and book chapters on motivation and behavior change and the application of the TTM to a variety of problem behaviors. Dr. DiClemente is coauthor of a self-help book based on this model of change—*Changing for Good*—and several professional books—*The Transtheoretical Approach: Crossing Traditional Boundaries of Therapy, Substance Abuse Treatment and the Stages of Change: Selecting and Planning Interventions*, and *Group Treatment for Substance Abuse: A Stages-of-Change Therapy Manual*. For the past 20 years, he has conducted funded research in health and addictive behaviors. He has directed an outpatient alcoholism treatment program and serves as a consultant to private and public treatment programs. Dr. DiClemente was recently given the 2002 Distinguished Contribution to Scientific Psychology award by the Maryland Psychological Association and was one of five winners of the 2002 Innovators Combating Substance Abuse award given by the Robert Wood Johnson Foundation.

Preface

How a society views individuals who engage in addictive behaviors has an important influence on addiction and recovery from addiction. If addiction is seen as a moral failing, it will be condemned. If seen as a deficit in knowledge, it will be educated. If the addiction is viewed as an acceptable aberration, it will be tolerated. If the addiction is considered illegal, it will be prosecuted. If viewed as an illness, it will be treated. Social policies mirror these different views with strategies ranging from prohibition and criminalization to hospitalization and mandated treatment.

The United States has used an economic view of supply and demand with which to frame its policies. However, supply reduction has coexisted uneasily with demand reduction, and interdiction with treatment. For many policymakers addiction is viewed predominantly as a legal problem, and so interdiction and zero tolerance are considered the appropriate policies. Increasingly, then, the major responsibility for managing addictive behaviors and addicted individuals is given to the police, the courts, and the legal system. At the same time, there are a number of illness-oriented policymakers who see addictions as social epidemics or chronic medical or psychological conditions. They, along with the treatment community, promote policies to provide interventions to assist the individual addict and reduce the harm from addictions on society.

There are serious shortcomings in current perspectives and the efforts at interdiction, prevention, criminalization, and treatment that they support. Interdiction and elimination of the supply feeding addictive behaviors appear impossible as long as the demand from current and new consumers remains high. Attitudes about legal and illegal addictions vary significantly, causing confusion in messages and approaches to addiction and recovery. Punishment has become closely linked to treatment, mixing external pressure with internal motivation that often increases attendance at treatment programs but makes personal recovery more challenging. Attempts to reduce harm for addicted individuals are often banned because they are seen as supporting addictions. Inconsistencies in attitudes and approaches toward addictions abound. The reality is that it is difficult to balance concern for the individual who becomes addicted and the welfare of the society and its other citizens. Many in the political, legal, prevention, and treatment systems believe that new approaches are needed.

This volume offers such a new approach in the form of an alternative, integrative perspective for understanding addiction and recovery. My premise is that addiction and recovery should be viewed as a process of behavior change. Research colleagues and I have followed thousands of individuals, examining how they become addicted and recover. In that research it is clear that addictions are not static states turned off and on with a switch. Addictions are multidetermined and take hold over time. There is a path to experimentation and through casual use to abuse and dependence. Recovery is also a journey that takes time and effort and is often filled with false starts and failed attempts. While the factors that lead a particular individual into addiction and out of it are unique to that individual, the process of becoming addicted and of recovery follow a common path. The path is also common across individuals and across addictive behaviors. In this volume I want to illuminate that common path and illustrate how multiple factors and experiences can influence an individual's movement along that path. More specifically, this book isolates important dimensions of the process of change involved in starting and stopping an addictive behavior; it highlights similarities in the process across addictions; and it sees both addiction and recovery in a larger life context. When viewed as a process of behavior change, addictions can be managed more effectively.

This book views addiction through the dimensions of the Transtheoretical Model (TTM) of intentional behavior change that James Prochaska and I have been refining in research and writings over the past 20 years. The TTM emerged from our seminal research examining how smokers were able to free themselves from their nicotine addiction and has been primarily applied to recovery from addictions. Although the model as described here is similar to descriptions in prior works, this is the first time I offer as complete, detailed, and precise a version. This book is also the first full application of the model to the process of becoming addicted. Other specific adaptations and changes to the model presented in this book include the following: a detailed explanation of the tasks for each stage of change and illustrations of how the stages and processes of change interact to produce movement through the stages of addiction and the stages of recovery. I have incorporated an extensive consideration of the context of change and how issues in multiple areas of life functioning interact with addiction and recovery to both help and hinder change. I hope the views offered in this volume will empower communities and enrich programs and policies to prevent addiction and promote recovery.

This book is organized into four parts. Part I introduces addiction and recovery as a process of change. It begins in Chapter 1 with a brief review of perspectives that have been used to understand addictions over the past 100 years, highlighting their insights and blind spots. These different models point to biological, psychological, and social influences and attempt to understand how risk and protective factors create addiction or promote recovery. Some are unsatisfactorily one-dimensional. Many are multidimensional but fail to explain how diverse dimensions interact over time to produce addiction or recovery. Most are rather static in how they see addictions start or stop and offer a limited view of the path into and out of addictions. Chapter 2 describes our current understanding of the process of behavior change as embodied in the TTM. This dynamic, developmental, and multidimensional change perspective offers an integrative framework for understanding change and the problems of addiction and recovery. The stages of change highlight the specific tasks of Contemplation, Preparation, Action, and Maintenance that mark the individual's progress toward addiction and the addicted person's pathway to recovery. Ten *processes* of change derived from different behavior change theories describe key mechanisms that move individuals through the stages. Five areas of functioning comprise the *context* of change that contain the risk and protective factors, resources, and barriers that influence process activity and movement through the stages. Finally, critical *markers* of change track an individual's decisional balance and self-efficacy/temptation as he or she moves through the stages of change. This multidimensional, integrative TTM offers a panoramic view of addiction and recovery. In Chapter 3, Part I concludes with a description of the fully developed, established addiction that represents the final stage in the path to addiction and, at the same time, the starting point of the stages of recovery.

Part II, comprising Chapters 4 and 5, goes back to the beginning and describes the road to addiction. I propose that a similar process and the same TTM dimensions mark the path to addiction as they do for recovery. Stages in the process of becoming addicted include moving out of Precontemplation for engaging in an addictive behavior and into serious consideration and experimentation with that behavior, then to preparing to engage regularly, and finally to developing a regular, problematic pattern of engagement. Stage transitions that lead to addiction also involve shifts in the processes and markers of change as well as in contextual risk and protective factors. The end point of these stages of addiction is the well-maintained addiction described in Chapter 3.

Part III describes in detail each of the stages of recovery from an addiction. Clearly, once an individual has achieved a "well-maintained addiction," the challenge lies in how to free oneself from this state. Chapters 6–10 describe each stage of recovery, discuss critical goals and tasks of each stage, and outline how the change dimensions of the TTM interact in the transition from one stage to the next. Stable maintained recovery, the opposite of the well-maintained addiction, represents the end point of recovery and the end of this section.

By linking these stages of addiction to the stages of recovery we can examine the entire journey of addicted individuals from their first steps toward the addiction through their struggle to free themselves and their path to successful recovery. This panoramic view of the process of change offers a detailed, dynamic, integrative framework with which to understand prevention and treatment. In Part IV, Chapters 11 and 12 examine the implications of a change process perspective for preventing addiction and promoting recovery. Innovative approaches are needed that target prevention efforts to interfere with the process of becoming addicted. Moreover, when communities, families, and treatment programs are aware of the path of recovery, they can better assist addicted individuals as they cycle and recycle through the stages of recovery.

Although we have learned a great deal about the biological, psychological, and social factors that influence addiction and recovery, there are still many interesting, challenging, and exciting questions to answer concerning the interaction and integration of these factors. The book concludes with Chapter 13, "Research on Addiction and Change." Bringing together the problem of addiction with the process of change creates a synergy that can enliven research and enlighten evaluation so both tell us much more about how individuals become enslaved by addictions and how they find their way to recovery.

It is my hope that this book will be useful to all who deal with addictions, especially treatment providers, prevention specialists, researchers, and policymakers. Examples and descriptions offer insights into a variety of addictive behaviors, including smoking and nicotine addiction, alcohol abuse and dependence, legal and illegal drugs of abuse, gambling, and eating disorders. Prevention and treatment specialists from many different disciplines that deal with addictions will find information and insights to enrich their work. Researchers in these areas will discover a wealth of new ideas and concepts to examine and a more detailed view of the process of addiction and recovery. Policymakers, service provision organizations, and funding agencies and foundations will find views that challenge current practices and argue for a more complex and extensive view of addiction. Understanding the challenges and goals of each stage will enable them to offer assistance and develop policies and programs that mirror the process of change. The ultimate goal of this book is to assist professionals to help individuals to move out of the path leading to addiction and to help those already addicted along the road to recovery.

Note: Descriptions of all the case and case examples in this volume represent fictional individuals. Although my experiences are represented in each of these examples, they do not represent any one individual, and in all cases significant descriptors have been altered so as to avoid any connections to patients I have seen.

Acknowledgments

The ideas and dimensions described in this book are the result of years of collaborative thinking and research that have involved hundreds of colleagues, research assistants, and graduate students, and thousands of clients, patients, and research volunteers. Although it is impossible to name them all, I want to thank each of them for their contribution to my understanding of addiction and the process of change.

My views of the process of change were initially developed and refined in a wonderful, collaborative synergy with my colleague and friend James Prochaska. Jim's intellect, energy, and enthusiasm have made our collaboration rich and productive from our initial working together at the University of Rhode Island through the 10 or so years of coordinated, multisite research. Our discussions about the research and the model that have taken place by ocean and pool and in conference and family rooms have truly been a peak experience in my life. Our thoughts and contributions blended to create the Transtheoretical Model (TTM). I acknowledge his contribution to the concepts and thoughts in this volume and am proud to have our names linked as developers of the model. However, I take responsibility for the description of the TTM of change in this work and for any limitations or problems in presenting these ideas.

The research and writings that examined and refined the TTM have been accomplished with the collaboration and contribution of many colleagues. Wayne Velicer, John Norcross, Joe Rossi, Ellie McConnaughy, Joe Fava, and a great group of investigators and graduate students at the University of Rhode Island have been involved in much of the seminal work. I was fortunate to have colleagues at the Texas Research Institute of Mental Sciences who also supported my research. I want to thank in particular Dr. Jack Gordon, who helped me open the first alcoholism treatment clinic that used the TTM as its guiding framework, and the many individuals who accompanied us on that journey. I also want to

thank colleagues at the University of Texas School of Public Health and
M. D. Anderson Hospital, who collaborated in a variety of research projects examining various dimensions of change with addictive behaviors,
especially Patricia Dolan-Mullen. I continue my good fortune in finding
creative collaborators in Maryland and around the country who have
joined with me to design research and produce publications that examine the process of change, including Alan Bellack, Maureen Black,
Melanie Gold, Steve Havas, Bankole Johnson, Carl Soderstram, and
Chudley Werch. The experience of being an investigator on Project
MATCH also contributed greatly to refining ideas and providing data
that were instrumental in gaining a better understanding of the change
process in recovery from alcoholism. The colleagues involved in this project are a very special group of professionals who represent the most
productive and best scientific collaboration I have ever experienced. I am
appreciative of all their support. Several of them have worked closely
with me exploring motivation and the dimensions of the TTM and de-
serve special thanks, including Gerard Connors, Dennis Donovan, Bill
Miller, and Allan Zweben. Gerard and Dennis recently have worked
with me on a book that describes how the stages model can be used in
planning substance abuse treatment. Finally, I want to thank my many
colleagues and friends at the Texas Research Institute of Mental Sciences
(TRIMS), the University of Texas Medical School, the University of
Houston, and now at the University of Maryland, Baltimore County
(UMBC), for their many years of support for my work.

I met Mary Velasquez in my days at TRIMS, where she volunteered
on one of my first research projects. She has been a wonderful collabora-
tor and helped coordinate much of the Houston research on the model.
Now a colleague at the University of Texas Department of Family Medicine, she continues to extend and promote the use of the model with addictions and other health problems by providing workshops and developing innovative research. Her most recent contribution is the group
treatment manual for substance abuse based on the stages and processes
of change. I am grateful for her dedication, support, and long-standing
friendship.

When I moved to the University of Houston I was very fortunate to
have Joe Carbonari join with me to develop the alcohol-focused measures and to provide the statistical sophistication to evaluate many complex questions about the process of change. Together with many students and staff at the Change Assessment Research Program, we worked
together on Project MATCH and many other research endeavors. He
has contributed valuable insights and analyses in the search for understanding addiction and change.

From the very beginnings of my research on the TTM at TRIMS to today, I have been blessed with graduate and undergraduate research assistants who have contributed lots of hard work as well as insights, challenges, and significant support. Although they are too numerous to name, I want to thank them for their help. In their theses and dissertations, graduate students at the University of Houston and UMBC have explored many questions about the process of change and addiction. I want to mention those who have been involved most directly in research that examined aspects of addiction and change. At the University of Houston in the Change Assessment Research Program there were Scott Fairhurst, Amy Grossman, Sheryl Hughes, Elizabeth O'Connor, Nancy Piotrowski, Alaina Suris, Angie Stotts, Catherine Perz, Tom Irwin, Teresa King, Jennifer Rothfleisch, Ken Sewell, David Pena, Rosario Montgomery, Kelly Wright, and Kirk Von Sternberg. At UMBC in the HABITS laboratory I have a wonderful group of graduate students who also are contributing to our knowledge of addiction and change, including Rebecca Lee, Jill Daniels Walker, Deborah King, Lori Bellino, Hildi Hagedorn, Nancy Haug, Angela Marinilli, Manu Singh, Shannon Whyte, Amanda Keevican, Janine Delahanty, Melissa Nidecker, Jennifer Malson, Leigh Winsko Gemell, and Deb Schlundt. There is a saying that good graduate students are worth their weight in gold. If that is true, I am a very rich man.

The research that I have done to develop my understanding of addictions and the process of change could not have been accomplished without two key ingredients, money and participants. I want to thank the National Cancer Institute (NCI), National Institute of Alcohol Abuse and Alcoholism (NIAAA), National Institute of Drug Abuse (NIDA), and National Heart, Lung and Blood Institute (NHLBI), as well as the Centers for Disease Control and Prevention (CDC), the Centers for Substance Abuse Treatment and Prevention (CSAT; CSAP), and the Robert Wood Johnson Foundation for funding research and dissemination projects related to the TTM. I also want to thank the many research participants who took the time and made the effort to participate in the research while they were on their journeys to and from addiction. I am constantly intrigued by their paths into addiction and inspired by their stories of recovery.

I am grateful to the many individuals around the world who have used the TTM in their research and clinical practice and have shared their ideas and findings with me and in their professional publications. I also want to thank the many nameless reviewers of grant applications and professional publications. The questions they asked and problems they pointed out have clarified and enriched my thinking and writing about the model.

Finally, I would like to thank Barbara Watkins, my editor at The

Guilford Press. She has been wonderfully patient and encouraging throughout the multiple drafts of this volume. Her feedback has been invaluable. She took the time to understand the ideas I was trying to communicate, which made her insights, edits, and comments tremendously helpful. She pared redundancy, assisted in clarity of expression, and guided the organization of this work. I am grateful for the sharpness of her thinking, her ability to see the forest when I was getting lost in the trees, and the incredible amount of time she dedicated to this project. She has my respect and gratitude for all she contributed.

Throughout my life journey and my work on this book I have had wonderful support and encouragement from my parents, family, and friends. I want to thank all of them, and particularly my father, mother, brothers, and sisters for their caring and closeness. My wife, Lyn, and my daughters, Cara and Anna, have had to bear the main burden that this work and the many years of revisions took in terms of days and evenings away from the family and times of frustration and stress. I am grateful to them for their love and comfort, their understanding and sacrifices.

Contents

PART IV. DESIGNING INTERVENTIONS TO MATCH THE PROCESS OF CHANGE

Part I

UNDERSTANDING ADDICTIONS IN TERMS OF CHANGE

Chapter 1

Models of Addiction and Change

A theoretical perspective provides a useful heuristic to advance our knowledge of any phenomenon and our ability to influence its existence, development, and growth.

Addictions have plagued society throughout history, as is evident from the Greco-Roman philosophers' call for moderation and condemnation of bacchanalian excesses to our 21st-century preoccupation with alcohol, drugs, food, and gambling. Explanations for addiction often have consisted in blaming individuals for their excessive engagement in these behaviors. Scientific theories and models for explaining and understanding addictions have existed for only the past 100 years. Although our explanations have become more sophisticated, our understanding of addiction is far from complete.

WHAT IS AN ADDICTION?

Traditionally, the term *addiction* has been used to identify self-destructive behaviors that include a pharmacological component. The most stringent application would limit the term addiction and the companion label of *addict* to individuals with a *physiological* dependence on one or more *illegal* drugs. This definition usually includes a strong physiological craving, withdrawal symptoms, and the need for more of the drug to get the same effect (American Psychiatric Association, 1980). In the strictest application of this definition, heroin, marijuana, cocaine and nonprescribed barbiturates and sedative–hypnotics would be the only addictions, because their use is illegal and they meet the definition of physiological dependence. However, within the last 20 years the scope of the term addiction has expanded to include any substance use or reinforcing behavior that has an appetitive nature, has a compulsive and repetitive quality, is self-destructive, and is experienced as difficult to modify or stop (Orford, 1985). Expanded use of the term addiction includes problematic relationships, excessive work behaviors, and even what some are calling *positive addictions* (e.g., exercise, meditation). Treatment professionals, addicts, and the general public are confused by the shifting scope of meaning for the term. Moreover, among scientists and practitioners in the field there is real concern about the continuing expansion of the application of the term. If what is labeled addiction becomes too broad, the word addiction will become devoid of meaning. However, a broader range of behaviors labeled as addictions would be justified if common features exist across a similar set of behaviors that increase our ability to understand addictive problems and expand society's capacity to intervene.

The definition of addiction used in this volume is purposefully broad and can include an array of behaviors without making every human problem or pathology an addiction. In this book addictions are understood as learned habits that once established become difficult to extinguish even in the face of dramatic, and, at times, numerous negative consequences. The critical dimensions for an addiction are (1) the development of a solidly established, problematic pattern of an appetitive—that is, pleasurable and reinforcing—behavior, (2) the presence of physiological and psychological components of the behavior pattern that create dependence, and (3) the interaction of these components in the life of the individual that make the behavior resistant to change. Each of these aspects is critical for identifying an addiction. Addictive behavior patterns are repeated and become predictable in their regularity and excess. Dependence is the second necessary and critical dimension to define addiction. The term *dependence* indicates that the pattern of behavior involves poor self-regulatory control, continues despite negative feedback, and often appears to be out of control. Moreover, reinforcers for engaging in this behavior become very strong. Often the addiction becomes prepotent in the life of the individual and an integral part of the individual's way of life and coping. Reinforcers are both physiological and psychological and combine to create a very powerful reward system that clouds awareness of problematic consequences related to the behavior and makes change difficult and, at times, seemingly impossible. In fact, failure to change, despite the outward appearance that change would be both possible and in the best interest of the individual, is considered a cardinal characteristic in defining addictions (American Psychiatric Association, 1994). In my view, change is the antithesis of addiction. The polarities of change and addiction, then, can be viewed as central themes for understanding how people become addicted and how they can free themselves from an addiction.

This definition of addiction is broad but not so broad as to become meaningless. Most psychological and psychiatric problems are not appetitive in nature, that is, activities that are engaged in because of their inherent pleasurable and reinforcing effects. Moreover, most disorders do not require engaging in repetitive, intentional behaviors in order to become established as a problem. For example, there is nothing inherently pleasurable in a psychotic break or a depressive episode. Nor do these chronic psychiatric conditions require that the individual engage in some purposeful activities in order to create these disorders. Addiction should not be used to describe most psychopathology. However, the scope of appetitive behaviors that become destructive and difficult to stop can include problematic behavior patterns related to eating, sex, drugs, and money. Habits most clearly associated with addiction include tobacco dependence, alcohol abuse and dependence, substance abuse, a range of eating disorders (including obesity and bulimia), as well as compulsive gambling (National Academy of Sciences, 1999). The clear similarities across these behaviors, which in their excessive forms are labeled addictions, include the following elements:

1. They represent habitual patterns of intentional, appetitive behaviors.
2. They can become excessive and produce serious consequences.
3. There is stability of these problematic behavior patterns over time.
4. There are interrelated psychological and physiological components to the behavior.
5. Finally, in every case individuals who become addicted to these behaviors have difficulty stopping or modifying them.

These elements represent the essential criteria used to diagnose an addiction (American Psychiatric Association, 1994).

The central defining elements of addictive behaviors involve the compulsive and out of control nature of current behavior patterns and the level of difficulty encountered in changing them. However, most traditional models for understanding addictions have concentrated on etiology and understanding the origins of these behaviors, rather than on how to change them (U.S. Department of Health and Human Services, 1980). The thinking behind this emphasis on etiology reflects a belief that the best way to understand and, ultimately, to change addictions is to understand why and how they began. In most disease models, understanding etiology is critical because it often uncovers the source of the problem—a virus or a contaminated environment and a mode of transmission—which when attacked or resolved leads to the eradication of the problem. However, when it comes to addictions, single-cause etiological models have been woefully inadequate to explain either adoption or cessation of addictive behaviors (Donovan & Marlatt, 1988; Glantz & Pickens, 1992).

There was a wonderful poster produced by the National Institute on Alcohol Abuse and Alcoholism in the late 1970s. The title read "The Typical Alcoholic American." Pictured were over 20 individuals who differed by age, race, occupation, and socioeconomic status and included an American Indian, doctor, housewife, elderly female, construction worker, and many others. Clearly, the point was that there is no typical alcoholic and that stereotypes need to be discarded to adequately address alcohol problems. Understanding addiction requires complex models to explain the diversity as well as the similarities among individuals who exhibit the addictive behaviors and who become addicted. If complexity were required for understanding any single addictive behavior, like alcohol, it would be even more important when examining multiple addictive behaviors, wherein heterogeneity among people and types of behaviors will be even greater. Any search for similarities and commonalties must account for the diversity and heterogeneity of the individuals who become addicted and also must respect the distinct and specific nature of each of the addictive behaviors.

TRADITIONAL MODELS
FOR UNDERSTANDING ADDICTION

Many different theories and models of addiction have been proposed. Several broad categories can be used to summarize these models. The most prominent explanatory models include (1) social/environment models, (2) genetic/physiological models, (3) personality/intrapsychic models, (4) coping/social learning models, (5) conditioning/reinforcement behavioral models, (6) compulsive/excessive behavior models, and, finally, (7) an integrative biopsychosocial model. Each of the models proposes a way of understanding addiction or a specific addictive behavior that focuses primarily on how addictions develop. Then, based on this etiology, the models propose suggestions for prevention and cessation as well as for intervention and treatment (Brownell & Fairburn, 2002; Leonard & Blane, 1999; Rotgers, Keller, & Morgenstern, 1996; U.S. Department of Health and Human Services, 1980). The following review of these explanations, although brief and cursory in comparison to the more extensive discussions offered in the previously cited books and monographs, will highlight strengths and weaknesses of each type of model in summary fashion. Supportive facts and interesting anomalies highlighted in the review will make the case for a more integrative model based on the process of human intentional behavior change.

Social/Environment Models

The social/environment perspective emphasizes the role of societal influences, peer pressure, social policies, availability, and family systems as mechanisms responsible for the adoption and maintenance of addictions. Certain types of drug use and individual addictive behaviors occur more frequently in some subgroups. This has encouraged researchers to examine subcultures related to drug use (Johnson, 1980) and to explore the importance of environmental-contextual influences in the search for risk and protective factors (Clayton, 1992). Patterns related to specific drug-use behavior support interesting, well-defined sociocultural connections (Connors & Tarbox, 1985; McCarty, 1985).

Social influence and support are often evident in the social context for use. Cocaine use has spawned the "crackhouse" where cocaine addicts gather; heroin addicts have created their "shooting galleries"; inhalant abuse often is concentrated among Hispanic youth. These phenomena, along with the fact that drug users and abusers often have more family and friends who use drugs, make a clear case for the importance of social context in the acquisition of addictive behaviors (Jessor & Jessor, 1980). In addition, conformity to some social norms as well as deviance from others are offered by some investigators as explanations for addictions (Kaplan & Johnson, 1992). Illegal drug use, abuse, and dependence are viewed as deviant behaviors in many sociological models (Robins, 1974, 1979). Deviance then becomes an underlying cause while the particular addictive behavior may reflect a response to the social context of peers (Lukoff, 1980). Research with Vietnam veterans demonstrated that higher preservice deviant behavior predicted initiation of heroin use (Robins, Helzer, & Davis, 1975) and is consistent with data that shows a history of delinquency prior to onset of heroin use among heroin-dependent individuals (Glantz & Pickens, 1992). However, the enormous increase in marijuana use in the 1960s demonstrated that as use spreads across the population it becomes harder and harder to use deviance as an explanation for use or dependence (Robins, 1980). Moreover, social norms and deviance explanations are more difficult to use as the sole explanation for alcohol dependence, nicotine addiction, gambling and eating disorders.

Additional support for the social/environment perspective comes from data indicating that availability and social policies, such as restrictions in use and taxation, influence use and abuse of certain substances. Policies restricting cigarette smoking and advertising have made important contributions to the declining rate of cigarette consumption in the United States (Biener, Aseltine, Cohen, & Anderka, 1998; U.S. Department of Health and Human Services, 1990, 1993). Changing the legal age for consumption of alcoholic beverages has influenced use and abuse of alcohol (Connors & Tarbox, 1985). Macro-environmental influences also play an important role in the initiation and cessation of other addictions (Connors & Tarbox, 1985; Institute of Medicine, 1990; Schinke, Botvin, & Orlandi, 1991; U.S. Department of Health and Human Services, 1997). These explanations are certainly more feasible when the substances and behaviors are legal than when they are already considered illegal and banned in the society.

Some proponents of the social/environment models have concentrated on the more intimate environment of family influences as a central factor contributing to the onset of addictive behaviors. Family influences support both a genetic, nature-based pathway of influence and a family interaction or family system, nurture-based path (Merikangas, Rounsaville, & Prusoff, 1992; Sher, 1993). Advocates of family explanations point to problematic parental modeling of adult roles that can include difficulties with relationships, conflicted and broken marriages, and excessive use of alcohol and other drugs on the part of the parents as important influences on the child's experimenting with and continuing an addictive behavior (Chassin, Curran, Hussong, & Colder, 1996; Jessor & Jessor, 1977; Kandel & Davies, 1992; Stanton, 1980). Steinglass, Bennett, Wolin, and Reiss (1987) have proposed a more indirect route of transmission of alcohol problems through the child's adoption or rejection of family rituals and traditions. Stanton (Stanton, Todd, & Associates, 1982) and others (O'Farrell & Fal-Stewart, 1999) have indicated that family system interactions can be responsible for one or more family members engaging in addictive behaviors as a result of the roles that are adopted to keep the system functioning. The idea is that family homeostasis acts as a regulatory structure in which the deviate addictive behavior plays an important role in individual and family functioning. This explanation has been used with alcohol problems, and particularly in discussions about eating disorders and anorexia (Minuchin, 1974; Minuchin, Rosman, & Baker, 1978; Selvini-Palazzoli, 1974). Proponents of a family influence model differ dramatically on the amount of influence attributable to family genetic factors as opposed to family psychosocial factors (Cadoret, 1992; Crabbe, McSwigan, & Belnap, 1985; Merikangas et al., 1992).

The social/environment perspective has many advocates. Proponents have presented substantial evidence for the role of social and environmental factors in the adoption of various addictive behaviors. However, as Robins (1980) points out, a natural history of drug abuse can only describe the current historical perspective. His description was of the 1970s drug-use era. Drug use and abuse, including alcohol consumption, was very different in the 1920s and appears to have substantially changed again by the end of the 1990s. Social influences and trends shift, as do the popularity of different types of addictive behaviors. Shifting social trends in addictions argue for an important role for social and environmental influences, while at the same time clearly offering evidence against viewing the social/environment perspective as a fixed explanation for all addiction at all historical points in time. It is also clear that even when there are substantial trends or social influences facilitating the development or cessation of a certain behavior, a large number of individuals do not follow those trends. Of the two inhalant drug abusers that I first saw in treatment, one was a southern White male in his 20s, the other a Hispanic teen. The latter fit the stereotype of an inhalant abuser in Texas, the former did not. Social and environmental influences clearly make a contribution both in the acquisition and cessation of addictions at a population level but often fail to explain in any comprehensive manner individual initiation or cessation.

Genetic/Physiological Models

The most convincing information concerning the role of genetics in addictions is available in the area of alcohol abuse and dependence. Family studies indicate increasing risk ratios for individuals as the number of alcoholic relatives rises and as the number and severity of familial alcohol problems rise (Shuckit, 1980, 1995; Shuckit, Goodwin, & Winokur, 1972). Twin studies as well as in-depth assessments of children of alcoholics seem to support the importance of genetics as a contributing factor to alcoholism (Hesselbrock, Hesselbrock, & Epstein, 1999). Although the role of genetics for other drugs of abuse is not always so clear, most scientists acknowledge a genetic influence on susceptibility to substance abuse (Crabbe et al., 1985; Hesselbrock et al., 1999). The National Institute on Alcohol Abuse and Alcoholism (NIAAA) is conducting several large-scale collaborative trials to investigate the possible mechanisms of genetic influence. However, it is clear that the search is not for a single "alcoholism gene" and that the solution will be polygenetic and complex (Begleiter & Porjesz, 1999; Gordis, 2000; Johnson, Van den Bree, Uhl, & Pickens, 1996; McGue et al., 1992).

For a long time physical dependence and addiction were understood as synonymous. Traditional markers to define drug dependence were both tolerance—the need for more of a substance to achieve the same effect—and a clear withdrawal syndrome, which included physical reactions like nausea and a craving for the substance. Proponents of the genetic/physiological explanation of addictions have used these physiological signs as critical indicators that addictions are biological entities and medical problems. However, not all drugs of abuse produce classic dependence syndromes of tolerance and withdrawal. Alcohol, nicotine, and heroin seem to produce such physiological dependence, whereas cocaine, amphetamines, and hallucinogens do not appear to do so. The latest revision of the *Diagnostic and Statistical Manual of Mental Disorders* (DSM-IV) of the American Psychiatric Association (1994) changed the definitions of drug abuse and dependence so that this distinction between abuse and dependence based solely on physiological tolerance was practically eliminated. However, the physiological component remains an important one in addictive behaviors, particularly as related to the ingestion of a psychoactive substance. There have been enormous advances in our understanding of the neurobiology of alcohol and drug addiction (Roberts & Koob, 1997). However, even for addictive behaviors that do not involve a substance such as gambling, it appears that the "rush" or "high" produced by the behavior is an important element (National Academy of Sciences, 1999). This physiological reaction and its potential for creating and reinforcing problematic patterns of behavior is often used as a reason for the inclusion of gambling under the rubric of addiction (McGurrin, 1992; Pickens, Elmer, LaBuda, & Uhl, 1996). However, physiological pathways are complicated and certainly not uniform in mechanism of action or type of involvement across addictive behaviors.

There are also some interesting anomalies that both support and challenge the genetic/physiological explanations of addictions. In the 1970s researchers became quite pessimistic about the prospect of getting smokers to quit and began to focus on developing a safer cigarette, one that did not contain nicotine. They attempted to create cigarettes using cabbage leaves and other organic materials. However, no one would smoke cigarettes that did not have the active nicotine effect! Similarly, methadone-maintained patients often lament the fact that it does not produce the "heroin high" that got them addicted, although it does help them avoid withdrawal. Clearly, physiological reactions to the ingestion of an active drug play an important role in the creation of some addictions. However, research studies also have produced visible alcohol or drug effects using placebos that contain no active substance. These studies appear to contradict a dominant role for physiology and argue for the importance of expectations or social context in contrast to the actual physical effect (Brown, Goldman, Inn, & Anderson, 1980; Collins,

Lapp, Emmons, & Isaac, 1990; Fromme & Dunn, 1992; Schulenberg, Wadsworth, O'Malley, Bachman, & Johnston, 1996; Southwick, Steele, Marlatt, & Lindell, 1981). In bar laboratory settings, many investigators have shown that drinkers will act as if they are intoxicated even when given simulated non-alcohol-containing drinks (Collins, Parks, & Marlatt, 1985; Goldman, Del Boca, & Darkes, 1999).

The physiological effects of tolerance and withdrawal as well as the movement away from an explanation of addiction as morally reprehensible behavior has led to addictions being understood within a medical model. This perspective has also been promoted in the materials describing the 12 steps and 12 traditions of AA that talk about the disease of alcoholism, which they liken to a chronic allergic reaction (Alcoholics Anonymous, 1952). Others believe that alcoholism is a disease that is not completely physiologically based (Miller & Kurtz, 1994; Sheehan & Owen, 1999). The disease model has been instrumental in shifting society's view of alcohol dependence from one of moral deviance and sinful behavior to one that promotes understanding and treatment. However, there are many criticisms of this use of a disease model for understanding alcoholism (Donovan & Marlatt, 1988; Miller & Rollnick, 1991). It is also interesting to note that proponents of the disease model for alcoholism will not always use the same explanation for drugs of abuse and have some difficulty when the concept is extended to behaviors like gambling.

For all addictive behaviors there appears to be a role for physiological mechanisms and, potentially, for genetic factors in the behavior's initiation, problematic long-term use, abuse, and dependence. However, there are many questions and concerns about assigning sole causality or primacy to genetic/physiological factors (Newlin, Miles, van den Bree, Gupman, & Pickens, 2000). Because so many different individuals can become addicted to so many different types of substances or behaviors, biological or genetic differences do not explain all the cultural, situational, and intrapersonal differences among addicted individuals and addictive behaviors (Cadoret, 1992).

Personality/Intrapsychic Models

Addictive behaviors have often been conceptualized as a symptom of more historical, intrapsychic conflicts, often labeled disorders of personality. Proponents of this perspective point to the frequent correspondence between drug abuse and a diagnosis of antisocial personality disorder or its predecessor, juvenile delinquency, as evidence of drugs being a symptom of a larger psychological problem (Robins, 1980; Weiss, 1992). The search for the alcoholic or prealcoholic personality has persisted for years, with mixed and unconvincing results (Cox, 1985, 1987; Nathan, 1988; Sutker & Allain, 1988). Some prealcoholic personality characteristics seem to be related to later alcohol dependence: impulsivity, nonconformity, antisocial behavior, independence, and hyperactivity (Cox, 1985; Hesselbrock et al., 1999). However, these relationships may be true more for male than female alcoholics and are not always present in every male alcoholic. In the related eating disorder arena the literature on anorexia nervosa often describes a typical adolescent female with serious issues regarding autonomy, control, and self-esteem (Cooper, 1995; Wonderlich, 1995). Psychoanalytic perspectives have characterized both alcoholics and persons with eating disorders as individuals who have had conflicts at the oral stage of psychosexual development and were fixated at this stage (Freud, 1949; Khantzian, 1980; Leeds & Morgenstern, 1995). Even the perspective of Alcoholics Anonymous describes a personality dimension when it calls alcoholism the result of a defect in character and a deficit of will (Alcoholics Anonymous, 1952; DiClemente, 1993a).

Many theorists explicitly state or implicitly believe that some internal mechanism or conflict drives what can be considered a "proneness" to addiction (Smart, 1980). Sometimes these conflicts can be the result of environmental problems but most often are seen as internally derived and leading to a dysphoric, meaningless life style (Greaves, 1980). Psychological dimensions, which can be conceptualized as temperaments or traits, have also been employed as predictors of addiction. Antisocial traits, low self-esteem, alienation, religiosity, and high novelty seeking, activity level, and emotionality have been identified as precursors or predictors of later addiction (Jessor & Jessor, 1980; Kaplan & Johnson, 1992; Pandina, Johnson, & Labouvie, 1992; Steffenhagen, 1980; Tarter, 1988; Wills, McNamara, Vaccaro, & Hirky, 1996). These traits are thought to produce the internal setting in the individual where availability or peer pressure can induce not only experimentation and use but also abuse and dependence.

Although it would seem logical to assume a role for internal personality dynamics in the addiction process, the evidence to date does not support the existence of an addictive personality that predictably and reliably will result in dependence on any or all of the addictive behaviors. There is a subgroup of "addicts" diagnosed with multiple drugs and other addictions who demonstrate a tendency to engage in multiple addictive behaviors (gambling, drug use, and alcohol dependence). This group would seem to be a prime location for discovering personality dynamics. However, there are individuals with similar traits or profiles who do not engage in any or all of these behaviors. As with the sociological and genetic factors described previously, personality factors appear to contribute to the development or establishment of an addictive behavior problem. However, personality factors or deep-seated intrapersonal conflicts do account for a possibly important but small part of the needed explanation for addiction (Nathan, 1988).

Coping/Social Learning Models

Often addictions are considered to be the result of poor or inadequate coping mechanisms. Unable to cope with life stresses, addicts turn to their addiction for escape or comfort. From this perspective, individuals use substances as alternative coping mechanisms and rely on their addictions to manage situations, particularly those that engender feelings of frustration, anger, anxiety, or depression (Wills & Shiffman, 1985). Appraisal-focused coping, problem-focused coping and emotion-focused coping are considered important domains of coping responses (Lazarus & Folkman, 1985; Moos, Finney, & Cronkite, 1990). One's ability to cope with stress—in particular, with anger, frustration, boredom, anxiety, and depression—has been identified as a critical deficit area in many theories or models of addiction (Pandina et al., 1992). In particular, emotion-focused coping has been identified as an important dimension. Alcohol, for example, has been viewed as addictive because of its tension reduction (Cappell & Greeley, 1987) or stress response dampening (Sher, 1987) effect. Because alcohol's effects on stress and tension are quicker and often more effective in dealing with a stressful event than other, natural coping responses, alcohol becomes the preferred, and possibly the only, coping mechanism.

The social learning perspective emphasizes social cognition and not simply coping. Bandura's social cognitive theory tends to focus more on cognitive expectancies, vicarious learning, and self-regulation as explanatory mechanisms for addictions (Bandura, 1986; DiClemente, Fairhurst, & Piotrowski, 1995; Maisto, Carey, & Bradizza, 1999). There is a growing literature focused on how expectations about the effects of a specific substance or addictive behavior are related to use, abuse, or excessive engagement. Alcohol expectancies have been found to be predictive of initiation of use and to the progression to problematic use (S. Brown, 1985; Connors, Maisto, & Dermen, 1992; Goldman, 1999). For example, individuals who believe that alcohol will make them more attractive, less inhibited, better lovers and more fun to be around would be more prone to use alcohol and to get in trouble with alcohol, particularly in social settings (Goldman et al., 1999).

The social learning perspective also emphasizes the role of peers and significant others as models. Advertisers who use sports figures to promote a product clearly employ social influence principles. Alcohol and cigarette promotions in baseball and football stadia offer more subtle examples of the power of modeling as an influence on substance use. The influence of expectancies is not limited to substances of abuse. The popularity of lotteries and the well-promoted big payoff to a lucky individual as well as our societal devotion to being thin play a clear role in promotion of gambling and eating disorders, respectively.

Coping and social learning perspectives have become quite popular among addiction researchers and clinicians. However, many successful businessmen and athletes who appear to have good general coping skills, or at least skills good enough to become successful in a competitive environment, get ensnared by addictive behaviors. Generalized poor coping cannot be the only reason individuals become addicted. That seems particularly true for people who engage in the behavior because of the positive enjoyment effects and not simply the relief of problematic emotions (Orford, 1985). However, even if coping defects are not the critical reason for the acquisition of addictive behaviors, one important consequence of addiction is a narrowing of the addicted individual's coping repertoire. Thus, coping responses may be more important as a way to remediate the consequences of an addiction than as a contributor to its acquisition (Shiffman & Wills, 1985; Schinke et al., 1991).

Conditioning/Reinforcement Models

There is a substantial body of research demonstrating the reinforcing properties of each substance of abuse (Barrett, 1985). Animal studies show that many of the same principles that define conventional reinforcers appear to operate in the ingestion of psychoactive drugs (Thompson & Pickens, 1972, cited in Barrett, 1985). Animal's responses in order to obtain psychoactive drugs seem to operate according to schedules of reinforcement (Barrett, 1985). Reinforcement theory seems an appropriate explanation for subtle physiological effects of substances as well as for the gross motor drug-seeking elements of addictive behaviors. The classic example of the power of reinforcement has been the slot machine; its variable-ratio reinforcement schedule creates a stable, hard-to-extinguish pattern of behavior. Reinforcement models have been used to understand the initiation of addictive behaviors as well as their stability, which makes them difficult to modify. Reinforcement models focus on the direct effects of the addictive behavior, such as tolerance, withdrawal, and other physiological responses/rewards, as well as the more indirect effects described in opponent process theory (Barrett, 1985; Solomon & Corbit, 1974). According to this latter theory, the appearance of an effect (dysphoria and withdrawal) that is opposite to the main effect sought by the user drives the continued use of that substance. Reinforcing effects appear to play an important role when addictive behaviors are viewed as goal-directed, operant behaviors. However, even proponents of this model describe drug taking and other addictive behaviors as complex, multidetermined behaviors (Barrett, 1985).

Many theories and theorists also have used Pavlovian conditioning to understand addiction. The ability of substances to produce tolerance and withdrawal effects in laboratory animals has been at the center of basic research on substance abuse. Demonstrating tolerance effects in animals set the stage for testing Pavlovian conditioning paradigms with these animals. It was not long before anticipatory drug-related behaviors could be linked to cues associated with the actual drug use. Situational cues could then elicit initial drug reactions and lead to "relapse" or resumption of the addictive behavior (Hinson, 1985). Several phenomena in the drug culture also support the important role of conditioning and cues in the acquisition of and recovery from addictive behaviors. The "needle high" of the heroin addict, who only needs to insert a needle with saline solution to get a partial replication of the actual drug-taking experience, supports a conditioning model, as do cocaine addicts who begin to sweat and get anxious at the sight of any bolus of a white substance, be it sugar or flour. In fact, many addictive behaviors seem to operate in a situation-specific manner. Travel to a gambling center like Las Vegas, Tahoe, or Atlantic City is often critical for compulsive gamblers. Many smokers have places or settings where they do not smoke. Certain types of food ("junk") or eating settings (home vs. restaurant) seem most related to eating disorders. Drinking behavior and bars are significantly linked. Situational cues and classical conditioning have an important role to play in understanding addiction and change.

More recently, classical conditioning approaches that originally focused only on physiological responses have been expanded to include cognitions and psychological mechanisms in the repertoire of cues and responses (Adesso, 1985; S. A. Brown, 1993; S. A. Brown, Goldman, & Christiansen, 1985). This has led to an integration of conditioning and social learning perspectives. For example, expectancy effects can vary in strength and magnitude depending on the presence of various cues. In fact, there is a growing body of evidence that shows that many behaviors thought to be direct effects of alcohol or drugs (e.g., increased aggression, disinhibition, etc.) can be produced by placebo doses in the right setting with the appropriate cognitive expectation (Collins et al., 1985).

There is substantive evidence for the role of conditioning and reinforcement effects in addictions. However, models that use only these two principles to explain acquisition and recovery appear to have difficulty explaining all the phenomena of addiction and change. Once addicted, even severe punishing consequences seem to be unable to suppress or extinguish the behavior. Even after long periods of abstinence, extinction appears problematic under certain conditions. For example, some women smokers stop smoking during pregnancy only to have the addiction reappear after the birth, despite 6–9 months of abstinence (Stotts, DiClemente, Carbonari, & Mullen, 1996). They appear able to suspend cigarette use at will across situations because of anticipated negative effects on the fetus. As with the previous models, the conditioning/reinforcement ones offer some insight, particularly into the creation of substance use problems and into the situational cues that can promote relapse after a quit attempt, but they do not explain all initiation or successful change (Marlatt & Gordon, 1985; Orford, 1985)

Compulsive/Excessive Behavior Models

The difficulty stopping or successfully modifying addictive behaviors and the overdetermined and repetitive nature of most addictions has led some theorists and practitioners to link addiction with ritualistic compulsive behaviors like repeated hand washing or cleaning rituals. The commonalties include the sense that the behavior is out of the control of the individual and appears to be trying to satisfy a psychological conflict or need. This same perspective can encompass both the compulsive and excessive types of models (Orford, 1985).

Those who compare addictions to compulsive behaviors most often come either from analytic perspectives, where addictions are seen as reflecting deep-seated psychological conflict, or from a biologically based view that compulsive behaviors represent a biochemical imbalance reflected in brain neurotransmitters. Proponents of the first explanation would envision the solution in terms of analysis or conflict resolution. Proponents of the latter would explore psychoactive pharmacological treatments to bring the addictive/compulsive behaviors under control. Although these views are similar to those described earlier under personality or physiological models, the compulsive behavior explanation seems to argue that the actual behavior, be it drug taking, eating, or alcohol consumption, is less important than the compulsive mechanism that somehow became attached to this behavior.

Orford (1985) has conceptualized addictions as excessive appetites. According to him, the appetitive nature of the behaviors or activities creates the potential for excess. Thus, eating, sexual activity, and gambling as well as alcohol and drug use share not only a potential for excess but also a similar process leading to excess. This process of moving to excess is described primarily as a psychological one, wherein the appetitive activities have many interactive determinants that are important in diverse areas of functioning and that become involved in a "developmental process of increasing attachment" best understood by a "balance-of-force social learning model" (pp. 319–321). Understanding both treatment and change of excessive behaviors would require personal cost–benefits analyses and a decision-making process as well as self-reconstitution.

Although the compulsive and excessive behavior models share a number of common explanatory components, they can differ dramatically in their suggested cures or treatments. Once again, the connection between the addictive behavior and the psychological functioning of the individual appears highlighted in this perspective as in the personality/intrapsychic models. However, the compulsive model seems to disregard the unique contribution of the various types of possible addictive behaviors. The excessive model, on the other hand, seems quite similar to a social learning perspective. Although it highlights the appetitive nature of the activities as a central dimension, the excessive model does not specify this appetitive process and how it can explain or underlie all addictions and, at the same time, predict unique addictions. Both compulsive and excessive behavior models appear to add a new twist to some previously described ones, adding some explanatory potential.

A Biopsychosocial Model

Discontent with the partial explanations offered by the previously described models spurred some thoughtful individuals to propose an integration of these explanations (Donovan & Marlatt, 1988; Glantz & Pickens, 1992). They indicate the integration of biological, psychological, and sociological explanations by calling their model biopsychosocial. This model proposes that addiction is best understood as the result of a confluence of factors representing these three broad areas of influence.

Donovan (Donovan & Marlatt, 1988) argues for the biopsychosocial model, stating that "addiction appears to be an interactive product of social learning in a situation involving physiological events as they are interpreted, labeled, and given meaning by the individual" (p. 7). The common features among addictions and the inadequacy of any single factor to explain addiction highlight the need for a more complex, multicomponent model across addictions. Thus multiple causes, systems, and levels of analyses are needed to understand the addiction process (Donovan & Chaney, 1985; Galizio & Maisto, 1985; Leonard & Blane, 1999). The biopsychosocial model argues for this multiple causality in the acquisition, maintenance, and cessation of addictive behaviors. Proponents of this model often use the commonalties in the relapse process as an argument supporting the need for a biopsychosocial model (Brownell, Marlatt, Lichtenstein, & Wilson, 1986; Marlatt & Gordon, 1985).

Although the proposal of an integrative model represents an important advance over the more specific, single-factor models, proponents of the biopsychosocial approach have not explained how the integration of biological, psychological, sociological, and behavioral components occur. This model does allow researchers from different traditions to agree on complexity and to use a common term. Most of the current models that explain the development of substance abuse problems emphasize risk and protective factors, identify factors from several biopsychosocial domains, and highlight an interaction of these risk and protective factors (Chassin et al., 1996; Sanjuan & Langenbucher, 1999; Schulenberg, Maggs, Steinman, & Zucker, 2001; Windle & Davies, 1999). However, without a pathway that can lead to real integration, the biopsychosocial model represents only a semantic linking of terms or at best a partial integration. As such it often allows individuals to use an integrative term while paying only lip service to aspects other than their primary area of interest. Biologically and physiologically oriented researchers talk about the *bio*psychosocial model whereas social influence advocates discuss the biopsycho*social* model, and so on. This appears particularly true when the model is used for prevention or treatment considerations. It is difficult to intervene in multiple areas at the same time, and many of the risk and protective factors are not amenable to change (family of origin, geographic location, parental absence). Often the primary interest area of the clinician or researcher is highlighted, with inadequate attention given to other aspects. The biopsychosocial model clearly supports the complexity and interactive nature of the process of addiction and recovery. However, additional integrating elements are needed in order to make this tripartite collection of factors truly functional for explaining how individuals become addicted and how the process of recovery from addiction occurs.

CHANGE: THE INTEGRATING PRINCIPLE

This brief and cursory review of the most prevalent models of addiction and related research demonstrates several important facts. First, addiction seems to involve multiple determinants that represent very different domains of human functioning, reaching from elements deep inside the individual, like self- esteem and biology, to broad-based societal influences. Second, the search for a single explanatory construct at a single point in the life of an individual appears fruitless. Finally, integrative perspectives such as the biopsychosocial model are beginning to dominate clinical and research discussions of addiction. Unlike the biopsychosocial model, however, a truly integrative framework should provide the glue to bring together the various research-supported explanatory models. Moreover, such a perspective should lead to a comprehensive view of addiction that could orchestrate the integration of the multiple determinants.

The diverse etiological perspectives for understanding addiction discussed above most often offer partial, often one-dimensional views of the problem of addiction. The social/environmental model envisions addiction arising mostly as a reflection of the type of social environment (poverty, lack of education and opportunity, and so on) surrounding the individual who becomes addicted or highlights the influence of labeling and other social phenomena. The genetic/physiological model searches for answers in the biological dimension. The personality/intrapsychic model views addiction as a failure of character and will. The coping/social learning model sees addiction as a function of personal coping behavior and the influence of role models, peers and parents. Conditioning/reinforcement models search the environment for the cues and reinforcers that create an addiction. There are clear case examples that would support one or another of these elements as a critical aspect or causal influence in addiction or recovery (Wholey, 1984). However, it bears repeating that no single source of influence has been found that can explain any single addiction, let alone all the various types of addictions (Glantz & Pickens, 1992). There is also no single developmental model or singular historical path that can explain acquisition of and recovery from addictions (Chassin, Presson, Sherman, & Edwards, 1991; Jessor, Van Den Bos, Costa, & Turbin, 1995; Schulenberg et al., 2001).

The Transtheoretical Model (TTM) of intentional behavior change attempts to bring together these divergent perspectives by focusing on how individuals change behavior and by identifying key change dimensions involved in this process (DiClemente & Prochaska, 1998; Prochaska & DiClemente, 1984). It is the personal pathway, and not simply the type of person or environment, that appears to be the best way to integrate and understand the multiple influences involved in the acquisition and cessation of addictions. Beginning and quitting addictive behaviors involve the individual and his or her unique decisional considerations. A person's choices influence and are influenced by both character and social forces. There is an interaction between the individual and the risk and protective factors that influence whether the individual becomes addicted and whether he or she leaves the addiction. The transitions into and out of addictions do not occur without the participation of the addicted individual. The individual is involved in how these influences are processed and whether their impact will be strong enough to overcome contrary values and become incorporated into her or his value system. Acquisition of an addictive behavior and recovery from addiction require a personal journey through an intentional change process that is influenced at various points by the host of factors identified in the etiological models just reviewed.

As often occurs, finding a resolution to conflicting models is best resolved with a "both–and" answer instead of an "either–or" type of question. The stages of change, processes of change, context of change, and markers of change identified in the TTM offer a way to integrate these diverse perspectives without losing the valid insights gained from each perspective. This is the essence of an integrative transtheoretical perspective. The TTM of intentional human behavior change (DiClemente & Prochaska, 1998; Prochaska & DiClemente, 1984) will be the integrating framework offered in this book.

Using the process of intentional human behavior change as the integrating construct has many additional advantages. First of all, implicit in the concept of human behavior change is a developmental perspective. Change in humans takes place over time, at different points in the life cycle, and, most often, involves a sequence of events. Addiction and recovery occur in the context of human development and of an individual's life space, which include both physiological and psychological events and transitions (Deas, Riggs, Langenbucher, Goldman, & Brown, 2000; Jessor et al., 1995; Kandel & Davies, 1992). In fact, the current developmental perspective on addiction is completely consistent with a process of change view on addictions. Schulenberg and colleagues (2001) characterize a developmental-contextual framework as one that "emphasizes multidimensional and multidirectional development across the life span, with stability and change occurring as a function of the dynamic interaction between individuals and their contexts" (p. 22). Furthermore, a change-process perspective avoids static explanations for what appears to be a rather active process. Addiction and recovery are dynamic in nature, include periods of perturbation and disruption as well as of stability, and are vulnerable to acceleration and deceleration. Finally, placing addiction into the larger context of an intentional, human change process can increase our ability to identify and explore similarities across addictive behaviors and allows us to compare modifying addictive behaviors with modifying other health and mental health behaviors.

In the next chapter I examine in greater depth the process of human intentional behavior change and the core dimensions of the TTM. The model has been labeled transtheoretical (across theories) because from its inception over 20 years ago, key elements used in creating the model were derived from different theories of human behavior and diverse views of how people change (DiClemente & Prochaska, 1998; Prochaska & DiClemente, 1984). Thus the model is an eclectic and integrative one that owes a debt of gratitude to many theory builders and researchers in the behavioral sciences past and present. In the following chapters I will describe how this theoretical framework can be used to understand better the process involved both in the creation of an addiction and in the recovery from addiction.

Addiction + Recovery are dynamic in nature

Chapter 2

The Process of Human Intentional Behavior Change

The Transtheoretical Model offers an integrative framework for understanding and intervening with human intentional behavior change.

HISTORY AND OVERVIEW OF THE MODEL

The TTM emerged out of the perceived need to find an integrative framework that could bring together fragmented approaches to treating problematic behaviors. Many competing theories of therapy were being used (Bandura, 1986; Bergin & Garfield, 1994; Freud, 1949; Rogers, 1954; Skinner, 1953). Like the models of addiction reviewed in the first chapter, treatments based on these theories presented a patchwork of diverse views concerning how people change. The initial elements of the model came from an analysis of these theories of therapy and highlighted potential common processes that could be identified across the various perspectives (Prochaska, 1979; Prochaska & DiClemente, 1986). The model took shape in early experimental investigations into how nicotine-addicted smokers were able to quit smoking (DiClemente, 1978; DiClemente & Prochaska, 1982; Prochaska & DiClemente, 1982, 1983, 1984). What began as an attempt to bring together and integrate treatment approaches, however, soon turned into a broader exploration of intentional behavior change with a focus on how people change addictive behaviors (Prochaska & DiClemente, 1983, 1986, 1992; Prochaska, DiClemente, & Norcross, 1992; Prochaska, Norcross, & DiClemente, 1994).

Most early research on the TTM consisted of naturalistic studies that simply followed individuals who were at different points in the process of quitting smoking to see how they did it and whether there were ways to track that process (DiClemente & Prochaska, 1985; Prochaska & DiClemente, 1986). Results of these early studies supported segmenting the process of change into different steps or stages. We also discovered interesting connections between these stages and the activities and experiences of individuals moving through the different stages (Prochaska, DiClemente, Velicer, Ginpil, & Norcross, 1985; Prochaska, Velicer, DiClemente, Guadagnoli, & Rossi, 1991). The common processes that we identified differed significantly as individuals moved through the stages of change (DiClemente & Prochaska, 1998; Prochaska & DiClemente, 1986). When we studied individuals who quit the addiction on their own and compared them with those who sought treatment for help in quitting, a similar process and path of change emerged (DiClemente et al., 1991; Prochaska et al., 1992). In addition, data from our research group and those of colleagues indicated that the same stages and processes of change could be assessed across various addictive and health behaviors (DiClemente & Prochaska, 1998; Prochaska & DiClemente, 1985).

As the research progressed and expanded, it became evident that this process of change is a generic one. There is a common pathway involved whenever an individual moves through an intentional change process (DiClemente & Prochaska, 1998; Horn, 1976). Research studies have demonstrated that the various elements of this change process as described in the TTM are important for all three types of behavior change: (1) *creating patterns of behavior* like exercising regularly, drinking alcohol, and smoking cigarettes (Kohler, Grimley, & Reynolds, 1999; Marcus, Rossi, Selby, Niaura, & Abrams, 1992; Pallonen, Prochaska, Velicer, Prokhorov, & Smith, 1998; Werch & DiClemente, 1994); (2) *modifying habitual behavior patterns* like changing to a low fat diet, eating more fruits and vegetables, or engaging in protective sexual behaviors (Curry, Kristal, & Bowen, 1992; Feldman et al., 2000; Glanz et al., 1994; Grimley, Riley, Bellis, & Prochaska, 1993); and (3) *stopping problematic patterns* of smoking, drinking, drug use, gambling, or other addictions (Connors et al., 2001; DiClemente, 1999a; Isenhart, 1994; Prochaska et al., 1992; Shaffer, 1992). Although the challenges differ in creating, modifying, or stopping a behavioral pattern, the process appears to be remarkably similar.

The dimensions of change identified in the TTM can be used to describe this similar path that leads into and out of the habitual patterns of behavior called addictions. The model consists of four broad dimensions of change and their interactions (see Table 2.1). These four dimensions are the stages, processes, markers, and context of change. The *stages of change* divide the process of change into distinct segments. Each stage is defined by specific tasks that need to be accomplished to a greater or lesser degree if movement forward to the next stage is to happen. The stages depict a person's movement through the process of change in terms of the motivational and temporal aspects needed to create a successfully sustained pattern of behavior. The *processes of change* represent the internal and external experiences and activities that enable a person to move from one stage to the next. Engaging in these processes provide the means for the individuals to accomplish the stage "tasks." Thus the processes create and sustain movement through the stages. The *markers of change* are signposts that identify where a person stands in two key change-related areas: decision making about the change, which is called the *decisional balance,* and the strength of one's perceived ability to manage the behavioral change measured by the *self-efficacy/temptation* status. The *context of change* surrounds the change process and often interacts with it. The context consists of five broad areas of functioning that represent both the internal workings of the individual and important interactions with environmental influences. Issues, problems,

TABLE 2.1. The Four Dimensions of the Transtheoretical Model of Intentional Behavior Change

Stages of change

Precontemplation — Contemplation — Preparation — Action — Maintenance

Processes of change

Cognitive/experiential	Behavioral
Consciousness raising	Self-liberation
Self-reevaluation	Conditioning/counterconditioning
Environmental reevaluation	Stimulus generalization/control
Emotional arousal/dramatic relief	Reinforcement management
Social liberation	Helping relationships

Markers of change

Decisional balance	Self-efficacy/temptation

Context of change

Areas of functioning that complement or complicate change.
1. Current life situation
2. Beliefs and attitudes
3. Interpersonal relationships
4. Social systems
5. Enduring personal characteristics

resources, and liabilities within these areas can help or hinder movement through the process of change.

Each of these dimensions holds some explanatory potential for understanding the process of change. Changing a single behavior, like smoking, drinking, or gambling, is a complex activity that takes time and energy to work through the various tasks of change and to move the markers of change in the desired direction. Various events and issues occurring in the context of change often influence completion of tasks and progress toward change. Although each dimension is interesting and informative in its own right, the interaction of these dimensions holds the key to understanding and exploring the process of human intentional behavior change. Processes of change seem to make sense only in the framework of the stages. Markers are related to specific processes of change and appear differentially important at different stages of change. Accomplishing stage tasks, engaging in appropriate processes of change, and shifting markers toward change are affected by the unique constellation of contextual factors.

STAGES OF CHANGE

By definition, the end-state of an addiction is a well-established way of behaving that is consistent, stable, and resistant to change (see Chapter 1). Change requires dissolution of this established pattern and involves a shake-up or perturbation of the status quo for some period of time until a new pattern can be established that replaces the old. Then, once again, there is a period of stability until change is again needed or wanted.

Patterns of behavior are not usually created, modified, or stopped in a single moment in time or with a single flick of a switch.[1] There are steps or segments to the process that the TTM labels *stages of change*. These stages depict the motivational and dynamic fluctuations of the process of change over time. Each stage represents specific tasks that

---

[1]See Miller and C'deBaca (2001) for a discussion of a process they call *quantum change*, which they view as different from movement through the stages. It is not clear, however, that this represents a completely different process of change. They identify an insight change that seems to be related to accelerated decision making and a behavior change process that encompasses multiple problems, similar to a conversion, which may be simply a dramatic, accelerated movement through the process of change. This would be an interesting area for research. In any case, often the accounts of individuals interviewed for this book indicate that the "quantum change" may not represent a completely intentional behavior change process because it can involve the intervention of a higher power or a force seen as external to the individual.

facilitated change

tasks

must be completed and goals that need to be achieved if the individual is to move forward from one stage to the next (Table 2.2).

The road that leads individuals to change an established behavior pattern begins in the Precontemplation stage, where they have no current interest in change. A person moves through the Contemplation, Preparation, and Action stages before arriving at the Maintenance stage. Maintenance becomes the final stage in the transition to the new pattern of behavior and ultimately can lead to the termination of the change process. The stages of Precontemplation and Maintenance represent periods of greater stability, whereas the stages of Contemplation, Preparation, and Action represent periods of greater transition and instability. The following sections describe each stage in an ideal linear sequence. However, movement through the stages is most often recursive and cyclical, with individuals moving back and forth through the early stages and recycling through the stages after a failed attempt to change. Although there is a logical, linear sequence through these stages of change, the actual path is often circuitous (Prochaska et al., 1992).

Precontemplation Stage

Precontemplation represents a status quo. An individual in the Precontemplation stage is satisfied with, or at least unwilling to disrupt, a current behavior pattern. Precontemplators are not considering change in the foreseeable future most often defined as a period of 6 months to a year. This applies whether change means adopting, modifying, or stopping a behavior. Change is seen as irrelevant, unwanted, not needed, or impossible to achieve (DiClemente, 1991; DiClemente & Velasquez, 2002). It matters little if the current behavior pattern involves cigarette smoking, eating a high-fat diet, physical inactivity, using illegal drugs, or abstaining from sexual activity. As long as the current pattern of behavior seems functional for the individual or no compelling reason arises to disrupt this pattern, an individual can remain in precontemplation for extended periods of time, even a lifetime. However, over the course of a lifetime social pressure, aging, illness, personal concerns, human development, shifts in values, and other types of influences move us to consider change for some finite number of our behavior patterns. It is the shift in concern about the behavior and in awareness of some reasons for change that spurs consideration of change and movement to the next stage. The task for Precontemplators is to become conscious of and concerned about the old pattern of behavior and/or interested in a new behavior. From a change perspective it is more important to recognize an

TABLE 2.2. Tasks and Goals for Each of the Stages of Change

Precontemplation

The state in which there is little or no consideration of change of the current pattern of behavior in the foreseeable future.

Tasks: Increase awareness of need for change; increase concern about the current pattern of behavior; envision possibility of change.

Goal: Serious consideration of change for this behavior.

Contemplation

The stage wherein the individual examines the current pattern of behavior and the potential for change in a risk—reward analysis.

Tasks: Analysis of the pros and cons of the current behavior pattern and of the costs and benefits of change. Decision-making.

Goal: A considered evaluation that leads to a decision to change.

Preparation

The stage in which the individual makes a commitment to take action to change the behavior pattern and develops a plan and strategy for change.

Tasks: Increasing commitment and creating a change plan.

Goal: An action plan to be implemented in the near term.

Action

The stage in which the individual implements the plan and takes steps to change the current behavior pattern and to begin creating a new behavior pattern.

Tasks: Implementing strategies for change; revising plan as needed; sustaining commitment in face of difficulties.

Goal: Successful action for changing current pattern. A new pattern of behavior established for a significant period of time (3–6 months).

Maintenance

The stage wherein the new behavior pattern is sustained for an extended period of time and is consolidated into the lifestyle of the individual.

Tasks: Sustaining change over time and across a wide range of different situations. Integrating the behavior into the person's life. Avoiding slips and relapse back to the old pattern of behavior.

Goal: Long-term sustained change of the old pattern and establishment of a new pattern of behavior.

individual's current views on change and address his or her reasons for not wanting to change than it is to understand how the status quo came to be.

Contemplation Stage

Consideration of the value and need for change represents movement into the Contemplation stage. With this, the individual enters into a period of instability. Consideration of change entails struggling with ambivalence about leaving one behavior pattern and moving to another (Miller & Rollnick, 1991). Although behavior change does not always appear to be a rational or logical process, human beings need a compelling rationale to leave the status quo. The Contemplation stage involves a process of evaluating risks and benefits, the pros and cons of both the current behavior pattern and the potential new behavior pattern. This evaluation involves not only generating rational considerations but also an emotional weighing of each consideration. If change is to move forward, the evaluation process results in a decisional balance that supports change (Janis & Mann, 1977). Human behavior change requires significant effort. It takes time and energy to practice a new pattern of behavior to make it firmly established. The reasons in favor of change need to be important and substantive enough to move the individual into deciding to make the effort to change. The task for Contemplators is to resolve their decisional balance considerations in favor of change. The decision to change marks the transition out of the Contemplation stage and into preparation.

Preparation Stage

The Preparation stage of change entails developing a plan of action and creating the commitment needed to implement that plan. To change a behavior, one needs to focus attention and energy on breaking the old pattern and creating a new one. Planning is the activity that organizes the environment and develops the strategies for making change. Commitment is essentially a matter of finding the time and energy to implement the plan. One of the most frequent reasons given as to why individuals do not change is that they lacked the time and energy to do it. But it would be difficult to implement and sustain any change plan without a firm choice and sustained commitment. Being prepared to take action requires some type of plan of action and the dedication or commitment to follow through on that plan. The tasks for Preparation stage individuals are to summon the courage and competencies to accomplish the change.

Action Stage

The implementation of the plan represents the Action stage of change. Acting to stop the old pattern of behavior and beginning to engage in the new one is the action stage. Most people equate this one stage with change. It represents a clear, visible shift from the first half of the change process that focused on intentions, considerations, and plans to the second half of the process, actual behavior change. Getting off the couch and beginning a regime of jogging, throwing out the cigarettes and going through nicotine withdrawal represent activities consonant with the action stage. Action is the initial behavioral step on the path to creating a new pattern of behavior.

However, the new behavior must be sustained over time in order to create the new habit. A behavior cannot simply be done several times and automatically become established. The old pattern retains its attraction and returning to it is often easier than sustaining a new pattern. It takes a long time to establish a new pattern of behavior. Three to six months is usually the time frame we have given for duration of the Action stage. This period of time seems adequate for creating, modifying, or quitting behaviors that have a high frequency of occurrence, like starting regular physical activity or quitting cigarette smoking. The Action stage may take longer for less frequent patterns of behavior like stopping infrequent binge drinking, or beginning monthly breast self-exams or annual colorectal cancer screening (Rakowski, Ehrich, Dube, & Pearlman, 1997). The tasks for Actors are to begin effective action that is continued in the face of barriers and challenges to making the change. Once the new behavior pattern is established in the routine of the individual, the task of behavior change shifts to one of continuing the change over the long haul.

Maintenance Stage

To become habitual the new behavior must become integrated into the lifestyle of the individual. This is the task of the Maintenance stage of change. During this stage the new behavior pattern becomes automatic, requiring little thought or effort to sustain it. It truly becomes an established, habitual pattern (Brownell et al., 1986). However, during maintenance there is still an ever-present danger of reverting to the old pattern. In fact, the new behavior becomes fully maintained only when there is little or no energy or effort needed to continue it and the individual can terminate the cycle of change (Prochaska, Norcross, & DiClemente, 1994). The new behavior then becomes the status quo, and once again there is little or no desire or intention to change, whether that be going back to the former pattern or moving onto another new pattern. The task for Maintainers is to sustain and integrate the behavior change into the total life context so that it becomes normative, familiar, and integral. This new sustained pattern of behavior, then, signals another period of stability.

This sequence of stages identifies the critical tasks that need to be accomplished in moving from one behavior pattern to another (Table 2.2). Movement through these stages represents successful change. However, successful *linear* movement through the stages in a short period of time appears to be the exception, not the norm (Prochaska et al., 1992). Individuals who enter the instability of Contemplation, Preparation, and Action can stay in a single stage, like Contemplation, for a long period of time (Carbonari, DiClemente, & Sewell, 1999). At times they can move backward as well as forward through the early stages. Some move into Preparation and develop a plan, but fail to initiate the plan effectively. Many act but fail to sustain the behavior change and return to an earlier stage in the process of change. Movement through the stages of change is more cyclical and circuitous than the linear description of movement presented here (See Figure 2.1).

Some critics have questioned whether the stages represent distinct

Stages of Change Model

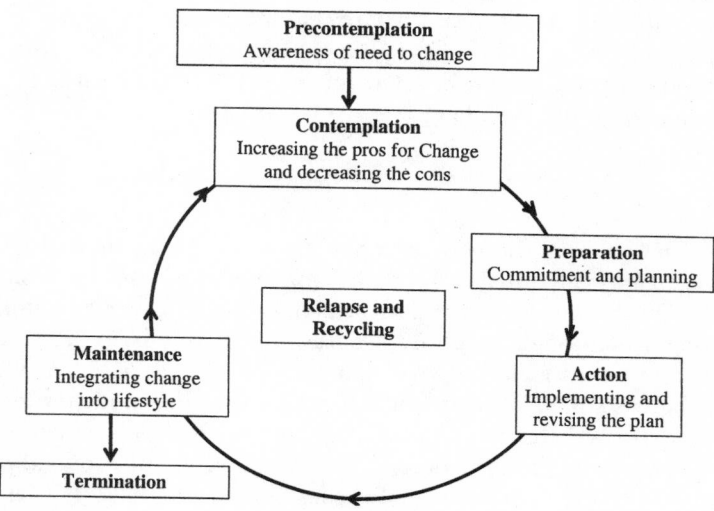

FIGURE 2.1. A cyclical representation of movement through the stages of change.

states, separate categories, or "real" stages (Bandura, 1997; Joseph, Breslin, & Skinner, 1999). These authors believe that the term *stages* should be reserved for states that are completely distinct, that have an irreversible linear sequence (caterpillars become butterflies but butterflies never become caterpillars), and that can be completely isolated. The stages described in this model do not meet all these criteria. As illustrated, the stages can be recursive in nature (Carbonari et al., 1999; Connors et al., 2001; Prochaska & DiClemente, 1998).

In addition, it is sometimes difficult to classify an individual into one of these stages accurately (Carey, Purnine, Maisto, & Carey, 1999; Littell & Girvin, 2002; Sutton, 1996, 2001). Capturing the individual in the process of completing the tasks of each stage can be difficult because the tasks are not always completed and individuals can move back and forth through the stages. All measurement of the stages approximates where an individual is in the process of change. It is particularly difficult to isolate the early stages, where there is no clear behavioral marker or time period that can be used to define the stage. Moreover, in situations involving illegal drug use, there may be reason for the individual to deceive. However, when there is no such reason, a straightforward assessment of the status of the individual appears to work well to divide individuals into subgroups that are consistent with other dimensions of change (DiClemente & Prochaska, 1998). The research indicates that activities and experiences shift over time as individuals move through the change process. Measurement difficulties exist, but there continues to be great value in the concept of the stages and in dividing the process of change into meaningful segments in order to better understand the process of change (Connors et al., 2001; Prochaska & DiClemente, 1984, 1992, 1998; Prochaska et al., 1992).

The stages of change delineate important tasks that need to be accomplished in order to move forward in the process of change. However, each of these tasks can be accomplished to a greater or lesser degree. An individual may feel pushed out of Precontemplation and engage in a cursory consideration of change. Another may want to change but fail to make a firm decision based on a solid risk–reward analysis. Success represents a resolution of each stage's tasks in a way that supports engagement in the tasks of the next stage, and so on. Movement back and forth as well as recycling through the stages represents a successive learning process whereby the individual continues to redo the tasks of various stages in order to get them right.

Described in this manner, the stages of change seem most like the stages of development described by Erik Erikson (1963). Erikson viewed the psychological growth and maturation of an individual as a series of bipolar tasks (trust vs. mistrust; industry vs. inferiority) that build on one another, that become important at different points in maturational development, and that can be more or less successfully resolved as the individual moves through life. How one resolves early stage issues affects how successfully the individual will be able to address the later stage tasks. Similarly, the tasks of each of the stages of change involve activities and issues related to initial motivation, decision making, efficacy, and coping activities that have an ongoing influence on the change process. These tasks can be accomplished quickly or slowly, and can be performed more or less completely. From this perspective the quality and completeness of the execution of the stage-specific tasks would impact success in the subsequent stages of the process of change.[2]

How does one move through the stages of change? Each stage has important tasks that need to be accomplished at least to some degree before there is movement into the next stage. The more specific question is how individuals accomplish the tasks of each stage in order to move from one stage to the next.

PROCESSES OF CHANGE

Processes of change represent the internal and external experiences and activities that enable individuals to move from stage to stage. The processes are the engines that create and sustain the transitions through the stages and facilitate successful completion of the stage tasks. The processes of change are the province and responsibility of the individual making the change and initiating, modifying, or stopping the behavior. There is an important distinction between the processes of change and the techniques of prevention, counseling, or therapy that are taught to intervention and treatment specialists. It is the consciousness raising of the client, for example, and not the techniques of the therapist that represent a process of change. The techniques employed by counselors are intended to engage or empower individual processes of change in the client (Velasquez, Maurer, Crouch, & DiClemente, 2001). However, counselors can perform powerful techniques in treatment without being successful in engaging the client in the specific processes of change targeted by that technique. Prevention and treatment techniques are not to be confused with processes of change. These processes of change have been identified in individuals who make substantive changes without the assistance of formal treatment or with minimal self-help approaches (DiClemente et al., 1991; Prochaska & DiClemente, 1986; Snow,

---

[2]See the final chapter of Connors et al. (2001) for a discussion of this issue.

Prochaska, & Rossi, 1994). It is clear that the entire process of intentional behavior change is more extensive and more comprehensive than any single intervention, treatment event, or course of therapy.

Although we do not have a complete understanding of all the activities and experiences that are involved in movement between stages of change, we have identified a number of important ones (DiClemente & Prochaska, 1998; Prochaska & DiClemente, 1986; Prochaska, Velicer, DiClemente, & Fava, 1988). These processes are the same as behavior change principles identified by different theories of behavior change and systems of psychotherapy.[3] There are two broad types of processes involved in intentional behavior change (Table 2.3).[4] One type represents those cognitive and experiential processes involving thinking and feeling. The second type involves processes oriented toward taking action; they involve behavioral commitment and actions to create or break a habit. All of these processes operate in similar ways but in different directions for the various types of behavior change: initiation, modification, and cessation.

The cognitive/experiential processes of change identify ways of thinking and feeling that create change. These include consciousness raising, emotional arousal, self-reevaluation, environmental reevaluation, and social liberation. The process of consciousness raising increases awareness, whether about the current or the new behavior or about a need to change. Consciousness raising has been highlighted by most behavior change theories as a fundamental process. It is a prime target for most prevention and treatment programs. The process of emotional arousal involves emotional and value-laden experiences with the new or old behavior. These emotionally arousing experiences can either enhance the value of the current or new behavior or decrease the value or need for these behaviors. Emotional experiences interact with and contribute to the consciousness raising and the reevaluation processes. Several emotion-based theories of change, like the existential and Gestalt therapies, and techniques, like psychodrama, consider emotional arousal to play a

---

[3]There is a detailed description of how these principles are related to therapy theories and approaches in Prochaska and DiClemente (1984), DiClemente and Prochaska (1998), and Prochaska and Norcross (1999).

[4]These two larger groupings are second-order factors identified in factor analyses of the 10 specific processes of change in studies of smoking, weight control, psychological distress, and drinking (Carbonari & DiClemente, 2000; Prochaska & DiClemente, 1985; Prochaska et al., 1988; Snow, Prochaska, & Rossi, 1994). Individual processes as well as the larger second-order factors have been used in various studies to evaluate change and stage movement.

TABLE 2.3. Processes of Change

Cognitive/experiential

1. *Consciousness raising:* Gaining information that increases awareness about the current behavior pattern or the potential new behavior
2. *Emotional arousal:* Experiencing emotional reactions about the status quo and/or the new behavior
3. *Self-reevaluation:* Seeing and evaluating how the status quo or the new behavior fits in with or conflicts with personal values
4. *Environmental reevaluation:* Recognizing the positive and negative effects the status quo or new behavior have upon others and the environment
5. *Social liberation:* Noticing and increasing social alternatives and norms that help support the status quo and/or change and initiation of the new behavior

Behavioral

1. *Self-liberation:* Making choices, taking responsibility for, and making commitments to engaging in a new behavior or a behavior change
2. *Stimulus generalization or control:* Creating, altering, or avoiding cues/stimuli that trigger or encourage a particular behavior
3. *Conditioning or counterconditioning:* Making new connections between cues and a behavior or substituting new, competing behaviors and activities in response to cues for the "old" behaviors
4. *Reinforcement management:* Identifying and manipulating the positive and negative reinforcers for current or new behaviors. Creating rewards for new behaviors while extinguishing (eliminating reinforcements) for current behavior.
5. *Helping relationships:* Seeking and receiving support from others (family, friends, peers) for current or new behaviors

pivotal role in change. Cognitive/experiential processes also include self-reevaluation, a reassessment process whereby one reevaluates the current or new behavior. This process involves consideration of how the behavior fits with current or aspirational values, beliefs, and goals. Many theories of change, particularly those that focus on cognitive factors believe that this type of self-reevaluation is critical to successful behavior change (Beck, Wright, Newman, & Liese, 1993; Ellis & Dryden, 1987). The environmental reevaluation process assesses the utility of the behavior in the current environment. Theories of change that emphasize role expectancies, perceived norms, and social influence focus on environmental reevaluation (Bandura, 1997; Goldman, 1999; Goldman et al., 1999; Rogers, 1995). Finally, an awareness of societal values and society's promotion or proscription of the behavior also play a part in the thinking and feeling processes. This social liberation process promotes realization and acceptance of social norms and societal sanctions, and engages the individual to view change as possible and to experience viable alternatives. Programs attempt to engage social liberation when they encourage advocacy to make individuals aware of norms (Mothers Against Drunk Driving), offer successful or unsuccessful models to promote change (Alcoholics Anonymous or juvenile offender visits to prisons), or create alternative activities like an alcohol-free parties.

Behavioral processes of change include self-liberation, stimulus generalization or control, conditioning or counterconditioning, reinforcement management, and helping relationships. Self-liberation involves making a choice and commitment to modify current behavior patterns and to engage in the new behavior. Humanistic and existential approaches to change have championed self-liberation as a process of change and emphasized the responsibility and personal choices involved in creating change. Two behavioral processes focus on creating and modifying the connections between cues and stimuli in the environment and specific behaviors. Wolpe (1958) describes in detail the processes of stimulus generalization or stimulus control and conditioning/counterconditioning. Changing connections between stimulus and response can be achieved by either increasing (stimulus generalization) or decreasing (stimulus control) the number and nature of the stimuli connected with the specific behavior, or substituting one behavioral response to a stimulus for another (conditioning or counterconditioning). Another behavioral process, reinforcement management, involves understanding, creating, or changing the environmental contingencies that reinforce a behavior pattern as described by Skinner (1953). This reinforcement management process investigates and utilizes the powerful rewards and reinforcements for a behavior that can be biological, psychological, and/ or social. Finally, the helping relationships process represents having and seeking support from others for the current or new behavior. Helping relationships and social support have often been viewed as having an important role in change by various theorists and researchers (Rogers, 1954; Sarason, Sarason, & Pierce, 1990). Having or creating a support system for engagement in a behavior seems to be an important element in initiation, modification, or cessation of behaviors.

These cognitive/experiential and behavioral processes of change are critical ingredients for creating movement through the stages of change (DiClemente & Prochaska, 1985; Prochaska & DiClemente, 1985). This range of processes derived from various theories is what makes the TTM "trans" theoretical. In addition, there are predictable interactions between types of process activity and successful movement through specific parts of the stages of change sequence. Cognitive and experiential processes are more important in negotiating passage through the earlier stages of Precontemplation and Contemplation. Behavioral processes of change are more important in the Preparation, Action, and Maintenance stages of change (DiClemente & Prochaska, 1998). As we learn more and more about the process of human behavior change, it appears that change-process activity matched to movement through the stages produces more successful change (Perz, DiClemente, & Carbonari, 1996). The secret to successful human intentional behavior change appears to be doing the right thing (specific process activities) at the right time (specific stages) in the process.

MARKERS OF CHANGE

From the beginning of this exploration into the process of intentional behavior change our research team looked for markers and mechanisms identified in other theories and perspectives that could help delineate the process (DiClemente, 1981; DiClemente & Prochaska, 1982; Prochaska & DiClemente, 1983, 1984). In addition to the stages and processes of change, two related constructs have been examined consistently in research using the TTM. They are decisional balance and self-efficacy/ temptation. Decisional balance identifies the relationship between the pros and cons for change (Janis & Mann, 1977) and has emerged as an important marker of movement through the early stages of change (Prochaska, Velicer, et al., 1994; Velicer, DiClemente, Prochaska, & Brandenberg, 1985). On the other hand, self-efficacy, Albert Bandura's concept describing an individual's confidence to perform a specific behavior, emerged as an important predictor of action and long-term success (Bandura, 1977, 1997; DiClemente, Carbonari, Montgomery, & Hughes, 1994; DiClemente et al., 1995; DiClemente, Prochaska, & Gibertini, 1985; Velicer, DiClemente, Rossi, & Prochaska, 1990). There are other potential markers and mechanisms that can interact with the process of human intentional behavior change, like intrinsic and extrinsic motivation (Curry, Wagner, & Grothaus, 1990; DiClemente, 1999a), rationalization and harm minimization (Daniels, 1998), and beliefs and barriers to change (Werch & DiClemente, 1994). However, I will focus, as has most of the research, on decision making and self-efficacy, which are considered important markers of movement through various stages in the process of change for addictions.

Decisional Balance

There is a sizable literature on decision-making theory (Mellers, Schwartz, & Cooke, 1998). The research and theory on decision making that is most connected to the TTM has its roots in the work of Irving Janis and

Leon Mann. They propose a rational decision-making model that identifies the weighing of the pros and cons of change and the resultant decisional balance as important components in making a decision to take an action (Janis & Mann, 1977). Through the early stages of change, an individual's decisional balance is an important marker of movement (Prochaska, Velicer, et al., 1994)

For any contemplated change, the current and the new behavior has its own set of pros and cons. An individual's personal reasons for and against the current behavior and for or against the new one result in an overall decisional balance. For example, in Precontemplation for recovery, the reasons against abstinence and in favor of continued drinking are greater than the pros of stopping and the cons of continued drinking. The decisional balance is in favor of the status quo. In Contemplation there is greater overall balance between the positives and negatives. If the individual is to continue to move forward, the pros for change and the cons for the status quo must increase. This will tip the overall balance in favor of the change (Miller & Rollnick, 1991; Prochaska & DiClemente, 1986; Prochaska, Velicer, et al., 1994; Velicer et al., 1985). Decision making is the desired outcome of this balancing process and marks the transition between the Contemplation and Preparation stages. Thus, the pros and cons of change become important markers that can be used to evaluate an individual's status with regard to a behavior change. In the latter stages of Action and Maintenance the decisional balance continues to favor and support change, but individuals often see the original factors involved as less important than they did earlier (Prochaska & DiClemente, 1986). The saliency of decisional considerations for stopping problematic behaviors like smoking decrease as the change becomes established (Prochaska et al., 1991). However, these considerations may continue to play a significant role in starting and modifying behaviors (Lee, 1998).

Self-Efficacy

Self-efficacy is the term used to describe an individual's confidence about performing a specific behavior (Bandura, 1977, 1986, 1997). Bandura's unique insight was to describe how efficacy expectations (Can I do it?) differ from outcome expectations (what I expect to happen after I perform the behavior). He highlighted the important role of efficacy self-evaluations in predicting performance of a behavior and identifying individuals who would or would not persist in performing that behavior (Bandura, 1997). Efficacy evaluations can represent an individual's self-reported confidence to abstain from a problematic behavior as well as to perform a desired one. Self-efficacy has been studied extensively in the context of addictions because of its potential to discriminate those who may be vulnerable to relapse, thereby contributing to relapse prevention (Bandura, 1997; Brownell et al., 1986; DiClemente et al., 1995; Marlatt & Gordon, 1985). Research exploring the TTM often has examined the role of self-efficacy in the prediction of behavior change over the past 20 years (Carbonari & DiClemente, 2000; DiClemente, 1981; DiClemente, Carbonari, Daniels, et al., 2001; DiClemente, Prochaska, & Gibertini, 1985; Velicer et al., 1990).

Self-efficacy has been examined among individuals at each of the stages of change. It seems a stronger and more important predictor once the individual begins to engage in the behavior change and as a predictor of maintenance of that change. Efficacy evaluations have been strong and effective predictors of individuals who are able to sustain the actions needed to instigate and maintain the behavior change over time (Bandura, 1997; Carbonari & DiClemente, 2000; DiClemente, Carbonari, Hughes, & Montgomery, 1994; DiClemente et al., 1995). Self-efficacy, then, emerges as an important marker of the transition from the Preparation stage though the Action and Maintenance stages. However, self-efficacy does seem to play a role in earlier stages as well. Individuals who have little confidence in their ability to perform a behavior like abstaining from alcohol may become stuck in the Precontemplation stage, feeling hopeless about the possibility of change (DiClemente, 1991; DiClemente & Hughes, 1990; Daniels, 1998). Therefore, efficacy evaluations may be able to play a role in discriminating different subgroups of Precontemplators (Daniels, 1998).

Efficacy evaluations interact in an interesting and logically consistent manner with the experiential and behavioral processes of change. For individuals in earlier stages of change, higher levels of efficacy are related to increasing use of experiential and behavioral change processes. The reverse is true in the later stages of change (DiClemente et al., 1985). In the Action and Maintenance stages the greater one's sense of confidence to perform the behavior, the less one uses or sees the need to use behavioral processes of change.

Temptation

Self-efficacy has a companion marker, temptation. Efficacy evaluations are typically measured across a range of situations or cues connected with engagement in the addictive behavior. Temptation represents the strength of the desire or inclination to perform the behavior in a particular situation (how tempted are you to smoke, drink, eat, or use drugs in this situation). Temptation and self-efficacy are assessed using the same set of cues or triggers. Usually temptation is negatively correlated with an individual's self-efficacy or confidence to abstain from that addictive behavior. For example, someone who is not at all tempted in a specific situation to engage in a particular addictive behavior is usually totally confident of being able to avoid it. However, this is not always the case. Some individuals going through treatment experience strong temptations to use drugs in certain situations but are confident in their ability to resist that temptation.

Temptation to engage in the behavior serves as a companion marker to self-efficacy to evaluate movement through the stages of change (DiClemente, Carbonari, et al., 1994; DiClemente et al., 1995). Measuring varying levels of temptation across relevant situations can be useful in developing change plans during Preparation stage activity and in predicting successful Action and Maintenance stage activities. Temptation and self-efficacy, although related, are not mirror images of one another. The relation of an individual's temptation to his or her level of confidence (self-efficacy) has been an interesting relationship to examine in the Precontemplation stage (DiClemente & Hughes, 1990) and to use as a predictor of success in the later stages of change (Carbonari & DiClemente, 2000; DiClemente, Carbonari, et al., 2001). Both temptation and self-efficacy will be included in the discussion of addiction and change.

THE CONTEXT OF CHANGE

Any single pattern of behavior occurs in the context of an individual's entire life. Therefore, changing a habit always has important implications for multiple areas of that life. A holistic perspective is needed in order to understand fully the process of human intentional behavior change. The contribution of life context in the process of change is represented in the TTM by five areas of functioning: current life situation, beliefs and attitudes, interpersonal relationships, social systems, and enduring personal characteristics (DiClemente & Prochaska, 1998; Prochaska & DiClemente, 1984). Issues, problems, resources, or liabilities in each of these five areas can facilitate or hinder successful change of any specific pattern of behavior.

These areas also represent the focal content areas emphasized in different theories of psychotherapy. Cognitive therapies view the level of beliefs and attitudes as the most critical place to intervene in order to get significant change. Family therapists concentrate on shifting the family system. Psychodynamic therapists focus on the enduring intrapersonal dynamics that they assume control successful long-term change of any single problem behavior. Thus, each area can be considered the primary focus or key targeted mechanism of change identified by different theories of therapy and behavior change. Once again, in its attempt to be integrative, the TTM highlights potential interactions among diverse theoretical emphases.

Originally these areas of functioning were called levels of change (Prochaska & DiClemente, 1984). The concept of levels was used to indicate that the five areas extended in hierarchical order from the most current and obvious area of problems (symptoms and life situations) to maladaptive cognitions, interpersonal conflicts, and family/ system conflicts, and ultimately to the most historical and deeply rooted types of issues (enduring personal characteristics or intrapersonal level). Problems occurring at the top levels were viewed as more easily changed and most often the focus of attention (symptomatic). Problems at the bottom of the hierarchy were those seen as most difficult to change and requiring more extensive interventions (Prochaska & DiClemente, 1984).

I have relabeled this aspect the context of change because these areas surround as well as interact with an individual's movement through the process of changing any single behavior pattern. These five areas could be organized in many different ways because they include psychological dimensions of symptoms, cognitions and intrapersonal conflicts, interactive dimensions of interpersonal relationships and larger social systems, and a situational dimension that focuses on the current environment and status of the individual. The hierarchical nature of these areas is not compelling. I keep these areas in the same order as they appeared in earlier versions of the model for consistency. However, I prefer to see these five areas in the broad context of the individual's life surrounding any single change of a pattern of behavior.

The distinction between an individual's behavior targeted for change and the context of that change is a matter of chosen focus. It can shift. The behavior change target is most often in the foreground, with the contextual areas in the background of the individual's attention. When the individual tries to quit drinking, other problems such as with his or her marriage or family are considered later. However, this relationship can shift when problems come to the foreground along with the target behavior. For example, while trying to change the alcohol problem, family or marital problems often arise, demanding attention. At other times the relationship resembles that of the perceptual shift between figure and ground. When one area comes into the foreground, other problems, even what was considered the most important target behavior, recede into the background. The relationships among areas of functioning and the addictive behavior will be a central theme in our discussion of movement through the stages of human intentional behavior change.

The five general areas of functioning identified are the following:

1. *Current life situation.* This area includes the current internal and external environment in which the change is to take place. The emotional and mental status of the individual as well as the current living situation is included in this area of functioning. The targeted addictive behavior is typically viewed as a problem symptom in the current life situation. Assessment of the current levels of anxiety and depression, the living situation, financial and educational resources, intellectual ability, and coping skills serves to identify examples of strengths and/or problems in the life situation that can interact with movement through the stages of change. Research demonstrates that, in general, individuals who have more resources and fewer problems in their current life situation have a better prognosis for a successful transition through the stages.

2. *Beliefs and attitudes.* An individual's current belief system and basic values provide the cognitive framework in which the change is to take place. Basic beliefs about how change should happen, about what is needed for successful change, as well as general beliefs about self and world, religion, god, and family interact with the process of change in many ways. Once again, assessing how beliefs are involved in changing the specific behavior pattern in question can assist in understanding why one individual may get stuck in Contemplation, rush to Action, or fail in Maintenance of the behavior change (Prochaska & DiClemente, 1984).

3. *Interpersonal relationships.* This area includes dyadic interactions in the person's life. Usually this includes interactions with significant individuals, like spouses, special friends, and lovers. These interactions can foster or hinder movement through the process of change in many ways. Interpersonal influence is often an important consideration in decision making as individuals' contemplate changing a particular behavior. Several of the key decisional considerations included in the pros and cons for change identified by Janis and Mann (1977) were the evaluation and approval of others. In addition, interpersonal problems can play a decisive role in the decision to make a change and often influence whether that change is sustained over time (DiClemente, Dolan-Mullen, & Windsor, 2000; McBride et al., 1999).

4. *Social systems.* Various social systems in which the individual exists can influence the process of change. The individual's family system as well as the social network and societal and work systems would be included in this area of functioning. These systems may offer support for or interfere with the change. Social systems influence through persuasion, modeling, social norms and social reference (Bandura, 1986) as well as by providing incentives or barriers for change (Chassin et al., 1996; DiClemente & Prochaska, 1998; Prochaska, Norcross, & DiClemente, 1992).

5. *Enduring personal characteristics.* This area encompasses basic personality characteristics and conflicts that influence the change process. For example, being more impulsive or obsessive can hinder or promote decision making, influence planning, and affect implementing the plan and taking action. Issues of personal identity, self-esteem, conscientiousness, extraversion, agreeableness, and neuroticism could all play a role in complementing or complicating change (Costa & McCrae, 1992; DiClemente, 1994).

These five contextual areas of functioning can influence the process of change. For example, a man who is sedentary needs to become more physically active. He can be assisted in moving through the stages of change by living near recreational facilities and having a value system that emphasizes physical health (Lee & DiClemente, 2000). In addition, if he has a partner who is active, a social network that encourages physical activity like golf, tennis, or swimming, and has a more outgoing personality, these could also facilitate his adopting a regular physical activity regimen. On the other hand, a cold climate, negative attitudes about sweating, a sedentary spouse and family, and a phlegmatic personality could interfere with that change. Similar factors can play a role in quitting an addictive behavior like cigarette smoking. Having a spouse and friends that smoke, believing that good health is genetic and unaffected by personal habits, and having a job that supports frequent breaks for smoking impedes consideration of change. Problems of being overweight, anxious, or depressed further interfere with quitting. But areas of functioning can also facilitate quitting smoking. A new job that has many smoking restrictions, a spouse who quits, a family member who gets lung cancer could help the transition into Contemplation for smoking cessation. Likewise, some areas of functioning can influence decision making and movement to Preparation and Action for smoking cessation: a parent who quit at one's current age, an age-40 transition, a new love interest who is allergic to smoke, or the birth of a child.

Resources and liabilities in these five areas of functioning can promote or hinder movement and affect the probability and speed of transition from one stage to the next. However, not every problem is relevant to changing a particular behavior. For example, sedentary spouses or negative attitudes about sweating may have no relevance to quitting smoking. The central question to ask is whether these five areas of functioning influence transitions through the stages of change for the specific targeted behavior. If issues in one or more of these areas of functioning are complementing or complicating the process of change, they may have to be addressed, augmented, neutralized, or modified in order to facilitate movement.

In any case, as individuals initiate, modify, or stop a behavior, changes in other areas of functioning almost certainly will occur. Creation and cessation of any habitual behavior have ramifications for other areas of functioning. Becoming a regular smoker, for example, sets in motion shifts in social networks. It can influence choice of partners, choice of residence, and beliefs about addiction. Change of any one habitual pattern of behavior reverberates through the entire personal lifespace and social network of an individual. The context of change helps us to identify factors that complement or complicate the process of change (DiClemente, 1994).

One final point should be made concerning these areas in the context of change. When the focus of change shifts from the original target to a problem in one or more of these contextual areas, the context problem can also be viewed through the stages of change. Individuals may be more or less ready to address the context problem. For example, individuals may have to change where they live or whom they live with before they can progress further in changing an addictive behavior. Thus, a living situation can be a specific target for behavior change along with, or sometimes prior to, being able to move successfully through the stages of change for an addiction. Chapter 7 discusses this in more detail. The important point to remember is that contextual areas make movement through the process of change more complicated because each of these areas can facilitate or frustrate completion of stage tasks and can, at any time, increase in salience or severity to become a primary focus of change efforts.

SUMMARY

The stages, processes, markers, and context of change outlined in the TTM offer a template for examining intentional human behavior change in various areas of an individual's life. Initiating or modifying habitual patterns of behavior are difficult endeavors that take time and energy. All of us have behavior change success stories and many tales of behavior change failures. The framework of the TTM attempts to outline the important steps, tasks, activities, experiences, and contextual influences that can help us to understand the differences between success and failure in the movement through the process of intentional behavior change. Although originally conceived in the context of psychotherapy and change of psychological problems (Prochaska & DiClemente, 1984), this model has been used extensively to examine health and addictive behavior changes (Connors, Donovan, & DiClemente, 2001; DiClemente & Prochaska, 1998; Prochaska et al., 1992; Weinstein, Rothman, & Sutton, 1998). The next chapter begins to apply this model to addictive behaviors in more detail.

Chapter 3

The Well-Maintained Addiction
An Ending and a Beginning

An addiction is the end state of a process of change whereby the addictive behavior becomes habitual, problematic, and difficult to dislodge.

DEFINING THE WELL-MAINTAINED ADDICTION

The path to becoming addicted ends in addiction. Addiction represents the final Maintenance stage of the process of change, and this explains why it can be so difficult to dislodge. Once individuals complete the Maintenance tasks and incorporate the addiction into their lives, they leave the process of becoming addicted and enter the Precontemplation Stage for the change process that ends in recovery (Figure 3.1). So it is appropriate to begin to understand the addiction and recovery processes of change with this stage. Addiction occurs when the individual becomes both *regularly* and *dependently* engaged in the addictive behavior. Both characteristics must be present and, as we have seen in Chapter 1, both terms must be defined clearly to understand the well-maintained addiction.

A Regularly Occurring Pattern of Behavior

A clear pattern of engaging in the target behavior or constellation of behaviors signals either Action or Maintenance stages for that behavior (DiClemente & Prochaska, 1998). Repeated, habitual engagement in an addictive behavior indicates that the individual has a pattern of use that is predictable. Regular use can include periodic or intermittent engagement in the behavior as well as daily use. There are many different pat-

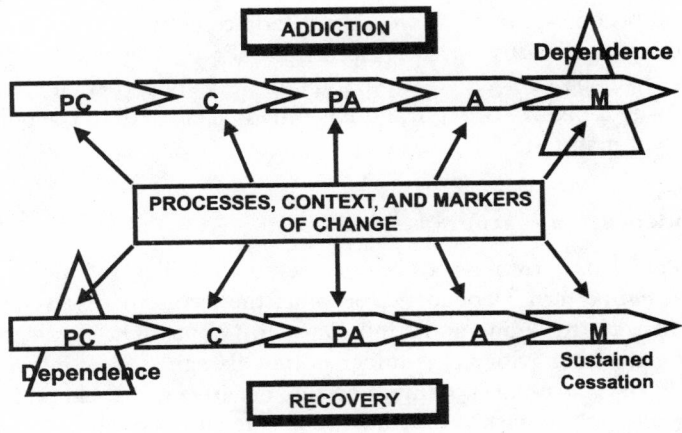

FIGURE 3.1. An overview the stages of addiction and recovery.

terns of frequency and intensity of engagement that can be considered habitual: individuals who travel to Las Vegas 10 times a year to engage in heavy betting; drinkers who predictably overdrink whenever attending a business meeting; cocaine users who go off to a crackhouse after every argument with a spouse. The face of addiction can vary by type of behavior as well as by pattern of engagement. If there is no pattern to the behavior or only sporadic use or engagement in the behavior, we are dealing with earlier stages of the process of becoming addicted. The Action stage and, even more critically, the Maintenance stage of a behavior are characterized by this repeated, consistent pattern of the behavior in question.

The addictive behaviors become so predictable that others in the immediate environment anticipate the behavior. Dunn and colleagues (Dunn, Seilhamer, Jacob, & Whalen, 1992) studied marital satisfaction of problem drinkers and their spouses on a weekly basis over several months. The findings of this study indicated that marital satisfaction decreased for spouses of the drinker *prior to* rather than after the period of heavy use. Family members of alcoholic and drug-addicted individuals learn to anticipate the behavior precisely because the addiction is patterned.

Once individuals begin to engage regularly in the addictive behavior, two paths are possible. One is a pattern of regulated use and the other a pattern of problematic, unregulated use. Some people develop a pattern of drinking beer or wine with meals that is regular but not problematic. Others develop a pattern of drinking to excess that causes problems and becomes an addiction. The difference between these two separate but related paths lies in whether or not the repeated pattern of behavior can be considered self-regulated and under personal control. That is why a pattern of regular use is only one element in the definition of the well-maintained addiction.

Dependence as a Marker of Addiction

For a regular pattern of use to be considered an addiction it must also be a *dependent* pattern. Dependence becomes the second necessary and critical dimension to define addiction. The term *dependence* indicates that the pattern of behavior (1) is under poor self-regulatory control or appears out of control, (2) continues despite negative feedback, and (3) has become an integral part of the individual's life and coping. Moreover, reinforcement for the behavior has become very strong and, often, is prepotent in the life of the individual. During this Maintenance stage of addiction these reinforcements are both physiological and psychological. This combination creates a very powerful reward system that clouds awareness of problems related to the behavior and makes change difficult and, at times, seemingly impossible. Note that individuals who develop a regular pattern of use which is under self-regulation and responsive to problematic feedback should be considered to be in the Maintenance stage of a self-regulated behavior, not an addiction. I discuss this path in Chapter 5.

Once individuals have developed this regular and dependent pattern of behavior—be it gambling; drinking alcohol; smoking cocaine, cigarettes, or marijuana; excessively dieting; or using illegal drugs—they appear locked into the behavior and are unwilling to consider change. The addictive behavior pattern can continue for long periods of time and for significant segments of people's lives. Many of the smokers in studies had been smoking regularly for over 20 years. They had been good at minimizing harmful consequences and creating lifestyles that allowed for smoking daily and continuously. These individuals certainly would qualify for having a "well-maintained addiction." The rest of this chapter examines some of the factors that contribute to the Maintenance of unregulated use, the final stage in becoming addicted.

BEHAVIORAL PROCESSES
CONTRIBUTING TO MAINTENANCE

As the individual moves into the Action and Maintenance stages of change, opportunities to engage in the addictive behavior seem to expand while activities and enjoyments in other areas of life contract. This phenomenon has been referred to as a narrowing of the behavioral repertoire and social circle, and it makes the addictive behavior more concentrated and central in the life of the addicted individual. As this happens, several behavioral and learning theory processes appear to be operating. The behavioral processes of conditioning, stimulus generalization, and reinforcement help to connect the addictive behavior to physiological, psychological, and environmental cues and various areas of the individual's life context. This makes the addiction an integral part of an individual's life and lifestyle. Other behavioral processes of change—self-liberation and helping relationships—play a critical role in creating the durable, extensive, problematic, and dependent pattern of addiction. There is also a role for the cognitive/experiential processes, as discussed later in this chapter. However, it is the continued, repeated engagement in the behavior itself that creates the habit. The behavioral processes cement it into the very fabric of the individual's life. These are powerful processes that, once put in motion, often require little thought or effort.

Conditioning

All addictive behaviors have a physiological and psychological reaction that makes them enjoyable and exciting. They are appetitive behaviors (Orford, 1985). This makes them vulnerable to conditioning. The learning process called conditioning involves pairing a neutral stimulus with a stimulus that automatically or predictably evokes a reaction; after a few pairings, the neutral stimulus by itself will evoke the reaction. In the famous but possibly apocryphal Pavlov experiment with dogs, a bell was paired with food. After several trials, the bell by itself could trigger the dog to salivate without the presence of any food. The capacity of conditioning with an addictive behavior is particularly compelling when we examine various psychoactive substances. Otherwise neutral sights, sounds, scenes, and behaviors that tend to occur with the drug taking become capable of producing by themselves the drug's physiological reaction. Many behaviors and situations that previously were unrelated to the addictive behavior become potent signals that arouse physiological and psychological states that feed desire and temptation. This conditioning effect occurs over time, so that the greater the frequency and intensity of the behavior, the more cues and triggers are created by the conditioning process (Hinson, 1985).

There are many examples of conditioning effects. Heroin addicts who are unable to obtain the drug will often inject themselves with a saline solution containing no heroin to experience what is called a "needle high." Numerous cocaine-addicted individuals in early recovery report intense reactions and temptation upon seeing any white substance in a plastic bag or patterned in lines on the table. The conditioned connections between cigarette smoking and a cup of coffee, a drink at a bar, and the ending of a meal are well known by smokers (Orleans & Slade, 1993). Conditioning creates an increasingly complex web of cues that are closely associated with the behavior. The cues then trigger a felt need for the addictive behavior (Galizio & Maisto, 1985). The conditioning process begins in the Action stage of engagement and culminates in the Maintenance stage to create the firmly established addiction.

Stimulus Generalization

Stimulus generalization is a process whereby something learned in one specific setting or under one set of circumstances generalizes, or spreads, to other similar settings, cues, and circumstances (Barrett, 1985). The smoker who began by smoking only in social settings with friends who smoke then starts to smoke in social groups of friends where there are few smokers, and then begins to smoke alone at home. The drinker who regularly stops off at a bar after work for a couple of beers begins to visit the bar at lunch. The weekend marijuana user begins to smoke weeknights after work during a period of stress. These are all examples of the change process of stimulus generalization. As the behavior becomes paired with more and more parts of the individual's life, it becomes ingrained into the very fabric of that life. More and more situations, emotions, events, and places become opportunities, cues, or triggers for the behavior. Stopping an addiction once this generalization process has occurred often involves restricting access to the places and situations where the individual has engaged in the behavior. Generalization is a powerful process contributing to the spread of the behavior throughout the life of the individual.

Reinforcement

B. F. Skinner (1938) demonstrated the power of reinforcement in shaping the behaviors of pigeons. In essence his theory states that behaviors followed by a reward, that is, those that are reinforced, tend to recur more often than those not so rewarded. These rewards can provide positive (experiencing something pleasurable or rewarding) or negative (experiencing relief or removal of something unpleasant) reinforcement. As described earlier, all addictive behaviors have positive physical and psychological rewards. In fact, reinforcing potential is an important characteristic in deciding which drugs have an addiction capacity. But the rewards of addictive behaviors can be obvious or subtle. The most obvious reinforcers are the high emotional arousal experienced by the cocaine user; the mellow, relaxed effect of marijuana use; the excitement of a run of luck at a gaming table; and the release of inhibitions after a couple of drinks in a social situation. Subtler but powerful reinforcers provided by addictive behaviors include release from tension, assistance in avoiding difficult emotions, almost imperceptible easing of self-doubt, and a real sense of belonging. Positive reinforcements create the reasons in favor of the addictive behavior, and negative reinforcements, including avoiding withdrawal and loss of the addictive behavior, add to the costs of giving up the behavior. Understanding the reinforcements for any particular individual can offer a clear picture of how the addiction developed and how the behavior is maintained. Unfortunately, even the addict is sometimes unaware of how many important reinforcers there are of the addictive behavior.

One of the most important negative reinforcements for the addictive behavior is the way further use remedies the unpleasant physical reactions that are consequences of the previous use. Feelings of depression follow a cocaine high later that day or in the days following (Weaver & Schnoll, 1999). But more cocaine can temporarily remedy the depression. Negative physical reactions following the mood-altering experiences of addictive behaviors are common and often referred to as withdrawal effects. They occur after a period of using and during a period of nonuse. Individuals who are moving into the Maintenance stage soon learn that the addictive behavior has the wonderful reinforcing property of reducing these negative physical symptoms. The "hair of the dog" remedy for an alcohol-induced hangover is a classic example of negative reinforcement. Relieving or escaping the negative effects creates negative reinforcement of the addictive behavior.

As an individual's addiction becomes well maintained, this negative reinforcing effect becomes more powerful. Regular cocaine users begin to find that "normal" life, experienced without the influence of cocaine, has lost its color and excitement. Events and activities that used to produce pleasure pale in comparison to the high experienced with cocaine. More and more cocaine is needed simply to avoid the depression and disillusionment that accompany a life without cocaine. Dependent, heavy-drinking individuals are in danger of grave physical withdrawal symptoms, including delirium tremens, if they quit drinking abruptly. Thus, drinking to avoid withdrawal becomes an important and compelling reinforcement for continued heavy drinking.

Both positive and negative reinforcement created by the physiological and psychological effects of the behavior play an important role in the development of the well-maintained addiction. Solomon and Corbit

(1974) examined this effect and developed the opponent process theory, which states that, in addition to the positive effects of engaging in the addictive behavior, it is the rebound effect attached to the substance use through a reinforcement process that make addictions so durable and resistant to extinction. These reinforcements play an important role in addiction's Maintenance stage, and physiological reinforcers are particularly potent. The strength of these physiological reinforcement effects during Maintenance probably accounts for the extensive emphasis initially given to physiological factors in the early definitions of addiction. These definitions equated addiction with physical dependence defined as tolerance and withdrawal. However, many addiction specialists have recognized the limitations of using physical dependence as the defining factor in addiction. All the reinforcing effects and not simply the physiological ones are important in creating a well-maintained addiction.

Self-Liberation

Although the processes of conditioning, stimulus generalization, and reinforcement often operate at the threshold of awareness, the addicted individual continues to make choices. These choices interact with the conditioning and reinforcement processes to support engagement in the addictive behavior. There are choices to seek substances, to frequent the places where there is access, and to stay around individuals who engage in similar behaviors. It takes choice and commitment to continue to obtain effective access and to seek the addictive behavior when there are negative personal and social consequences that begin to emerge. The state of being addicted does not take all choice and decision making from the individual. However, choice becomes compromised as more and more areas of life become infused with the addictive behavior and reinforcements provided by it become the most salient ones in the individual's life. The addicted individual appears to be functioning more on autopilot than choosing. Nevertheless, a chosen commitment to the addictive behavior continues.

Helping Relationships

Once a person begins to regularly engage in the addictive behavior, by necessity he or she begins to associate with other persons who are like-minded and have similar patterns of behavior. These groups of individuals create a support system for engaging in the behavior and offer companionship. They become a normative group against which to measure oneself. College binge drinkers report more friends who drink and perceive more drinking on campus (Quigley & Marlatt, 1996). Often individuals who are referred to treatment by courts or families will protest that they do not drink any differently than their peers. This is not usually a lie. These individuals associate with others who are drinking at a similar frequency and intensity. Many times they will assert that they are able to drink with fewer consequences and even less quantity than those around them. If they have a problem, then so do the entire cohort of their friends! Drinking, drug use, gambling, and smoking each create an environment and a support system that encourages continued engagement in the addictive behavior. In moving from Action to Maintenance of an addiction, the behavioral process of helping relationships operates to support the addiction. Fellow users will confirm that families, courts, other friends are overreacting and that there is no problem. Social support for engagement is often a strong component in creating the well-maintained addiction (Beattie & Longabaugh, 1999).

What emerges in this view of the Maintenance stage is the importance of the behavioral processes of change in creating a solidly established, dependent pattern of an addictive behavior that escapes self-regulation and is labeled addiction. The behavioral processes of conditioning, generalization, and reinforcement play crucial roles in developing the regularity of the behavior pattern and in encouraging maintenance of this pattern in the face of negative consequences. Self-liberation plays a role as the individual continues to make choices and commitments that support continued engagement in the addictive behavior. Helping relationships are created that normalize problematic engagement. The addicted individual turns more and more for support to others who are similar in their pattern of behavior. However, the importance of the behavioral processes does not eliminate a role for experiential processes of change and some of the cognitive markers of change.

DECISIONAL BALANCE IN THE MAINTENANCE OF ADDICTION

Is continued dependent engagement in an addictive behavior a rational choice? What role does decision making play in this Maintenance phase of addiction? These are important and controversial questions. Many models of addiction reviewed in Chapter 1 consider the individual's behavior to be no longer under voluntary control once she or he is addicted. In the medical and disease models, the disease takes over and the physiological craving is overwhelming. The problem is an allergy-like condition or a defect in character or will that no longer allows for choice when faced with the prospect of engagement (Sheehan & Owen, 1999). These perspectives have been promoted to counter the overemphasis earlier in this century on addiction as simply a moral problem easily cured by straightening up and doing the right thing (Donovan & Marlatt, 1988).

However, addiction need not be viewed as either totally within or totally outside individual choice and rational functioning. As anyone who has been addicted can attest, once engaged in regular, dependent use, the prospect of living without this particular behavior seems illogical and impossible. On the other hand, there are virtually hundreds of little decisions that are made daily and weekly to ensure access to the behavior. Arranging schedules, making excuses, sneaking off for periods of time, and minimizing consequences are all part of the process of protecting continued engagement in the addiction. Although self-regulation is compromised as individuals move from Action to Maintenance stages, this does not mean that there is a total absence of choice or freedom. When I was a smoker, I remember deciding to leave my warm home to go out driving in the middle of the night in the dead of winter searching to find an "open all night" grocery to get a pack of cigarettes. The choice was spurred by the realization that I would have to go to sleep and, more importantly, wake up the next morning nicotine deprived and craving a cigarette; it seemed a reasonable thing to do at the time. Once addicted, individuals continue to make the little decisions that maintain the addiction and contribute to the stability of the behavioral pattern.

The Potency of Positives in Addiction

Our research into the decisional balance of individuals who are addicted and not interested in change is instructive. In almost all cases smokers and drinkers who do not want to quit endorse the pros of the behavior more strongly than the cons of the behavior (DiClemente et al., 1991; King & DiClemente, 1993; Prochaska, Velicer, et al., 1994; Velicer et al., 1985). This often seems unreasonable to the observer. However, the essence of addiction is that the behavior becomes integral to the individual's functioning in a way that only someone who has experienced it can really understand. Initially considerations like "this feels really good" or "I have never felt this relaxed or at ease" influence continued use. As personal coping and interpersonal environment become more involved, the individual sees the addictive behavior as more and more essential to well-being. Once negative reinforcement, like avoiding withdrawal, begins to kick in, considerations for continued engagement in the addictive behavior have become extremely powerful, often overshadowing many of life's other considerations. The reinforcing effects of physiological, psychological, and social aspects of addiction become a very potent force for continuing the behavior.

The addicted individual's decisional considerations, however, are not all positive. Regular, dependent engagement often brings negative consequences and bad experiences. Addiction does not make individuals completely irrational. Even addicted individuals who do not want to change can generate some negative, personal considerations about their addictive behaviors. Most smokers will report that smoking is a bad habit and can cause serious physical harm. Most drug addicts will admit that their drug use causes some problems. But they also see the negatives as not that bad, and the positives of continued use as substantial (Daniels, 1998; see also Chapter 4 on Precontemplation for recovery). This is their view even when, to an outside observer, the negatives are numerous and very serious. And so the basic decisional stance of the individual in the Maintenance stage of addiction is in favor of the behavior. One reason this balance can be sustained is the real strength of the many positives. But another reason is the puzzling impotency of serious negative consequences. That issue is discussed next.

The Impotency of Negative Consequences

As individuals move from the Action to the Maintenance stage of addiction, serious single consequences are most often followed by a series of other consequences. For example, cocaine use can interfere with attendance and performance at work and result in job loss. Drinking and the ensuing violent arguments with a spouse can cause divorce. Gambling can create such a large debt that theft or embezzlement follows. A disorderly conduct arrest may be directly attributable to intoxication. These are common negative consequences experienced by individuals in the Maintenance stage of addiction. Yet addicted individuals do not readily make the connection between the addictive behavior and its negative consequences.

Such consequences arrive as disconfirming evidence about the benefits of the behavior. But a variety of tactics can be used to deflect their impact. Psychoanalytic clinicians attempting to treat unwilling clients often call their tactics defense mechanisms (Freud, 1949). From a change perspective these tactics are Maintenance mechanisms that often involve the experiential processes of self-reevaluation and consciousness raising. Minimization, rationalization, projection, overintellectualization, repression, and avoidance are all ways of thinking and managing our experiences. They can be used to initiate change, but during this Maintenance stage of addiction are used to protect the commitment to the addictive behavior. Because all of us use many of these tactics in our daily lives to protect our beliefs, values, and ways of behaving, it becomes difficult to identify when they are creating harm. One person's rationalizations are another person's reasons.

A process described by Leon Festinger in 1957 can help to explain how individuals keep a decisional balance positive for a tightly held belief or way of life despite negative consequences. That process is called cognitive dissonance resolution, and it has been very helpful in understanding addiction (Miller & Rollnick, 1991, 2002). There are two common tactics for resolving the cognitive dissonance that are particularly relevant for maintaining addictions. They are deflection and disconnection.

The cognitive dissonance resolution tactic of deflection consists of attributing a negative consequence to technical problems and not to the addictive behavior. For example a technical interpretation of a driving while intoxicated (DWI) arrest would define it as a *driving* problem or as *getting stopped by the police.* So a solution might be to avoid driving when having consumed too much or to be more vigilant for police. Drinking is not the problem. This solution is reminiscent of the original dissonance studies in which true believers whose end-of-the-world prediction failed resolved the disconfirmation by seeing a miscalculation in the date as the problem, not the belief that the end is imminent. Deflection is a helpful mechanism in maintaining an addiction and avoiding the impact of consequences.

Seeing the consequences as unrelated to the basic behavior and blaming some other factor is called disconnection. It is at the heart of what has been called denial. While addicts are not immune to experiencing the consequences, they do possess an incredible ability to reinterpret the source of the consequences as unrelated or minimally related to the behavior. One professional basketball player was caught using cocaine by the National Basketball Association (NBA) random drug-testing program. Even after a suspension from his job and a 4-week stay in a drug treatment program, the basketball player insisted he did not have a drug problem. The real problem, he said, was the drug testing policy of the NBA and how it was unfair to players. He had a drug *testing* and not a drug *taking* problem. Disconnection of consequences from the addictive behavior is rather common. Smokers complain about pollution and pollen as the causes of their chronic coughs. Alcohol-dependent individuals will claim the problem is their wives' hypersensitivity to alcohol.

Deflection and disconnection as well as many traditional defense mechanisms are part of the self-reevaluation process of change. Reevaluations include reorganizing how one sees the behavior in terms of current values and beliefs. In maintaining an addiction these reevaluations are in the service of sustaining the addiction and keeping it a valued part of the individual's life. In order to do this the addicted individual must manage the decisional considerations and keep them tipped toward continued engagement in the addictive behavior.

A Possible Role for Self-Efficacy

A very different explanation for the impotency of negative consequences lies in the self-efficacy beliefs of the individual. As discussed in Chapter 2 as a marker of change, self-efficacy is confidence that the individual can perform a particular behavior. The greater the confidence and sense of effectiveness an individual has, the greater the probability that the individual will make the effort and persist in the effort to perform the behavior (Bandura, 1977, 1997). In a presentation at the University of Houston, Bandura described a particularly compelling example of persistence that he attributed to self-efficacy. He noted that many very famous authors and artists persisted in their endeavors despite overwhelming negative external evaluations. One author of an award-winning novel had received over 500 rejection letters before finding a publisher. Persistence in the face of such negative feedback in this case was attributed to a strong sense of self-efficacy.

What is a virtue for the talented writer is a vice for the addicted individual. This same type of persistence can be seen in the maintenance stage of addiction. Because the addicted individual is experiencing negative consequences, it appears to others that he or she is losing self-regulation. However, this individual often is completely convinced of his or her self-regulatory capacity. Many addicted individuals believe that they are in good control of their behavior. They believe that they are very efficacious in their ability to control the drinking, drugging, gambling, or eating. They just don't do it or don't want to do it. Unlike the award-winning novelist, the reality is that they cannot completely control the addiction or they would have done so, in light of the serious consequences. This overinflated sense of efficacy leads to what Bandura described as the "confident incompetent" (Bandura, 1977, 1986). This unrealistic confidence is an effective tool to deflect the impact of any negative consequences. These tactics reflect a critical deficit in accurate self-assessment and can help explain, at least in part, the inability of basic feedback to influence individuals in the Maintenance stage of addiction.

THE CONTEXT OF CHANGE
IN THE MAINTENANCE OF ADDICTION

Multiple problems in the context of change accelerate the path through the stages of addiction, complicate self-regulation, interfere with feedback mechanisms, undermine realistic assessment of self-efficacy, and multiply risk factors. If they did not exist prior to dependent engagement in the addictive behavior, they develop as a function of time spent in the

Maintenance stage of addiction. Once it is well maintained, the addiction becomes integrated into the entire life context of the individual. Issues and problems in other areas of functioning interact with and continue to fuel the addiction. Clinical depression, marital conflict, and parental interference become reasons for engaging in the addiction as well as problems in their own right. Problems within the personality structure of the individual and with basic values and beliefs also are exacerbated as the individual continues to engage in the addictive behavior.

As the addictive behavior becomes a predominant presence and an overriding value in the life of the individual, other areas of life are undervalued, problems in those areas seem less significant, and effective problem solving is compromised. Problems in the context of change increase the probability that the addictive behavior will have greater general coping value and interfere with the feedback system. As the problems in these various areas multiply, the relief provided by the addictive behavior becomes a potent negative reinforcer. As the addiction becomes well maintained, the research findings of Newcomb, Bentler, and colleagues (Newcomb & Bentler, 1988; Newcomb, Scheier, & Bentler, 1993) become most informative and relevant. They found that the addictive behavior and other life problems are mutually interactive. Life problems promote engagement in the addictive behavior, which in turn increases the number and intensity of life problems, which promotes engagement in the addictive behavior, which in turn . . . and so on. These findings describe the negative downward spiral of increasing serious consequences that is often experienced as individuals remain in the Maintenance stage of addiction. Continued engagement creates a context of life adapted to the addiction. By the time the individual has developed a well-maintained addiction, the problems in areas of functioning have become intertwined with the addictive behavior whether they preceded the addiction or not. These problems often impede the ability of the individual to move toward recovery.

The current discussion of dual-diagnosis problems offers an interesting example of these interactions. Many individuals who suffer from serious mental disorders also have significant problems with substance abuse and other addictive behaviors (Bellack & DiClemente, 1999; Regier et al., 1990). Although alcohol and drugs can be particularly disruptive for these individuals, they can serve as a coping mechanism, a distraction, or a way of joining with other individuals on the fringes of society. Symptoms of schizophrenia, depression, or bipolar disorders can precede, coincide with, or follow engagement in the addiction. However, as the addiction becomes well established in the lifestyle of a mentally ill individual, patterns of interaction emerge. Discontinuing antipsychotic medication produces symptoms that can be masked by alcohol and cocaine use. Drug use triggers loss of housing and produces homelessness. Lack of a structured environment increases engagement in the addiction and exacerbates the mental illness. Behaviors associated with either the addiction or the mental illness bring the individual to the attention of the police and create legal problems. Family members who can tolerate the mental illness become fearful and disgusted with the addiction and refuse to allow the individual to return home. Drugs and alcohol become more important as ways to cope with being homeless and on the streets.

CASE EXAMPLES AND OVERVIEW

The charts and files of every addiction treatment facility are filled with stories of well-maintained addictions. The fictional cases of Bill X and Beth Y illustrate several variations. Both have entered and spent time in the Maintenance stage of change. However, their addictions are integrated into their lifestyles to different degrees and for differing lengths of time.

Bill X is a 40-year-old insurance broker who has been successful in his work but recently has experienced a downturn in business. Bill was a heavy drinker in college and was very active in his fraternity. After college he began working for an insurance company and was very successful, getting one promotion after another. Drinking continued to be significant part of his life after graduation from college. Entertaining was an integral part of his work, and his social circle was filled with fraternity buddies who continued to go to sporting events and to meet in bars where the alcohol flowed freely. He met his wife at one of these gatherings. They married and have two children who are now 14 and 12 years old.

Although always considered a heavy drinker who could hold his liquor, his drinking and problems associated with his drinking have increased in the past 10–12 years. As he moved up in the company, he had more evening business activities and would extend these events into the wee hours of the morning, consuming ever-greater amounts of alcohol. His boss began giving him some feedback about his drinking and he reacted by changing jobs, going to a company that had been courting him for the past several years. With the advent of the children, his wife became focused on the home and the children and did not accompany him on many of his social outings with his friends. His social network became smaller and more alcohol-concentrated as some of his buddies no longer joined in the heavy drinking activities. Soon he was going to a neighborhood bar alone and creating a social network there. His wife was less tolerant of this activity and began complaining about his drinking. He responded at first by trying to spend more time at home but the children were not used to his being there and rebelled at his efforts to control their lives. Increased family conflict increased his desire and need to be out of the house, either at work events or at the bar. Instead of trying to resolve the conflicts, he escaped them and increased his drinking. One night, coming home from one of his heavier drinking episodes, he was stopped by the police and given a sobriety test. He failed and was given a ticket for drunk driving. He attempted to hide this from his wife and hired an excellent attorney who was able to have the charges dismissed. However, when his wife found out, she was furious and threatened to divorce him if he did not get stop drinking.

During this entire time, Bill continued to see himself as a heavy drinker who could hold his liquor. He felt justified in drinking heavily because of his work and felt that he did not drink excessively in comparison to others in his group. He believed that he could stop his drinking whenever he really wanted and that drinking was one of the few pleasures he allowed himself because work was very demanding and he had no other hobbies or pastimes. His conversations with others about his drinking tended to reinforce his views as he mainly had conversations with others who drank as heavily or more heavily. He believed that his wife was being unreasonable in asking him to change his entire lifestyle, that his children were ungrateful and spoiled, and that problems at work were simply the result of a business downturn that has little to do with him.

Beth Y is a 28-year-old divorced mother of two children who is struggling to keep her job as a manager in a retail department store, take care of her children, and have a relationship with a man she met over a year ago. Although she had experimented with a variety of drugs while she was in high school and both drank and smoked cigarettes, she had not become involved with illegal drugs to any great extent until 5 years ago. Her ex-husband began to use crack cocaine about that time and introduced her to it. She started off just using with him on weekends when she was off work. It was a great high and helped her to get away from the hassles of work and the kids. Because her parents lived nearby, she could ask them to baby-sit so she and her husband could go out and have some fun. Her husband quickly became a heavy user, started getting into trouble with the law, and lost his job. He would spend lots of time away from home and with other women. Beth confronted him over and over and nagged him about the money problems until she could no longer put up with it. With the aid of her parents, she divorced her husband and was attempting to begin her life over.

About a year ago she met Mel and really fell for him. Mel was similar to her first husband but had a good-paying job and seemed more responsible. Mel also used cocaine on occasion, and they began to use together to relax and chill out. Beth's parents were very involved in taking care of the children since her ex left, so she could get away and go out with Mel some evenings as well as on the weekend. She began to spend more and more time at his place, where there was rather easy access to the cocaine. What began as periodic social using soon became a daily activity, but only after work or on the weekends. She began to have some problems at work because she was becoming more impatient with her fellow workers and was more irritable. As she spent more and more time with Mel, her use increased but she continued to get to work and spend some time with the kids. She believed that she deserved some happiness after all the stress and hard work. The cocaine became her way to relax and to have fun. Other activities seemed less exciting, and she even cut down on her drinking. Her increased use of cocaine has gone on for the past 9 months but she has been able to hide it from her parents. They think that Mel is not a good influence and have been asking her about him, but they are unaware of the cocaine use. She defends Mel and her right to have a relationship that makes her feel good. The children have also begun to complain that they do not see her. She believes that they are jealous of her relationship with Mel and complains that their father does not help take care of them at all. She begins to spend more and more time away and over at Mel's.

Both these cases represent individuals who have entered the Maintenance stage and illustrate behaviors, thoughts, and activities in the dimensions of change that represent the Maintenance stage of addiction (see Table 3.1). Bill X has maintained the addictive behavior over a longer time, accomplished the tasks of integrating it into his life, has a decisional balance and efficacy beliefs that support continuation of heavy drinking, and clearly has engaged in the behavioral processes of change to create a well-maintained alcohol addiction. Beth Y is in the midst of the Maintenance stage of cocaine addiction. She has flirted with cocaine before, but this time she is engaging in behavioral processes that narrow social interactions and support the cocaine use. Problems are minimized and deflected. Context of change issues complicate and, at the same time, interact with her increasing use of cocaine. Consequences are still at a minimum currently but could increase dramatically if job problems or family pressures increase. Both Bill and Beth are now faced with the challenge of changing the addiction and beginning the road to recovery.

SUMMARY

Understanding addiction as an end stage of the path of change provides a dynamic, behavior-based, process-oriented view that is in marked contrast to the more traditional static, person-based views. Addiction is a

TABLE 3.1. The Maintenance Stage of Addiction: An Overview of the Dimensions of Change

Stage task

Sustaining a regular, dependent, problematic pattern of behavior over time (more than 6 months) so that it becomes integral.

Change processes at work

Behavioral processes contribute to developing regularity of the behavioral pattern and encourage continued use in the face of negative consequences:

Reinforcement: Behavior has physiological and psychological rewards—for example, positive reactions and feelings as well as removal of negative feelings—that increase frequency and create a pattern of behavior.

Conditioning: Situations, activities become associated with the behavior, creating a web of cues that trigger the desire to engage.

Stimulus generalization: The web of triggers spreads to more and more settings, circumstances, and emotions in the person's life.

Self-liberation: The person makes choices to engage, ensuring access and opportunities to engage even as self-regulation is compromised.

Helping relationships: The person associates more and more with others who engage, support, and encourage the behavior. This social system normalizes this problematic behavior.

Markers of change

Decisional balance: Weighted strongly toward engagement because of potency of the positives, impotency of the negative consequences, and increasing loss of alternative rewards.

Self-efficacy: Possible false sense of self-control and/or sense of hopelessness about the ability to change that justify maintenance of the status quo.

Context of change

Multiple increasing problems—preexisting and/or consequent problems—function to complicate self-regulation, interfere with feedback mechanisms, undermine self-efficacy, and multiply risk factors.

---

well-maintained pattern of regular, dependent engagement and requires Maintenance stage activities in order to sustain the behavior. The critical dimensions of self-regulation and self-control have become disabled as the individual moves from the Action stage to Maintenance. Once in Maintenance, the individual often finds it easier to continue the problematic behavior than to change. As time in this Maintenance stage extends beyond the minimum Action stage criterion of 3–6 months, the addictive behavior becomes more entrenched in the life of the individual.

Engaging in the addictive behavior becomes the norm. The ties between this behavior and other aspects of the life of the individual grow stronger. For the well-maintained addict, repeated engagement in the addictive behavior seems to relieve more of life problems than it creates. Actually, the addiction becomes a constant companion, a friend, and something to count on for a predictable effect or outcome. Some commentators on addiction describe it as a love relationship because of the intensity of the bond and the commitment to the behavior (Peele, 1985).

The behavioral and cognitive/experiential processes of change contribute to establishing this habitual pattern of behavior that becomes integral to the individual's functioning. The behavioral processes of change contribute cues and reinforcements. Choices and relationships sustain engagement as the behavior extends into many areas of functioning, creating a context that supports the addiction. The decisional balance remains supportive of the addiction because of the many benefits. When negative consequences in various areas of functioning occur as a result of the addiction, a variety of tactics can be used that provide supportive self-evaluations, resolve cognitive dissonance, and create a false sense of self-efficacy that keep the negative consequences at bay. It takes effort, energy, and thought to create the well-maintained addiction. This maintained behavior pattern then takes on a life of its own and is often viewed as having a life separate from the individual engaging in the behavior. Once entrenched in the Maintenance stage of addiction, the individual seems incredibly attached to the behavior and very resistant to change, which describes perfectly the first stage in the process of recovery that we have labeled Precontemplation for changing the addictive behavior. Thus the end-state of the process of addiction becomes the beginning state for the process of recovery.

Many individuals never engage in some addictive behaviors. Others engage but do not become addicted. The reality is that the well-maintained addiction is achieved by relatively few of the people who experiment or engage in addictive behaviors like drinking alcohol. Understanding how these few individuals make their way along the path to develop the well-maintained addiction is the focus of the next section of this volume.

Part II

THE ROAD
TO ADDICTION

The Journey through
the Stages of Addiction

Exploring the Precontemplation, Contemplation, and Preparation Stages of Becoming Addicted

Thinking plays a role before, during and after someone becomes addicted. Expectations, intentions, and experiences protect some from becoming addicted and lead others to rush toward addiction.

The stages of intentional behavior change track individuals as they shift from being uninterested in an addictive behavior to becoming involved, attached, and finally addicted. The end of this change process is the well-maintained addiction as defined in the previous chapter. The process of becoming addicted involves creating a new habit as opposed to modifying or stopping an already established one. This examination of the process of becoming addicted offers a dynamic view of the personal path into addiction that highlights what influences movement toward addiction, how addictions are created, and ultimately what needs to be undone in recovery.

The road to addiction begins with an individual's exposure to the behavior and with personal views about the value of engaging in the behavior. Early stages of addiction identify the tasks and critical transitions that mark an individual's progress from not considering engagement (Precontemplation) to serious consideration and the creation of a positive decisional balance (Contemplation) and finally to initial engagement and setting the stage for regular engagement (Preparation). Individuals can move forward and backward through these early stages. Understanding the tasks of each early stage in some detail can elucidate the underlying process of becoming addicted and the important distinction between addiction and self-regulated, nonproblematic engagement in the addictive behavior. This chapter will describe the initial stages of this process of change leading to addiction.

PRECONTEMPLATION FOR STARTING AN ADDICTIVE BEHAVIOR

The defining characteristic of Precontemplation is simply that the individual is not seriously considering engaging in the addictive behavior in the foreseeable future, often defined as the next 6 months. This lack of interest can have its origin in a lack of knowledge or information, a value system that excludes consideration of the addictive behavior, or a considered decision not to engage in that behavior. Pressures to engage and protection from engagement vary depending on the age and developmental tasks of the individual in Precontemplation. A 40-year-old mother of three in the suburbs could be expected to have a different set of influences than a 16-year-old high school student in an urban public school when it comes to considering using Ecstasy. However, both would be in Precontemplation for Ecstasy if they have no current consideration of use.

Defining Characteristics of Precontemplation for Engagement

Precontemplators are individuals who have inherited or created decisional considerations that are weighted against engagement in the addictive behavior. Using cognitive/experiential change processes individuals have assimilated information and attitudes that support a negative view of the addictive behavior and counteract any positive views. Consciousness raising, self-reevaluation, environmental reevaluation, emotional arousal/dramatic relief, and social liberation have helped to develop this negative decisional balance. Moreover, the environment of the Precontemplator is often supportive of nonengagement, with few cues and stimuli related to the addictive behavior. For some the natural environment of home, school, work, or neighborhood is structured this way. Others have had to create such an environment by avoiding cues to use and seeking support systems that are incompatible with the addictive behavior. In either case the context of change provides protective rather than risk factors and Precontemplators generally have a strong sense of confidence in their ability to abstain from the behavior and to refuse invitations to consider use.

Precontemplation by Default or Design

How do individuals remain in Precontemplation for an addictive behavior? One strategy is to keep individuals ignorant of the behavior's existence. If individuals are never exposed to alcohol, heroin, cocaine, or gambling either directly or vicariously (through television, news stories, and so on) they would never think about engaging in these behaviors. However, in order for ignorance and unavailability to function as a protective mechanism, the addictive behavior has to be essentially nonexistent in the society or the society has to control access to all information about it.

There are some interesting examples of how information and accessibility interact in the society to promote consideration of an addictive behavior. Prior to the 1960s smoking peyote was limited to a very small ethnic or cultural subgroup in our society and was not even considered by the vast majority of North Americans as a potential behavior for initiation. This changed as word began to spread of its mind-altering properties and stories about its use became popular. Carlos Castaneda's (1984) Don Juan books exposed a large audience to the world of peyote-induced altered states of consciousness. In the context of the cultural messages about seeking greater self-awareness, this information spurred many to consider using this substance. Similarly, a few years ago adolescents in West Texas rediscovered the hallucinogenic and, at times, fatal effects of the Jimson weed. This weed had existed in that community for a long time, but a rekindled interest prompted a number of youth to begin experimenting. Rising awareness and interest moves individuals to consider adding the substance or behavior to their personal repertoire of activities, and so they move out of Precontemplation. This can happen in larger communities or among smaller subgroups of individuals.

Although ignorance may be a protective factor when there is little access, once information or availability arrives, ignorance is no longer blissful. New activities with potential for excitement are immediately attractive to many, particularly to adolescents. After exposure, ignorance means the person has little information with which to evaluate the behavior's uses or consequences. There are also no models clearly demonstrating appropriate use or problematic dependence. Thus Precontemplators, by virtue of ignorance or of lack of opportunity, may actually be more vulnerable to moving quickly to considering use and experimenting and to abuse and dependence. The introduction of alcohol to Native Americans or to the Alaska Inuit seems to be a good example of this accelerated initiation process (Castro, Proescholdbell, Abeita, & Rodriquez, 1999; Reback, 1992).

Ignorance of addictive behaviors probably accounts for only a small minority of Precontemplators. For example, information from the National Household Surveys on Drug Abuse indicates that only 25% of the population report no alcohol or drug use (Clayton, 1992). With the proliferation of state and multistate lotteries to generate revenue, there are few youths or adults who are ignorant of gambling and games of chance or the possibility of winning the lottery (DiClemente, Story, & Murray, 2000; National Academy of Sciences, 1999). The same is true of eating disorders, like bulimia, since examples of well-known entertainers have been described in news stories on TV and in the tabloids. Therefore, ignorance or unavailability of a particular addictive behavior is probably only relevant as a protective factor for some substances, for the very young, or within some subcultures.

Once exposed to information about an addictive behavior and given some access to that behavior, individuals usually must do something to remain in Precontemplation. For most people, low levels of exposure and a number of personal protective factors insulate them against moving into the Contemplation stage. Although research on protective factors is not as extensive as on risk factors, indications are that a modicum of academic and interpersonal success and certain values and attitudes help to keep the addictive behaviors incompatible with the person's self-perception (Chassin, Presson, Pitts, & Sherman, 2000; Jessor et al., 1995). The most often discussed and measured protective factors are religiosity or religious involvement, good family relationships and interactions, good self-control or self-regulation skills, peers in similar stages for adoption, parental monitoring, and economic and social stability (Chassin et al., 2000; Jessor et al., 1995). Each of these can serve as protective factors in the environment. They provide a context of change supportive of remaining in Precontemplation (Clayton, 1992). The presence of these factors helps to keep individuals in Precontemplation. Their absence puts a person at risk for moving into Contemplation and experimentation and for progression through Preparation to Action and from use to abuse (Clayton, 1992; Glantz & Pickens, 1992).

How do these personal protective factors help? Academic success, social stability, and religious values promote positive considerations of alternative behaviors and support negative considerations of engaging in the addictive behavior. Thus, when information becomes available or thoughts about use arise, they are dismissed, and when there is access to the addictive behavior, it is not considered seriously. Because of these protective factors, the individual has a positive self-evaluation and overall life satisfaction, and there is little need to consider risky addictive behaviors. There are few serious problems or issues that would encourage the individual to engage in self-reevaluation or consciousness raising about these behaviors. Personal self-efficacy to perform other satisfying behaviors is high. Efficacy to avoid the problematic addictive behavior is also strong. Temptation to engage in the addictive behavior is low or nonexistent. These factors promote a lack of interest in the acquisition of a new behavior that could disrupt the current patterns.

The TTM's processes of change are what move individuals from one stage to the next. In moving from Precontemplation to Contemplation individuals need to engage in consciousness raising, environmental reevaluation, and self-reevaluation processes of change related to the addictive behavior. Once exposed to that behavior, individuals remain in Precontemplation if they have little or no need to engage in these processes in order to reevaluate their decisional considerations. On the other hand, individuals with fewer protective factors and/or multiple risk factors find it more difficult to avoid a serious consideration of whether the addictive behavior could be an interesting one to try. The combined effects of environment, risk factors, and protective factors on the individual's thinking and self-evaluation engage cognitive/experiential processes of change, potentially shift decisional considerations, and, ultimately, determine whether or not there is movement out of Precontemplation.

The Role of Context in the Transition Forward through the Stages of Addiction

Risk and protective factors are found in the context of change and so highlight its role in the process of becoming addicted. Risk factors represent problems and issues in various areas of functioning that interact with thinking about and engaging in the addictive behavior. Protective factors are usually personal resources, positive factors, and external support in these areas of functioning that make movement toward addiction less likely. The context of change makes movement out of Precontemplation easier or more difficult for a particular individual, depending on the confluence of risk and protective factors in these various areas of functioning. The context influences movement forward or backward through all the stages of addiction.

Protective factors are not simply the opposite of risk factors. Jessor and colleagues (1995) identified a number of protective factors in the areas of current life situation, beliefs and attitudes, interpersonal relations, and social systems. Current life situation elements included positive orientation to school and prosocial activities like involvement in family, volunteer and school activities, sports, and clubs. Belief and attitudes included positive valuing of health and beliefs about health consequences of health risk behavior as well as a commitment to conventional values and intolerance of deviance. Interpersonal relationships and social systems included friends who model conventional behavior and positive relations with adults. This study found that these protective factors independently predicted less involvement in problem behavior, including drinking and use of drugs. In addition these protective factors interacted with an independent set of risk factors to lessen the impact of the risk factors on engagement in problem behaviors.

Protective factors, however, should never be viewed as making it impossible for individuals to progress toward addiction. The environment, for example, can have a great impact on individuals, even those who have many protective factors. Although Robins (1979, 1980) found that having some problems prior to going to Vietnam predisposed individuals to become hooked on drugs in Vietnam, even individuals with low levels of preexisting problems became addicted. During the 1960s many individuals who would have been classified as at very low risk to develop drug use or abuse because of their protective factors experimented and used illegal drugs, particularly marijuana (DiClemente, 1994). Although protective factors certainly make a difference in predicting the probability of engaging in an addictive behavior, they are not completely protective. In fact, for those of us in the treatment arena, it seems clear that, at an individual level, everyone is vulnerable to developing an addiction of one type or another.

Implicit in the discussion of risk and protective factors is the view of addictions as problematic coping responses. Addictive behaviors are needed less as adequate coping is available and stress levels are low to moderate (Shiffman & Wills, 1985). This coping model provides an important perspective and can serve as an overarching conceptual framework with which to understand the Precontemplation stage for initiation of addictions. Individuals who have the ability to make their lives work by achieving some successes in developmentally appropriate tasks and by developing solid relationships with parents and peers tend to be less likely to consider using or abusing substances or engaging in other addictive behaviors.

The protective factors of adequate coping skills and supportive environment to some degree do protect against some addictive behaviors. This seems particularly true for drug abuse (Jessor et al., 1995). High school students who are active and engaged in academic and other pursuits are less vulnerable to seeing drugs as a potentially useful or pleasurable activity. However, these factors do not seem to stop these students from considering and drinking alcohol. Thus, adequate coping may operate as a protective factor only with certain addictive behaviors. For alcohol consumption or other ubiquitous addictive behavior, coping skills may moderate the transition from self-regulated use to abuse and dependence rather than prevent consideration of engaging in an addictive behavior.

Nevertheless keeping low-risk youth in the Precontemplation stage for an addictive behavior is not as problematic as doing the same for individuals with multiple life problems or with families and environments that predispose to engaging in addictive behaviors. Risk factors for acquisition of an addiction extend throughout the various areas of functioning in the life context. The risk factors identified in the Jessor study (1995) included low school achievement and current feeling of hopelessness, depression, and alienation. Attitudes included low expectations for success and for achieving goals. Having friends with problem behaviors and a lack of compatibility between parents and friends also contributed, making social systems more vulnerable to use and abuse. In the areas of personal characteristics, low self-esteem and a low sense of confidence in one's ability to manage responsibilities also were identified as risk factors. These factors combined to predict problem drinking, delinquent-type behavior, marijuana involvement, and sexual intercourse experience. Again, risk factors predicted independently as well as interacted with protective factors.

It is not clear what is the best strategy to inoculate individuals against addiction. The goal of most current prevention efforts is to move individuals into Contemplation so that they can become Precontemplators by decision and design rather than default. Prevention programs like the "just say no" campaign, generic drug education and refusal programs, and "zero tolerance" efforts educate all youths about drugs while emphasizing the dangers of drugs. Most often these programs are implemented across an entire population regardless of risk or protective factors. These programs make youth knowledgeable about drugs in an effort to promote an informed decision not to use. (A more detailed discussion of these programs can be found in Chapter 11.) However, when given to some Precontemplators, such approaches may awaken them to the possibilities and make the addictive behavior more salient than it would be in the natural environment (Tobler, 1986; Werch, 2001). When availability is low and the references, cues, and models for engaging in the behavior are rather restricted, strategies that simply make the particular addictive behavior a nonissue may be best. Creating a highly visible and negative image of the behavior can have the effect of raising awareness of the behavior and making it desirable. This is particularly true during certain developmental periods. In adolescence, for example, negative messages from parental figures often have the paradoxical effect of making the behavior valued because it can contribute to the sense of independence or separation from parents (Chassin, Curran, Hussong, & Colder, 1996). At the same time, the best prevention strategy for high-risk youth or for any youth who will experience significant exposure and accessibility is probably to move them into the Contemplation stage so that they can make a conscious decision not to use. When the environment is filled with availability and opportunity to use, knowing about the addictive behavior and making a choice not to engage is a more protective stance than remaining in ignorance.

The point in time when movement into the Contemplation stage is desirable for high-risk or low-risk youth is not clear. Keeping individuals in the Precontemplation stage for adoption of the addictive behavior is not an easy task. Simplistic approaches may be part of the problem rather than contributing to the solution. Identification of subgroups of individuals with varying degrees of risk and protective factors seems to be the best way to think about dividing up the population and developing prevention strategies. Numerous studies have identified risk and protective factors for initiation of substance abuse, gambling, and other addictive behaviors. However, few have examined how these factors affect Precontemplators and their thinking about the addictive behavior. Until we learn about how prevention programs interact with the various environmental and family influences and impact processes of change with respect to the specific addictive behaviors in question, we will not understand the very first steps that individuals take toward addiction (DiClemente, Story, & Murray, 2000; Werch, 2001).

Several groundbreaking studies have begun to examine the process of change for acquisition of an addictive behavior. Pallonnen and colleagues (1998) examined adolescent smoking and compared these results to the more extensive research on adults. He found that both teens and adults appear to utilize identical cognitive and behavioral activities to change their smoking. Teens also looked similar to adults on the markers of decisional balance and temptation to smoke. There were some differences between adults and teens in their level of use for particular processes of change. However, adolescent smokers looked similar to adult smokers on these dimensions of change overall. In another study that focused on staging acquisition and cessation for adolescent smokers, Pallonen and colleagues (1998) examined Precontemplators for beginning smoking and those who were planning to try smoking. Those who had never smoked were most vulnerable to try smoking when they anticipated that smoking would help them cope and reduce negative mood or increase positive mood. Hudmon, Prokhorov, Koehly, DiClemente, and Gritz (1997) examined decisional considerations and temptations to try smoking among a multiethnic cohort of 5th, 8th, and 12th graders and found the predicted increase in temptation and pros of smoking and a steady decrease in cons of smoking across the stages of smoking initiation. These studies have identified various dimensions of change from the TTM as useful for examining and understanding smoking initiation. Similar measures should be used and monitored to evaluate the impact of prevention efforts aimed at those in Precontemplation for any of the addictive behaviors.

THE CONTEMPLATION STAGE FOR ADDICTION

Once individuals begin to consider engaging in an addictive behavior, they move into the Contemplation stage for addiction. Individuals in Contemplation are open to considering the positive and negative aspects of the behavior. They are amenable to listening to and thinking about advertisements and information about the behavior. Stories about how a particular famous athlete became involved in using cocaine or developed an alcohol problem may become particularly interesting to Contemplators. Looking toward various role models to see how they deal with the behavior, seeking information about how many peers engage in the behavior, and asking questions about possible consequences are all more likely at this time.

These activities do not occur necessarily within a concentrated period of time. For example, a 15-year-old male may look around one day and notice that two of his friends have begun to experiment with cigarettes. At that point he thinks that this behavior is stupid. Then he begins to notice more cigarette ads and how some of those people in the ads look interesting or "cool," "boss," "hip," or otherwise enviable. Several months later he may see one of his teachers at a mall smoking a cigarette and be surprised but intrigued. After months or possibly years of these infrequent but important considerations, he finds himself out having some fun with one of these friends who smokes and asks to try one of those "cancer sticks." The process is often a subtle one. More often than not there is not one single consideration or moment of truth but a building up of the pros for initiation and a lessening of the cons or negative considerations of the behavior (Hudmon et al., 1997).

Defining Characteristics

The tasks of the Contemplation stage of addiction are to gather information in order to weigh the pros and cons of engaging in the addictive behavior until a decision is reached either to move forward to Preparation or to return to Precontemplation. In Contemplation the cognitive and experiential processes of change are engaged and influence the positive and negative decisional considerations about the addictive behavior. Images, messages, modeling, and personal experiences about drugs, smoking, alcohol, and gambling are taken in and processed by the individual. Consciousness raising gathers important information and considerations. Self-reevaluation and environmental reevaluation compare and contrast the information about addictions with other salient and relevant information about the individual's life and current functioning. Personal experiences and vicarious experiences of peers who are positively or negatively affected by engaging in the addictive behavior create emotionally arousing experiences that contribute to decisional considerations. Societal prohibitions and norms engage the social liberation process of change, supporting the cons or paradoxically offering some pros for engagement to the more rebellious.

Decisional considerations shift back and forth, marking both Contemplation and ambivalence, and can move gradually or more precipitously either toward or against engagement. There are three outcomes for Contemplators who are processing all these considerations. The first would be to have the decisional consideration shift toward engagement and transition forward to the Preparation stage. The second would be have all these considerations, experiences, and evaluations create a decisional balance that is firmly against engagement and supports a transition back into the Precontemplation stage. The third is to remain in Contemplation and to continue information gathering with a decisional balance that is rather ambivalent and insufficient to support movement forward or backward in the stages of change.

Although behavioral processes of change and self-efficacy related to the addictive behavior are not as relevant in Contemplation, there is a role for temptation. As the pros for engaging in the addictive behavior increase, individuals become more tempted to engage. An increase in temptation to try the addictive behavior accompanied by an increase in the pros for engagement creates an increased risk for initial use or experimentation (Werch & DiClemente, 1994). Confidence to avoid the behavior decreases as temptation to use increases for those who are moving ahead through the stages toward addiction.

The Contemplation stage can include some initial experimentation with the addictive behavior. This experimentation offers a personal experience with the behavior that gets added to the information already in the decisional considerations. Initial experimentation seems to fit into this stage better than in the Preparation stage, since a large number of individuals who engage in limited experimentation find information about the addictive behavior that shifts the decisional balance away from considering any additional use. If you talk to individuals who tried a particular drug once and never touched it again, they will tell you that they tried it and so disliked the experience that they never thought about doing it again. Data from a recent survey of eighth-grade students found that 30% of them reported that they had tried alcohol once or twice and were not planning to try it again (Werch, personal communication, November 20, 2001). This also can happen with substances like hallucinogens, where the altered state is so scary or so bizarre that the individual never wants to experience that kind of loss of control again. A bad first experience can be considered a behavioral protective factor that interferes with the transition from the Contemplation stage to Preparation stage and prevents extensive experimentation or regular use.

Initial experimenters, then, are best considered Contemplators because many will not go on to engage in the behavior to any significant extent. However, initial experimenters whose experience with the drug or the behavior is positive, intriguing, or interesting will add this information to the decisional balance matrix, tipping it in the direction of continued experimentation and possible initiation. This personal experience seems to be critical for moving forward into the Preparation stage. I remember hearing about research done many years ago indicating that individuals who become alcoholics tended to remember their first drink of alcohol, whereas other drinkers, who did not have a problem, would not. Several cocaine abusers that I have seen in treatment have indicated that, even though they had tried other drugs and had been able to keep out of trouble with these drugs, the first time they tried cocaine they knew they were in trouble and would become hooked. The first experience is then a critical element in the process of decision making that promotes movement toward becoming addicted.

Thinking and Making a Decision about the Addictive Behavior

In the Contemplation stage, the individual begins to develop the personal rationale that will support the move toward use and possible addiction. Constellations of positive and negative considerations begin to develop, but accurate information is often missing for many individuals at this stage. If you ask teens, for example, the risks of using cocaine or the socially acceptable reasons for using alcohol, you can access the set of concepts that they have put together about these behaviors (Bandura, 1986; Brown, Goldman, Inn, & Anderson, 1980; Dunn & Goldman, 1996). Teens find these concepts confirmed and disconfirmed on a rather regular basis. A 16-year-old girl is told that cocaine causes death and physical injury, even the first time you use it. When she begins to talk with several peers who have done cocaine a number of times and appear to be among the "healthiest" kids she knows, she begins to question not only the "facts about cocaine" but also the source of those facts. She then modifies her decisional balance in ways that make her more likely to experiment with cocaine.

Active consideration of the behavior and initial experimentation appear important in the initiation of marijuana, according to research by Kandel and colleagues (Kandel & Davies, 1992). A longitudinal study of high school students contacted first in 1971 and followed for 13 years examined the onset of marijuana use and the progression to near-daily use. Interestingly, a very large number of this sample (78.4% of the men and 70% of the women) reported having used marijuana by the third follow-up in 1984 when they were age 28–29. This figure indicates the existence of a cohort effect when examining the process of change with different substances. It is unlikely that such a high percentage of 28- to 29-year-olds would now report marijuana use because this drug is not as popular or as accepted in our society at present.

To study onset of marijuana use, these same researchers examined all subjects who were not using by age 15–16 at the time of the first interview and looked for predictors of who would begin to use over the next 13 years. Because they were interested in social psychological processes of imitation and social reinforcement, there were no individual cognitive considerations like pros and cons included in this analysis. Factors that emerged as significant predictors of onset of marijuana use were high educational expectations, parental use of psychoactive drugs, and participation in delinquent activities. These factors increased the risk, whereas frequency of attendance at religious services decreased risk of initiating marijuana use. There were also some predictors that operated differently for males and females. For males, in contrast with females, a higher level of parental education decreased risk. On the other hand, closeness to parents decreased risk of initiation for females but not for males. Females seem to be influenced more by the number of friends using marijuana than are males. These findings seem to support a role for imitation and social influence. However, the differences between males and females seem to argue that it may not be the event or influences as much as the evaluation of the event by the individual that affects consideration and onset of use. Moreover, the majority (56.4%) of those who experimented with marijuana did not progress to regular use. These findings indicate an important role for personal decisional considerations in the initiation of addictive behaviors.

This personal cognitive evaluation process is often underestimated in the research on initiation. Adults, particularly those who have never left the Precontemplation stage, assume that the initiation process in addiction is an automatic one involving little or no thought. Because acquisition of many addictive behaviors occurs during adolescence, impulsivity and lack of thinking appear to be logical explanations. However, this is a rather naive position. Adolescents think. They do not necessarily come up with the same conclusions as adults, however. I can remember some of my own thinking as many of my peers began smoking. I considered it and even took a couple of puffs at one point. However, since my father was a smoker who quit during my early adolescence, parental statements about the problems of cigarette smoking influenced most of my thinking. In fact, I felt pride that I would not smoke despite the influence of my peers. This seems to me a conscious Contemplation process and a decision to not use at that time. Although my initial adolescent Contemplation of smoking ended in movement back to Precontemplation, I moved into Contemplation again in my early 20s. This time I became a regular cigarette smoker. I convinced myself that smoking had some social merit and could be of value in my interactions with new groups of colleagues. The self-reevaluation and environmental reevaluation processes were critical to my Contemplation and decision making.

For each addictive behavior there are separate decisional considerations. However, there can be overlap, and there even seems to be a pattern to the initiation of multiple addictive behaviors, particularly those that involve substances (Kandel, 1975). Once an individual has evaluated one addictive behavior positively, it is easier to use some of the same positive considerations (exciting, excellent, risky, cool, etc.) for other behaviors. It is also the case that peers who engage in one addictive behavior will model others and offer positive role models for engaging in a second or third behavior. However, it is also true that individuals do not often choose to engage in these other behaviors. Although this process of contamination has been identified, it has not been studied extensively. In particular, expectancies about the benefits for engagement across multiple addictive behaviors have not been examined. Most studies focus on the actual engagement in multiple behaviors (experimental use, abuse, dependence) and do not examine how participants are thinking about these behaviors (Glantz & Pickens, 1992; Winters, Fals Stewart, O'Farrell, Birchler, & Kelly, 2002).

The Context of Change and Contemplation

The context of change is filled with risk and protective factors that influence evaluations in the Contemplation stage. The same protective factors that help keep people in Precontemplation can provide important information and experiences for Contemplation. Academic achievement, positive relationships with adults, prosocial attitudes and activities, self-confidence, and healthy peer networks offer positive reasons for not engaging in the addictive behavior. They also provide support for a negative evaluation of the behavior in terms of its ability to add anything of value to the individual's life. On the other hand, risk factors like low self-esteem, problematic peers and relationships, lack of achievement and prospects for success in life contribute to more positive considerations for engaging in the addictive behavior. The reinforcing nature of the addictive behavior can be particularly appealing to one who is mired in a negative and unrewarding context. Thus, the context of change brings multiple influences to bear on decision making that can foster forward movement toward addiction or offer positive alternatives that promote lack of interest.

One of the central mechanisms responsible for initiation of addictive behaviors is peer or social influence. We are learning more about how social influence operates (Bandura, 1986; Cialdini, 1988; Werch et al., 2000). Social influence is not simply a matter of being coerced by peers into using a substance. How modeling by peers affects an individual is subtle and complex. Bandura (1986) describes a comparator process whereby the individual compares input from the environment with internal standards and norms. According to this theory each of us uses experiences of society and norms that we observe, adds other considerations and creates a set of personal norms and expectancies about our behavior. Influences from others to behave in a certain way are processed through this screen of personal norms and values. In making decisions it seems that each individual develops a very personal decisional balance sheet (Janis & Mann, 1977) that is a combination of environmental influences and personal considerations. It is in this context that vulnerability to social influence operates. Knowledge, attitudes, and beliefs interact with personal experience and social influence to create a dynamic matrix that develops and shifts during an individual's life.

In addition, decisional considerations relating to substance use are influenced by personal self-evaluation. The more negative this self-evaluation, the greater is the susceptibility to social influences (Schinke et al., 1991). Low self-esteem, low self-confidence, and a lack of a sense of personal control increase the need for social approval and so increase the influence of individuals who are models promoting a deviant but attractive lifestyle. Social influences pass through the screen of personal Contemplation to become a part of the decision making. All of these are the active ingredients that contribute to a decision to use or not to use.

Experimentation initiates the physiological and behavioral experiences that influence the decision whether or not to continue engaging in the addictive behavior. The first experimental use becomes a marker event about which researchers need to gain more information. One-time experimenters are very different from frequent experimenters. For the individual whose expectancies and reflections make her vulnerable to social influence, the press of peers engaging in the addictive behavior coupled with the positive aspects of the first experimentation promotes continued experimentation with the behavior. Once the first experimentation opens the way to continued experimentation and multiple use experiences, there is a decision to engage that indicates movement of the Contemplator into the next stage of addiction, Preparation.

PREPARING FOR REGULAR USE

The Preparation stage for initiation is marked by continued experimentation and an often gradual but deliberate setting of the stage for regular use. Whether that pattern of use becomes a "social," moderated one or a less controllable one, it is a pattern of use that marks the end of Preparation and the beginning of the Action stage of addiction. Preparation is another transitional stage, and the directional outcome of the process of change is not predetermined. When experiences with the behavior deliver positive reinforcements physiologically and psychologically, the pros of engaging in the behavior continue to grow and the cons diminish. "If something feels so good, how can it be bad?" is a typical comment of someone moving through the Preparation stage. At the same time, if there are few or no negative consequences associated with the behavior, it becomes harder and harder to believe all the negative statements by parents, school health programs, and media public service announcements. Protective factors are being undermined at the same time that positive experiences are enhancing the value of the behavior. Continued shifting of the decisional considerations to favor engagement sets the stage so that both cognitive and affective evaluations support acquisition of regular use.

Defining Characteristics

The Preparation stage of change represents a bridge on the road to addiction from the positive decisional considerations supporting engagement that were established in the Contemplation stage to the repeated involvement in the behavior that characterizes the action stage of change. During Preparation the decisional balance is tipped toward engagement and the individual is open to experimenting. Initial experimentation becomes more frequent. Decisional considerations supporting engagement are strong enough to create a commitment to engage in the behavior as opportunity arises. Temptation to use increases and there is a growing sense of confidence that the individual can engage without serious consequences. Self-efficacy to abstain from the behavior decreases. During the Preparation stage there is also increasing use of behavioral process as the individual becomes more extensively exposed to the addictive behavior. Cues in the environment become associated with engagement in the behavior. Primary reinforcers associated with the behavior increase. Secondary reinforcers that involve activities related to the addictive behavior begin to increase the desire for and the frequency of engagement. The stage is being set for a more regular, repeated engagement that can become a pattern of behavior. At any point in the Preparation stage the individual may have negative experiences or consequences that will force a reconsideration of the decision to engage. At that point the individual may go back to weighing the pros and cons and may return to the Contemplation or Precontemplation stages. However, if the commitment and reinforcement continue, the individual develops a plan of how to include this addictive behavior in his or her life. Beginning to engage in a repeated manner, so that the addictive behavior becomes patterned and habitual, marks the transition into the Action stage of addiction.

Experimentation and Early Engagement in the Addictive Behavior

We have some pieces of information about starting an addiction that can help us get a clearer picture of important aspects of the Preparation stage. A serious flirtation with the behavior contributes toward making a commitment to including this behavior as part of the individual's life. There have been many studies to confirm this fact. Laurie Chassin and her colleagues (Chassin, Presson, Sherman, & Edwards, 1990; Chassin et al., 2000) have found that even infrequent experimentation in adolescence doubles the risk of becoming an adult smoker. While engaging in the behavior, even at an experimentation level of use, is a good predictor of continued use and later use, behavior alone is not the only predictor.

Among preteens and adolescents experimental use is part of a complex picture. There are differences between current substance abusers classified as drug abusers before age 18 compared with a group diagnosed after 18. For the early-onset group, behavioral adjustment problems, antisocial tendencies (problems following societal rules), and hyperactivity are risk factors for initiation (Pandina, Johnson, & Labouvie, 1992; Tarter, 1988). The early-onset group also has more school performance problems, a central task of the adolescent years (Tarter & Mezzich, 1992), and problems in executive cognitive functioning (Giancola & Tarter, 1999). When connected to family disruption and adjustment problems, the risks of becoming addicted increase.

How can we understand risk factors in light of the stages of initiation and the context of change? It is becoming clearer to clinicians and researchers in the field that a multivariate and multicomponent array of influences are needed to explain adoption of addictive behaviors (Schinke et al., 1991). Social learning and social cognitive theory (Bandura, 1986) has been used to attempt to understand the phenomenon of initiation because it combines environmental influences with behavioral experiences and self-regulatory mechanisms in an interactive, mutual causality. Although it is difficult to isolate contributory factors in an interactive model, it is important to discuss them.

Researchers have examined the ontogeny of substance use across individuals in order to find the common elements that predict substance abuse. Their conclusion was that "the transition from use to abuse to dependence, reflecting a progression of severity, is actually highly individualized and is invariably not a linear process" (Tarter & Mezzich, 1992, p. 154). All of the preceding predictors create a probability estimate for initiation that never accounts for all of the variance. For example, as just mentioned, hyperactivity is a risk factor for the development of alcoholism. However, at most, 20% of hyperactive children develop alcoholism. Parental alcohol problems are associated with the increasing probability that the individual will develop drug abuse or dependence, yet the majority of individuals with histories of parental alcohol problems do not develop abuse or dependence (Cadoret, 1992).

The path through the Contemplation and Preparation stages of addiction is a winding one with no absolutely predetermined outcome. For each individual the confluence of family, environmental, and peer influences interact with personal views, norms and expectancies to create complex cognitive processing of information that leads to experimentation. Experimentation brings the individual into direct, first-hand experiential knowledge about the effects of the addictive behavior. The influence of the behavior itself begins to play a major role as the individual moves through the Preparation stage. The vagaries of this path through the early stages of initiation are best illustrated by looking at two fictional examples.

Sally Struggle, a 16-year-old high school sophomore who is a C student, has always had trouble with academics in school. She had to repeat an early grade and has always wanted to appear older than her chronological age. Her parents, Sid and Samantha, have serious marital problems and openly argue in front of Sally. She has two older brothers who have been somewhat overprotective of their little sister. Since age 14 Sally has dabbled with cigarettes and found a group of friends who are risk takers, older, and get in trouble with the law for vandalism. During the past 6 months several friends have begun to use cocaine when they go out on the weekend. Sally has thought about trying cocaine but avoided any experimentation until last month. During the past month she did break down and use twice. She is currently considering using again this weekend and spending more time with the couple of user friends since they are more "fun" to be around.

Suzy Smart, on the other hand, is a sophomore who is one year younger but is a B+ to A student. She is the oldest of four children, and her parents argue about finances but in general have a solid relationship. Recently Suzy has been having a great deal of conflict with her parents, marked by her rebellious stance about wanting to date an older male who is 18 and a senior. She has been sneaking out of the house to see him because her father has forbidden her to go out with him. During the past month she has been out with him and some of his friends, where they have been using cocaine. Suzy has taken a taste of the cocaine on two occasions. She is about to sneak out again this evening, telling her parents that she will be at the home of a friend. There is a party at the apartment of a close friend of her boyfriend. She knows that they will have some cocaine there. She is considering what will happen at the party.

Sally and Suzy represent two somewhat parallel paths into the Contemplation stage for cocaine use, and both seem poised to enter the Preparation stage. Sally's course seems a bit more gradual and less influenced by the single peer factor of a new boyfriend. Sally's use of cigarettes may also influence her decision making because she has already been breaking rules of conduct with regard to substances. Moreover, the marital problems in the family probably have curtailed communication and parental monitoring and represent complicating problems in the context of change. From both these perspectives Sally seems at greater risk for developing use and potential abuse and dependence.

It would be difficult, however, to predict the immediate decision of either Suzy or Sally. Both could easily move into the Preparation stage for adoption and move into some pattern of regular use. Once experienced, the highs of the cocaine use become another influencing factor. Physiology and psychology join together in the Preparation stage as they influence use. Because Suzy has fewer problems and more resources, it would be logical to predict that she would have a lower probability of developing problems. Such a prediction would be supported by the literature. However, do not put the entire bankroll on that bet. Often individuals like Suzy develop the more serious problem. The interaction of the factors come together in a rather unique way for each individual, and it is that interaction that results in the movement from Contemplation to Preparation to Action. We would need to know much more about the thinking and evaluations of both

Suzy and Sally in order to be able to understand this movement. An in-depth exploration of their attitudes and decisional considerations and the reinforcement value they place on various considerations would help to make our predictions more accurate. It is precisely at this point that the cognitive/experiential processes of self-reevaluation, social liberation, emotional arousal/dramatic relief, and environmental reevaluation become connected to the behavioral processes of conditioning and reinforcement. It is the complex interaction among these processes that can help to understand the probabilities of either Sally or Suzy using drugs.

These examples highlight three important aspects for understanding addiction. One is that additional considerations provided by contextual problems complicate the process of change and contribute to the prediction of more serious involvement in the addictive behavior. The second is that specific decisional considerations related to the specific addictive behavior provide critical information for the prediction of stage movement. The third is that no matter how much we are able to increase predictive ability, there will always be some uncertainty in the equation because the shifts from the one stage to the next depends on unique personal considerations and individual decision making that are constantly changing. We need probabilistic predictions, not absolute, deterministic perspectives to accommodate the process of initiation of an addictive behavior and to increase our ability to predict addiction (Collins & Horn, 1991).

The Context of Change and Preparation

Problems and assets in different areas of functioning complicate the process of change. If we can identify and understand the activity in change processes and markers during the Preparation stage, we can get a clearer picture of the influence that protective and risk factors play. Until the individual moves into the Preparation stage, risk and protective factors in the life context are more subtle and latent contributors to the change process. Once the individual gains a positive decisional balance, builds a commitment to engage in an addictive behavior, and begins to experiment, the influence of multiple problems in various areas of functioning have their greatest impact. The cases of Suzy and Sally presented earlier are examples.

Often serious family and personal adjustment problems are occurring as early use and engagement in the addictive behavior begins. At the same time, vulnerable adolescents or adults are experiencing less success in coping with the tasks of daily life. Even when experimentation occurs later in adolescence, poorer adjustment and diminished coping abilities are often involved. Problematic coping both precedes and follows the engagement in addictive behaviors, particularly for alcohol or drug abuse and dependence (Newcomb & Bentler, 1988; Shiffman & Wills, 1985). Coping deficits and other problems potentiate the processes of change and decision making that prepare an individual to begin to get involved in an addictive behavior. These deficits also contribute to the behavior becoming problematic early on in regular use. I will review potential complications and contributions involved in the transition from Preparation to Action from each of the areas of functioning identified in the TTM's context of change.

Current Life Situation

Environmental influences and current psychological symptoms are most relevant in this area as contributors to engagement in the addictive behavior. These influences and symptoms operate by making the experienced need for the addictive behavior greater or increasing its functional utility. For example, serious anxiety (psychological symptoms) or friends who are into rule breaking (environmental influences) contribute to a positive consideration of addictive behaviors and increase access. On the other hand, belonging to an active church youth group and having a group of peers who do not engage in drinking alcohol or doing drugs, even though there may be one special friend who does, can serve as protective factors.

Beliefs and Attitudes

Beliefs and attitudes concerning the specific addictive behaviors, core life values, and risk taking play a significant role. When positive expectancies about the addictive behavior are joined with positive expectancies about risk taking and a belief that nobody cares, the combination can greatly facilitate movement through Preparation and into Action. The family's belief system is an important influence during Preparation. While family prohibitions and adolescent rebellion can lead to experimentation, other family attitudes can set the stage for accelerated movement through the Preparation stage. For example, the individual may belong to a family "that can hold their liquor" or to one that uses pills whenever there is a problem. Beliefs about the nature of addiction and the power of the particular addictive behavior to "hook" an individual are also critical at this juncture. Beliefs and expectancies act as facilitative and inhibitory factors during the Preparation stage. "Marijuana is not addictive"; "One cannot become addicted to beer"; " Only certain types of people or families get addicted" represent beliefs and expectancies that can accelerate movement through the Preparation stage toward Action.

Interpersonal Conflicts and Issues

Interpersonal conflicts and issues have an enormous influence in the process of adopting an addictive behavior. Initiation of addictive behaviors occurs most frequently during adolescence when interpersonal sensitivity and conflict are a central focus of developmental tasks. These interpersonal conflicts are taken very seriously by the adolescent and are often underestimated or underplayed by surrounding adults. Emerging sexuality and romantic involvement increase the intensity and confusion surrounding adolescent interpersonal relationships. Feelings of alienation from peers, a sense of inadequacy about interpersonal skills and outright conflicts with various same-sex and other-sex peers can contribute significantly to the initiation of the addictive behavior. Risk taking and conformity behavior are both related to these types of conflicts (Newcomb, 1992).

The vulnerable adolescent has problems in interpersonal functioning. On the other hand, interpersonal effectiveness, a sense of belonging with at least one significant other, and having close friends can offer alternative reinforcements and options that make the addictive behavior less alluring. In my earlier examples, it is not coincidental that both Suzy and Sally have significant social and interpersonal pressures. These pressures are part of the process of movement through the Contemplation and Preparation stages.

Social Systems

As is also clear from the examples of Suzy and Sally, social systems complicate the process of change. Family system conflicts can both precede and follow initial movement from the Contemplation to the Preparation stage and can influence additional movement to the Action stage of addiction. Family history of alcohol or drug abuse not only suggests a genetic contribution but also offers modeling and facilitative belief systems as contributory factors (Stanton, 1997). Conflicts between parents or other family stresses create an atmosphere where the addictive behavior, be it using alcohol or drugs, offers a great escape from family tension. Sibling rivalry, hypercritical parenting, lack of parental monitoring, and other problematic family dynamics can create serious negative emotional states that can facilitate adoption of the addictive behavior. Family reaction to any indicators of initial experimentation or excessive use can also be an important event.

Other family system characteristics can hinder initiation. Religious affiliation, family cohesion, and parental involvement have all been identified as factors that can protect the individual from moving forward in the process of change. Messages about drinking and driving, discussing questions about drugs and alcohol consumption, intervening with initial bulimic behavior, and responding to any risk taking and excitement-seeking behavior on the part of the child are also important parental control dimensions (Sanjuan & Langenbucher, 1999). Parents give important messages to the adolescent about family attitudes. These messages can create either conflict or understanding. They can result in either rebellion or a more considered, measured perspective on the part of the adolescent.

Enduring Personal Characteristics

Adolescence is a period of individuation and development of the self where the seeds of enduring personal characteristics are planted. Most adolescents are too young to have developed long-standing, enduring personal characteristics. However, self-esteem, identity, and other intrapersonal issues are assuredly present and influencing decisions about whether to try and experiment with the addictive behaviors. It is clear from the literature that problematic psychological development often demonstrates itself early and contributes to the development of addictive behaviors (Chassin et al., 2000; Deas et al., 2000). Problems with self-esteem and self-concept occurring during adolescence as well as later in life influence initiation of most addictive behaviors (Steffenhagen, 1980).

Issues arising in each of these areas of functioning in the context of change contribute to the probability equation that could predict movement through the first three stages of initiation of addictive behaviors. The more intense and the more extensive the problems in each area of functioning, the greater is the probability of transitioning from the Preparation to the Action stage. Conversely, protective factors indicated by healthy development and a lack of problems in each of these areas can serve to interfere with this transition. The contextual areas of functioning offer a way of categorizing both protective and risk factors in the initiation of addictive behaviors. Linking the context with the stages of change offers a multidimensional, process perspective on how addictions develop. Focusing on the contribution of these influences to specific stage transitions from Precontemplation to Contemplation, from Contemplation to Preparation, and from Preparation to Action can help unravel the complex network of risk and protective factors that have been implicated in the process of becoming addicted.

SUMMARY

To summarize, the path of initiation begins with the entire population being Precontemplators for adoption either by default or design. Precontemplation represents the lack of any serious consideration for engaging in an addictive behavior due to either a naive ignorance or a more conscious decision. Moving from this Precontemplation stage to the Contemplation stage, wherein an individual considers the pros and cons of engaging in the behavior, happens to a large number of individuals. This movement out of Precontemplation for addictive behaviors, especially those involving drug and alcohol consumption, occurs primarily during adolescence, when these high-risk behaviors are particularly attractive. Adolescents are also facing issues related to the development of identity and the multiple problems associated with this development. Family issues, social influences, and peer models also play an important role during this Contemplation phase. Initial experimentation seems to shift the Contemplation process, either advancing it toward addiction or reversing direction.

Continued experimentation indicates that the decisional balance has shifted and that the addictive behavior is not considered to have enough of a negative valence to be avoided. This shifting in the decisional balance and continued experimentation lead the individual into the Preparation stage of addiction and more regular experimentation and repeated use. As the experimentation continues, it brings personal and physiological incentives as well as social influences and pressure that can move the individual through the Preparation stage. Successful negotiation of the first three stages of engagement in an addictive behavior increases the probability that individuals will adopt a more regular pattern of use that marks the Action stage. During this process of change and movement through the stages of acquisition for this single behavior, the dimensions of change and the context of the individual's life play important and varied roles influencing progression or regression through these stages.

Chapter 5

Repeated and Regular Use

Moving from Preparation to Action
on the Road to Addiction

The interaction of biology, psychology, and social influence has its greatest impact during the transition to a pattern of repeated engagement in an addictive behavior.

Once individuals engage in any addictive behavior with some regularity and create a pattern of use, they enter the Action stage for use, abuse, or addiction. In this stage important interactions occur among behavior, physiology, emotions, and cognition related to the addictive behavior. These interactions determine whether the Action stage will consist of self-regulated, nonproblematic use or whether it will consist of a problematic, excessive, and poorly controlled pattern of engagement.

The distinctions between use, abuse, and dependence can be controversial but they are also critical for understanding the process of addiction. This is particularly true for addictive behaviors that involve consumption of legal substances such as alcohol and nicotine. Engaging in any behavior that has an "addictive" potential always poses risks of excess and addiction. However, not everyone who engages in some regular pattern of use becomes addicted. The paths that lead either to self-regulation, abuse, or dependence are best understood as an interaction of multiple, interrelated factors that move individuals toward self-regulation or addiction. Although there are clear genetic contributions to these paths, we will focus on the factors where the individual is an active participant.

DISTINGUISHING USE, ABUSE, AND DEPENDENCE

As defined at the beginning of this book, addiction is a pattern of regular, problematic, dependent engagement in a behavior. Abuse has been defined as engaging in significant levels of the behavior and experiencing some serious consequences without meeting criteria for physiological and psychological dependence (American Psychiatric Association, 1994). The Action stage for becoming addicted involves establishing a problematic pattern of engagement for a period of at least 3–6 months. Those in the Action stage have not yet developed dependence on the behavior. They are abusers. Abusers' engagement may elude self-control but in a sporadic pattern interspersed with periods of regulated use or abstinence. They can remain in the Action stage for addiction for long periods of time and are always at risk for developing a more sustained problematic pattern that is addiction. Once a problematic pattern is sustained in the short term and becomes resistant to self-regulation, it meets the definition for dependence, and the individual moves into the Maintenance stage of addiction.

On the other hand, self-regulated use is defined as a controlled, modulated engagement in the addictive behavior with few or no negative consequences. This is not a problematic pattern. When excess or negative consequences do occur, they trigger a reevaluation of the use pattern and a reinstatement of self-regulation. For individuals able to self-regulate, the addictive behavior plays a minor role in their life and lifestyle.

Self-regulated engagement requires active use of the processes of change to maintain decisional balance, efficacy, and temptation at levels that ensure continued self-regulation. For example, there is a realistic and balanced view of the pros and cons of the behavior and an acknowledgment of the potential for negative consequences. If anything, the negatives of any excessive engagement outweigh the positives. Cognitive/experiential processes of consciousness raising and self-reevaluation are employed to seek information and evaluate any consequences. This provides the feedback needed for self-regulation. Behavioral processes of stimulus control and reinforcement management are used to avoid situations where excess could be promoted and to access other reinforcers so that the addictive behavior does not become predominant as a reinforcer. These processes support a growing sense of self-efficacy for avoiding excess and for controlling the behavior, as they help limit exposure to cues and decrease the strength of temptations to engage in the behavior. In addition, contextual areas of functioning either provide protective factors that support self-regulation or contain problems that are resolved in ways that avoid using the addictive behavior as a coping mechanism.

DEFINING CHARACTERISTICS
OF THE ACTION STAGE OF ADDICTION

In the Action stage for abuse and dependence, however, there is a different picture of what is happening. Decisional considerations are skewed toward a positive view of the behavior and support repeated engagement in the behavior. Behavioral processes of change (conditioning and reinforcement) are involved in establishing patterns of use and reinforcing engagement over a wide range of situations. Stimulus generalization rather than stimulus control is operative, so that more and more situations become attached to engagement in the addictive behavior. Reinforcements from the addictive behavior become prepotent in the life and functioning of the individual. Cognitive/experiential processes of change are used to normalize engagement and minimize problems associated with the engagement. Self-efficacy to control and avoid the behavior is weakened. The context of change is often filled with problems and issues that become attached to the addictive behavior. In fact, the context starts to become influenced and shaped by the addictive behavior as relationships, beliefs, attitudes, and social systems are modified to support repeated engagement in the addictive behavior. In the following sections we will examine aspects of the behavior, elements of the process, and the impact of the context on successfully completing the Action tasks that lead to becoming addicted.

TAKING ACTION TO CREATE AN ADDICTION

Many aspects of the addictive behavior, in the environment, and in personal considerations contribute to the loss of self-regulation and excess (Orford, 1985). Different theories concentrate on one or another of these areas and make it the defining aspect of addiction (see Chapter 1). But each of these aspects is important; it is the interaction among them that creates an addiction. In this section I examine aspects of behavior, environment, and personal considerations to see how they contribute to addiction.

Behavioral Elements

Quantity and Frequency

Frequency and quantity are often used as markers for the severity and depth of an addiction. Although we define the Action stage as any regular, problematic pattern of engagement, quantity and frequency make a difference. Doing several ounces of cocaine several times a week differs from one use per week of a lesser amount; smoking 5 cigarettes a day differs from smoking 25; and drinking five drinks in a 4-hour period twice a week certainly is different from a 12-pack of beer each night of the week. Even for non-substance addictions like gambling, the amount spent and the frequency of the behavior are important for defining the problem. This is not to say that less is always virtuous. Even small amounts of many substances can create significant problems, particularly if they are illegal substances or street drugs of unknown purity.

Is there an amount of behavior that should be judged as out of self-regulatory control? Although impairment and consequences should follow excessive engagement, there is not a simple correlation between quantity and consequences. The reality of physical tolerance, the legality of the behavior, and the great disparity among individuals in economic and other resources complicate the correlation between amount of engagement and negative consequences. Individuals who engage more often in the behavior of drinking alcohol, for example, actually appear to have better self-control after drinking large amounts of alcohol than others consuming less. In one alcohol treatment research project, graduate student interviewers were constantly amazed at how coherent some alcohol-dependent participants were after registering well above .20 on the Breathalyzer, over twice the legal limit of intoxication. Often gamblers who wager and win or lose thousands of dollars every visit to the casino could be considered problem gamblers simply by virtue of the amount of money bet. However, this amount of money gambled and lost would have different consequences if these gamblers were Michael Jordan and Larry Flynt rather than laborers making minimum wages.

Another critical dimension for determining self-regulation is how the individual and the immediate social peer group view the quantity and frequency of the behavior. As an individual's definition of non-problematic drinking becomes greater in frequency and larger in quantity, so does the propensity to move into problematic engagement in the addictive behavior. These personal definitions are important for problem realization and have led to many often-repeated and problematic definitions of alcoholism. Drinkers, for example, have their own definition of the amount or pattern of drinking they consider out of control. If the individual's drinking does not meet this definition, he or she believes that it is under control. Such definitions might include drinking before noon; drinking hard liquor instead of beer (because beer is not considered strong alcohol); and drinking alone instead of at bars because there is moderation in numbers.

The important dimensions of quantity and frequency are difficult to evaluate when the patterns of use are less regular. Individuals who engage in a pattern called "bingeing" can be as hooked by a particular addictive behavior as those who engage more frequently and regularly.

Some individuals, particularly those who are in the sales and advertising professions, have business events that predictably lead to excessive drinking or drug use. They can find it extremely difficult not to drink at those occasions and actually can have as much or more difficulty controlling this behavior as regular, high-quantity drinkers. Addiction treatment specialists consider an individual who consumed a significant quantity of any mind-altering substance on a daily or almost daily basis over time to have lost or, at the very minimum, to be in great danger of losing self-regulatory ability. However, binge patterns of engagement that occur only weekly or monthly can elude personal control and be very resistant to change as well.

Quantity and frequency of the addictive behavior are certainly important dimensions to consider in the transition from Preparation to Action. However, they are not the only or the most sensitive dimension to consider.

Physiology and Pharmacology

Quantity and frequency are important but inadequate to define addiction. This has led many researchers and clinicians to concentrate on the physiological responses and the pharmacokinetic action of the behavior or substance as the critical mechanism for addiction (Barber & O'Brien, 1999; Hinson, 1985; Liskow & Goodwin, 1987; Litten, Allen, & Fertig, 1996). The physiological response to a substance or an addictive behavior appears to play a central role in various stage transitions. Individuals who find the effects of the substance to be pleasing in the initial and ongoing experimentation come to rely more and more on this consistent physical effect during the Action stage. If I want a certain feeling or want to avoid certain feelings, these behaviors will make it happen (Pandina et al., 1992). Physiology and conditioned learning begin to interact so that the feelings associated with the wanting and the using get connected to more and more events, occasions, persons, and places (Barrett, 1985). As the effect becomes more and more useful to the individual, the probability of the behavior being repeated, patterned, and linked with other aspects of the individual's life increases. Physiology and habit begin to intertwine, creating a single woven fabric.[1]

---

[1]There is a fascinating new line of research in this area called pharmacogenetics that is examining how genes influence different pharmacokinetic functions and play a role in vulnerability to abuse and dependence. In addition, this field is looking for mediating factors that can help pharmacists make compounds that could be effective as either agonist or antagonists for the actions of specific drugs of abuse, including alcohol and nicotine.

There have been rather heated debates over the unique roles of physiological dependence compared with psychological dependence in the creation of addiction. One side believes that biology is the defining characteristic because addictions can be created in laboratory animals. The other offers that psychology is the primordial stuff of which addictions are made. An adequate resolution of this debate requires both sides to be declared winners. In human self-administration it is difficult, if not impossible, to have one without the other. Physiological effects and pharmacokinetics can identify which substances have addictive potential, but they do not determine which individual will become addicted (Hesselbrock et al., 1999). In the Action stage of the initiation of addiction both physiology and psychology contribute to the learning process and to the distinctions between use, abuse, and addiction. A multidimensional attachment to the behavior helps explain progress from self-controlled use to abuse and dependence. Both physiological and psychological factors play a significant role in this process (Montgomery, 1991). But there are also important environmental factors.

Environmental Influence: The Microsetting

Drug and alcohol use as well as engagement in other addictive behaviors are influenced by the immediate surroundings in which the behavior takes place, often referred to as the microsetting. The larger social, legal, cultural, and economic environment is called the macrosetting (Connors & Tarbox, 1985; McCarty, 1985). I discuss environmental considerations and the larger macroenvironment in the section on the context of change later in this chapter. In this section I focus on the microsetting, the topography, of the actual behavior.

The importance of the microsetting can be seen in the development of crackhouses, drug dens, and the ubiquitous presence of bars and pubs. Microsetting appeared to be critical in the dramatic reports about soldiers addicted to opiates in Vietnam who stopped heavy, dependent use immediately on their return to the United States (McCarty, 1985; Robins, 1979, 1980). The microenvironment contributes to the development and durability of the habit and thus to dependence (Kaplan & Johnson, 1992). Often the first uses of substances, particularly illegal substances, are done in clandestine locations or settings. The excitement of doing something risky becomes connected with the actual physiological responses to the substance, intensifying the experience.

The most extensive work in the area of microenvironment has been done in examining the influence of setting for alcohol consumption (Collins et al., 1985; Fromme & Dunn, 1992). In elaborately and carefully constructed laboratory bars, researchers have examined the influences of a variety of factors from the lighting and physical setting to the behavior of bar staff and the modeling of codrinkers using alcohol and placebo drinks. The evidence clearly supports the influence of the microenvironment on the quantity and frequency of the drinking pattern as well as on the reactions of the individual during and after consuming alcohol and placebo drinks (Goldman et al., 1999). The alcohol industry uses the influence of microsetting to foster consumption of alcohol. Most of us are aware of the influence of the bowl of pretzels or beer nuts at the bar on the quantity of the drinking. Offering games, food, and other forms of entertainment at bars are certainly meant to influence both the time spent at the bar and the amount of the substance consumed.

Although there are fewer controlled studies with other addictive behaviors, the influence of the microsetting is obvious in many cases. Often the environment is constructed to facilitate consumption or engagement. The lighting and absence of windows in the casinos in Atlantic City or Las Vegas are intentional prompts to lose track of time and spend increasing amounts of money. Free casino chips, low-priced airfare and accommodations, special clubs, and offering free drinks to players are carefully managed aspects of the setting geared to promote gambling behavior. Most of these prompts and incentives are directed at individuals in the Action stage of engagement when they are most influenced by the microsetting. Individuals in the Action stage of addiction are ready to engage in the particular addictive behavior at will and so incentives and cues can have their most profound influence. However, once these individuals enter the Maintenance stage, the behavior itself has become so intrinsically rewarding and so habitual that these microsetting "fringe benefits" will have less influence on the frequency or intensity of the actual behavior. They will only influence which bar or gambling establishment is frequented.

Setting, then, is another influence on the individual that influences self-regulation and progress to abuse and dependence. Where, when, and with whom individuals begin to engage in an addictive behavior can be very influential in the amount of exposure, the types of expectations developed, and the regularity and pattern of use. Beginning to drink in a bar where most of the patrons were regulars and drank to excess would be different from beginning to drink on identifiable occasions in various bars and social settings where moderation was the rule. Again, the best prediction model would be one that did not pit setting against physiology or psychology but that included setting as a parallel influence during this important Action stage of initiating addictions.

Societal rules and regulations also play a role in designing settings and creating microenvironments that are more or less conducive for the individual to engage in the behavior, a process that we have called social liberation. Laws that allow gambling slot machines at horse racetracks or in bars increase availability of different types of gambling. Making some behaviors illegal is another social strategy that can influence engagement in the addictive behavior and cause or prevent problems. Establishing laws dictating the age when individuals can buy products in certain settings can reduce consumption or create illegal activities and markets. Setting and environment play an important but not independent role in the progression to addiction.

Personal Considerations

Attitudes, Expectancies, and Beliefs

A belief may be characterized as a network of attitudes and expectancies related to the addictive behavior. Beliefs are larger than attitudes and expectancies and can include societal and global views about the behavior. Attitudes and expectancies are usually related to a more specific personal perspective. This section discusses all three factors, starting with attitudes.

ATTITUDES

Attitudes toward a particular addictive behavior usually are formed early in adolescence and adulthood, often prior to experimentation. Adolescents who begin to drink with the family at meals or special occasions and see little or no use of alcohol to cope with problems or emotions have a better chance of developing attitudes and expectancies that would support self-control in the use of alcohol. Those who begin their drinking career in a heavy-drinking fraternity or sorority with a pattern of always drinking to get drunk would develop different attitudes about how drinking fits into their lives. Children and adolescents who grow up in environments where alcohol is a reward for work, a way to socialize, or a mood manager could develop attitudes toward alcohol that more easily lead to abuse and dependence. (See Baer, 1993; also S. A. Brown, Creamer, & Stetson, 1987; Jessor et al., 1995; Mann, Chassin, & Sher, 1987.)

Parental or familial modeling of a specific substance may not be as important as the more generic message of parental behavior. Parents who drink a lot of alcohol are often shocked to hear their teens compare alcohol consumption to marijuana use or cocaine use. For the teens the leap is not so surprising because their attitudes about using drugs are connected to the larger picture of using mind- or mood-altering chemicals. The attitude conveyed may be a general one of better living through chemistry.

Teens are constantly involved in the processes of consciousness raising, self-reevaluation, and environmental reevaluation, where they are gathering information and evaluating that information to create their own opinions and attitudes. These attitudes, then, influence use or engagement. Attitudes developed by adolescents toward a specific addictive behavior can restrict consideration of use and promote self-regulated use or give permission for greater quantity and frequency and for more multipurpose use of the particular substance or behavior (Zucker & Gomberg, 1986). It is these attitudes that contribute to the decisional considerations in the earlier stages and then interact with actual use or engagement in the transition from Preparation to Action.

EXPECTANCIES

Expectancies exist prior to drinking initiation. These expectancies are fluid and capable of change. However, the more extensive the network of these expectancies and the more well developed, the more they can act as facilitators of drinking acceleration once drinking has begun. Expectancies are very influential in the evaluation of decisional considerations that influence movement from Contemplation to Preparation, Preparation to Action, and Action to Maintenance.

After reviewing the extensive research on the role of expectancies in the development of drinking behavior, Dunn and Goldman (1996) reported that even preschool children have some knowledge of alcohol and its effects. Even more interesting was the finding that by the third to fifth grade positive expectancies seem to develop in a pattern that is similar to those of adults (Dunn & Goldman, 1996). These positive expectancies may be related to the acceleration of alcohol use as these individuals enter adolescence (Mann et al., 1987). Research indicates that it is the positive expectations of socializing, fun, and partying that are related to initiation and acceleration of drinking (Fromme & Dunn, 1992; Fromme, Stroot, & Kaplan, 1993; Leigh & Stacy, 1993). The research on coping and substance use, however, seems to indicate that using the addictive behavior to cope with negative emotions predicts substance use problems and the movement toward abuse and dependence. To reconcile these apparently contradictory findings, it would be important to remember that many of the expectancy studies were conducted with adolescents. Positive expectancies may promote regular use during the Action stage of addiction. Using the addictive behavior to coping with negative emotions may predict the movement from active use to problematic drinking patterns and ultimately to abuse and dependence. How the mechanisms of expectancies and coping are related to the transitions from Preparation to Action and then to Maintenance could provide important information for understanding the process of becoming addicted. In order to adequately assess the impact of expectancies it may be critical to separate individuals into homogenous groupings with respect to drinking and development of dependence (Kaplan & Johnson, 1992). The more fine-grained analysis provided by the stage transitions can help to clarify the contributions of the various elements to specific transitions.

BELIEFS

Beliefs represent the individual's internalized view of generic, basic operating principles that are often influenced by or largely formed through family and sociocultural factors (Stanton, 1997). Beliefs are part of the larger context of change but are discussed in this section because of their close relationship with expectancies. Like expectancies and attitudes, beliefs about the addictive behavior are developed early in an individual's life. Often they are derived from the statements of meaningful adults and the practices of the individuals in the immediate environment. A belief that drugs are the work of the devil, that gambling is sinful, that excess demonstrates a defect in character would all have some impact on the process of initiation. The same would be true of beliefs that pleasure is a right, that frustration should not be tolerated, and negative emotions should be relieved in any way possible.

As with expectancies, it is tricky to attempt to predict how certain beliefs affect acquisition and addiction. Some very negative beliefs toward drugs (e.g., the work of the devil) may accelerate movement toward dependence, as discussed in Chapter 11. Experimentation can debunk a very negative belief, leaving no fall-back position. On the other hand, when such negative beliefs about drugs remain intact and in the context of a solid religious orientation to life, they could lead to a long-term protective mechanism.

Beliefs and expectancies are two-edged swords. They can serve as both risk and protective factors during the acquisition process. They both influence and are influenced by actual engagement in the addictive behavior. Beliefs and expectancies are influenced by both personal and environmental factors. They develop prior to experimentation with the addictive behavior based on the sociocultural environment. During the Action stage these beliefs and expectancies are informed by the behavior itself. The change processes of self-reevaluation and environmental reevaluation make these beliefs and attitudes more central to the lives of these individuals. It is easy to see how behavior, physiology, and microsetting can interact with the early expectancies about the addictive behavior. This interaction creates a new and more stable set of beliefs and expectancies that can either support or undermine the acquisition of the addictive behavior.

Reinforcement Value

According to Shiffman and Wills (1985), substance use can become a mechanism for coping with life stresses because it can minimize negative mood or maximize positive mood. Because of the potent physiological effects of addictive behaviors, they can easily become reinforcers and replace less quick or less effective methods of coping with stress or stressors. The more the addictive behavior begins to replace other coping mechanisms, the greater the probability that the individual will progress from use to abuse and dependence. The processes of reinforcement and contingency management replace adaptive reinforcers with more problematic ones. Smokers often report using their cigarettes and drinkers, alcohol, to manage stressful situations (Slade, 1999). Once again the physiological effect interacts with the psychological value of the behavior to create a durable and problematic pattern of behavior. In fact, one of the defining features of abuse and dependence is that the behavior begins to take over a larger and larger role in the life of the individual. As other coping mechanisms drop out, the individual begins to rely more and more on the addictive behavior to cope with problems.

This perspective is supported by the reports of individuals who relapse after some success at stopping the addictive behavior. Many studies that have examined relapse precipitants across addictive behaviors have found that negative emotions like frustration, anxiety, and anger are important occasions for triggering the need to engage (DiClemente et al., 1995; Donovan, 1996; Marlatt & Gordon, 1985; National Academy of Sciences, 1999). In fact, negative emotions often emerge as the central set of precipitant situations in examinations of self-efficacy for abstaining from most substances (DiClemente, Fairhurst, & Piotrowski, 1995). Thus the need to cope with negative emotions seems to be a driving force moving individuals toward dependent use of the substance or engagement in the behavior. The more individuals use the drugs or behaviors to relieve stress or noxious feelings, the more problematic becomes the use. I have often reminded my clients who are concerned about their drinking of the words of my colleague, Dr. Jack Gordon: "Alcohol becomes a problem when it begins to be used as a drug and not a beverage." During the Action stage of initiation, this process of increasing use for its coping effect is central for understanding the movement from use to abuse and dependence. The individual moves forward on the road to addiction as quick and efficient reinforcing effects of the addictive behavior begin to be chosen more and more frequently over less immediately reinforcing coping activities.

Many prevention researchers are guided by the coping and addiction connections. They suggest that development of social competence and a broad-based sense of self-efficacy can be an effective way to prevent substance use among early adolescents (Clayton, 1992, cited in Glantz & Pickens, 1992; Jessor et al., 1995; Pentz, 1985, cited in Shiffman & Wills, 1985). As described earlier, problems with social competence create a significant risk for development of addictive behaviors. Conversely, social competence may act as a protective factor, particularly in the Action phase of initiation. Thus, good social skills and abilities may not simply be a marker of reduced experimentation; they may act as a protective factor to prevent the transition to abuse and dependence once experimentation has begun.

CRITICAL EVENTS IN BECOMING ADDICTED

All of these factors—the addictive behavior, the environmental influences, and the personal considerations—come together during the Action stage to support engagement in the addictive behavior. They shape the personal history and experiences of the individual influencing self-regulated use or unregulated addiction. Several critical events occur during the Action stage that allow the more problematic aspects of behavior, environment, and personal background to coalesce and create a regular pattern of problematic engagement that ultimately leads to addiction.

The Sirens' Call: Regular Use without Consequences

One of the important mechanisms of a self-regulatory system is the feedback mechanism. Self-regulation is a self-correcting system that adjusts to changes in the environment and within the individual. When the human body experiences extremes of hot and cold, self-regulatory responses like sweating or heat conservation occur. Individuals who get food poisoning develop an aversive conditioned response and thereafter typically avoid that food. Speakers read listener facial expressions to adjust their delivery. Feedback, the accurate interpretation of that feedback, and an adaptive response are important elements in human communication and personal self-regulation (Miller & Brown, 1991).

During the Action stage feedback about the addictive behavior is critical for determining the paths of self-regulation and addiction. Feedback from first experimentation with a particular behavior may either inhibit or promote continued use. In order to move forward from Preparation to Action, individuals usually have had few or no negative experiences with the substance or have had positive experiences that seem to outweigh the negative. Action-stage individuals already have a positive mindset and decisional balance toward engagement in the addictive behavior. In the early stages of acquisition drinking, gambling, and using cocaine, for example, do not have many, if any, negative aspects. This is probably the norm for most individuals entering the Action stage. Although there are tragic stories of individuals in the early stages of use who died from an overdose, these cases are rare.

Lack of negative consequences plays a particularly important role in the continued and accelerating use during the Action stage. As use becomes more frequent and of greater intensity or quantity, the probability of negative consequences increases. As the individual drinks more alcohol at one sitting, experiences like hangovers, blackouts, and physical reactions such as vomiting are more probable and more severe. Gamblers who engage more frequently or bet more money increase the probability of losing significant sums of money. Quantity and frequency increase the opportunity for negative consequences to occur while at the same time creating the conditioning and positive reinforcement that make the addictive behavior more valuable to the individual.

As the individual experiences negative consequences, the self-regulatory process should engage and signal the need for a reduction in the problematic behavior or avoidance of it. Thus the drinker who has been sick states that she will never mix beer and hard liquor again or that eight beers or a bottle of wine is just too much to drink in one evening. The gambler who experiences serious losses begins to think that he must stay away from the casinos or gamble only to the limit he allows himself. This type of feedback and adaptive response could keep the behavior under self-regulatory control and allow the individual to maintain a pattern of nonproblematic drinking or gambling without progressing to abuse and dependence. If the individual experiences particularly dramatic consequences early in the Action stage, he or she may decide to stop the behavior completely and return to the Precontemplation stage for initiation. A female college student who became pregnant after a heavy drinking episode with a boyfriend and then had an abortion decided to avoid alcohol completely except on special occasions like weddings, when she would allow herself only one drink. She became a Precontemplator for any regular use.

Individuals who experience few negative consequences, who interpret any negative consequences as normal aspects of use, or who consider particular use experiences, like a hangover, as a sign of a good time will have greater difficulty keeping the behavior under self-regulatory control. Thus the lack of negative consequences or the minimization of these consequences acts as the sirens' call, leading the individual farther and farther into extensive engagement with the addictive behavior. This initial failure of the self-regulatory system increases the probability that this individual will engage in greater and more problematic use. At this point only more serious or more frequent consequences would have a chance to influence the progression toward addiction.

Narrowing Behavioral and Environmental Repertoires

If the addictive behavior supplies a significant amount of positive reinforcement (excitement, social ease, and pleasure) and/or a significant amount of negative reinforcement (relief from boredom, frustration, and negative feelings), individuals will tend to seek out and increase their engagement in the behavior. Unrelated activities and behaviors begin to take second place or fade out of the person's repertoire. The addictive behavior becomes more and more central to the life of the individual as life narrows around that behavior.

This narrowing of the behavioral repertoire often happens in work and family settings with positive and healthy behaviors as well. Since the arrival of our second child, my wife and I are preoccupied with taking care of and being with the children during our free time; non–child oriented activities have moved more and more into the background. The narrowing of the behaviors is simply a natural part of becoming preoccupied with a preferred activity.

Similarly, as an individual becomes more and more involved with an addictive behavior, it becomes a priority to seek opportunities to engage in the behavior and associate with others who share the behavior. Gamblers will often get to know others who like to play cards for money or go to the casinos. Drinkers and smokers will have more friends who drink and smoke. With the policy restrictions on smoking currently being enforced in the United States, enclaves of smokers can be seen huddled at the front doors of buildings or in parking lots engaged in at times animated conversation and probably mutual support.

At the same time the person's behavior and environment narrow around the addictive behavior, the world of the addictive behavior expands. The rewarding physiological effects of the behavior get paired with many different situations and events in the life of the individual. This is perhaps most clearly seen with cigarette smoking. Until recently, smoking was something that you could do everywhere. Individuals who began to smoke only at certain times and in certain places rather quickly learned to expand the behavior to a variety of places. They learned to smoke to relax, to relieve tension, and to enhance conversation. Smoking before going to sleep, after engaging in sexual intercourse, during a meal, with coffee after a meal, or at bars while having a drink became automatic for many smokers and became part of the picture of smokers reflected in television and movies. Although availability of opportunities has not been as ubiquitous as smoking, a similar expansion of engagement and narrowing of alternatives happens as marijuana, cocaine, or heroin use becomes more and more a focus in the life of the individual.

More Serious Consequences: A Silenced Alarm

Although initial engagement in the addictive behavior can have little or no consequences, repeated and regular use will almost always bring with it some rather obvious and serious consequences. It is unlikely that steady, heavy drinking does not bring some criticism or concern from others, does not create some problems in family or work functioning, or does not offer some potential for legal consequences like a DWI. As with initial consequences, how these later consequences are experienced and processed in the feedback and self-regulatory system will be critical as to whether they interrupt and foster self-regulation or sustain problematic engagement in the addictive behavior. If the potential for increasing negative consequences is accurately perceived and processed, the individual can stop or modify the behavior and bring it under self-regulatory control before it progresses further down the road to dependence and addiction. If the impact and potential of negative consequences is silenced, the probability of movement from abuse to dependence is greatly increased. Consequences that are rationalized or rejected, ignored or minimized will not provide the self-regulatory feedback that is so critical for interrupting the initiation process.

There are many ways that the feedback system becomes co-opted and made ineffective. Specious reasoning processes will effectively undermine accurate processing of feedback. Husbands who arrive at treatment because of their wives' insistence that they have a drinking problem often blame the wife's fundamentalist religion or alcoholic father for her hypersensitivity. Lateness to work after a prior evening's bout with cocaine or alcohol is attributed to not being "a morning person." Contentions that "I do not drink any differently than my friends so I cannot have an alcohol problem" will also mute critical reflection. Many current smokers will point to relatives who are advanced in age and still smoking as some type of personal protection against the rather well-established link between smoking and disease. This kind of reasoning and thinking increases as the individual becomes more and more attached to the addictive behavior.

As we all have experienced, it is rather easy to find positive reasons that outweigh or invalidate the negative when evaluating a behavior that we really want to do. Judgment becomes impaired and reasoning more erratic as the attachment to the addictive behavior becomes the dominant force in decision making. Consciousness raising and self-revaluation continue to be used to support engagement in the behavior. Reasons why the behavior is not a problem for the individual are continually sought. The process of self-evaluation is filled with harm minimization activities (Daniels, 1998).

This process is particularly problematic when it occurs in adolescence and early adulthood because feedback that comes primarily from adult figures is often suspect. Distrust makes it easier to discount criticism. Some acting out is expected during adolescence, and expressing individuality is an important developmental task (Kaplan & Johnson, 1992). Thus, peer influences become increasingly important. The social network and its values often get substituted for family values. Finally, adolescents have more flexibility in meeting the demands made by school, home, and work. It is not as problematic to lose a part-time job, to have a bad semester academically, or to be irresponsible at home. The structure of social expectations, the tasks of adolescence, and the expectations of significant others in the environment can make undermining self-regulation easier during adolescence and early adulthood (S. A. Brown et al., 1985). Thinking and judgment can get distorted and consequences ignored or silenced.

This active distortion of consequences and feedback is a critical turning point in the process of becoming addicted. Once the individual effectively neutralizes minimal consequences of early experimentation and then the more serious consequences during the Action phase, the road to addiction and dependence seems short and inevitable. That is why abuse is often a critical period in an individual's path toward addiction. As individuals move to abuse, they are faced with the dilemma of allowing the feedback of the consequences either to stop the abuse and increase self-regulation or to ignore the consequences and lay the foundation for the more serious dependence. Abusers who increase self-regulation can create behavioral strategies to avoid serious consequences, moderate behavioral excesses, or stop the behavior. Otherwise they seem destined to progress to dependence and addiction.

ACTION AND THE CONTEXT OF CHANGE

The influence of resources and problems in the context of change is critical during the Action stage of addiction. Situational problems and influences can increase the value of the addictive behavior for all the reasons detailed earlier. Beliefs and attitudes create the foundations for regulation or excess. Relationships, family and peer systems, psychological problems, and personality characteristics complicate the feedback about the addictive behavior and can accelerate the increases in quantity and frequency, consequences and pattern that make for an addiction. Because microsetting and beliefs have already been discussed, this section focuses on the interaction of personality dimensions, comorbid psychiatric problems, and various aspects of the family and social environment with the process of becoming addicted.

Personality and Psychopathology

Many would like to find the answer to the question of self-control or self-regulation within the character of the individual. Some individuals demonstrate great self-control. Conversely, others individuals seem to have little or no self-control. Research on alcohol consumption has searched extensively for an "alcoholic personality" to explain the difference between those who get addicted and those who can drink socially. As discussed in Chapter 1, this search has not been a particularly fruitful one. Most researchers today do not subscribe to the premise that one or two personality types predict alcohol dependence (McGue, Pickens, & Svikis, 1992).

However, there are several individual characteristics that have been associated with becoming addicted. Disinhibition, impulsivity, or behavioral undercontrol have been identified as a cluster of constructs related to risky behaviors on the one hand and harm avoidance on the other (Giancola & Tarter, 1999). These characteristics have been associated with early-onset alcohol and drug use (Shedler & Block, 1990; Sher, Walitzer, Wood, & Brent, 1991; Smith & Anderson, 2001). However, recent reviewers of this literature refuse to focus exclusively on these factors and prefer either an integration of personality and learning risk factors (Smith & Anderson, 2001) or an interactive model between personal characteristics, expectancies, environment, and other life problems (Bailey & Rachal, 1993) as a more complex portrayal of the influence of personality on addiction.

There are also chronic psychiatric conditions that have high comorbidity rates for addiction (Regier et al., 1990). Individuals with chronic mental illnesses appear to be at higher risk for developing an addictive disorder. A complex set of factors that include physiological and social dimensions related to the chronic mental illness creates this vulnerability. Alcohol and drugs of abuse often interact with the illness or the medication that is used to control the illness in ways that facilitate excessive use. In a recent study of the pros and cons for drinking among a group of chronic schizophrenic patients with alcohol problems, Hagedorn (2000) identified a set of unique considerations for the pros of drinking that included statements like "drinking makes me feel normal," "drinking helps me with my medication side effects," and "others like me better when I am drinking." Recent surveys have found that the smoking rate among schizophrenic patients is 3 times the average prevalence across the general population (DeLeon, 1996; Lohr & Lynn, 1992). However, it is not clear whether rates of abuse and dependence on addictive behavior in the seriously mentally ill represent a unique pathway to addiction or simply a more potent mixture of social environmental influence, greater coping value, and access (Rosenthal & Westreich, 1999). Once exposed to these addictive behaviors, individuals with serious mental illness may find it easier to increase use, more difficult to exercise self-regulation, and experience more consequences of use in a shorter period of time.

Family Influences

The role of the family already has been mentioned as an influence in the sections on behavioral topography and in development of attitudes, expectancies and beliefs. Particularly in adolescence, the family can influence the movement toward regular use and then to abuse and dependence. During the Action stage families can influence the process in several different ways: through reinforcement, lack of punishment, modeling, tacit approval, intense disapproval, and disengagement. Processes of reinforcement management, helping relationships, and social influence are most relevant to the interaction of the adolescent and the family. These interactions feed the adolescent's self and environmental reevaluation.

Family responses to the first use or experimentation on the part of a child can also foster continued use or interfere with movement into the Action stage. There seems to be no one magic way to respond. Proponents of a "tough love" approach urge serious consequences and referral for counseling or treatment. However, this message is most often directed at parents whose parenting styles have been overly accepting and easily manipulated by their children and who have adolescents who are already well on their way to being addicted. The message for adolescents who are experimenting and beginning to move into the Action stage needs to be carefully crafted so that it does not promote rebellion and foster movement toward addiction. Mothers Against Drunk Driving have encouraged frank and open discussions with adolescents about drinking and driving. They recommend that the parents include the option that if the teen does drink or is with others who are drinking and/or are drunk, they always have the option of calling for a ride. This strategy is a harm reduction one designed to prevent auto accidents and injuries. However, some have complained that this approach gives tacit approval to overdrinking and getting drunk. Consequences and communication are important considerations for preventing progress from experimentation to abuse and dependence. The exact amount of each is often difficult to determine. However, it seems clear that both too little (pampering and making excuses) and too much (overreaction and rigid overcontrol) can influence the salience and/or importance of the behavior and increase the probability of abusive and problematic use (Chassin, Rogosch, & Barriera, 1991; Chassin et al., 1996).

Interpersonal Relationships and Significant Others

Acceleration to regular use and to abuse and dependence often occurs after the individual has moved out of the familial home either to college or to another living situation where there is greater freedom of behavior. Although the influence of peers and special friends is important throughout adolescence, it is in these settings that the influence of significant others increases and becomes more influential in the initiation of the addictive behavior. An adolescent female dating an older, drug-using male presents a clear danger for initiation even if she remains in the home. However, that danger increases as the family ties weaken and the importance of this significant other increases. It is also true that many male drug experimenters have been tamed by the influence of a stable and loving female who would not put up with excessive behavior. In fact, I have heard many parents praying for just such an influence for their son or daughter to counter peer pressure for excessive use. Significant others can be both facilitating and inhibiting factors during this Action stage.

This type of influence does not stop once adolescence ends. There are documented cases of what I call defensive drinking problems—individuals who initially drink in moderation but who develop abusive and, at times, dependent drinking patterns after marrying an alcoholic. It seems that these individuals increase their consumption both to accompany the alcohol dependent partner and to cope with the negative feelings generated by living with this partner (Leonard & Mudar, 2000).

Social Support for the Behavior

General social support (having a network of friends and family) can be a protective factor, particularly in the early stages of initiation. It seems that if an individual has a broad social support system made up of some individuals who engage in the behavior but many others who do not, exposure to that behavior is more limited. It can be a protective factor retarding the movement from use to abuse. However, as individuals enter the Action stage and begin some pattern of regular problematic engagement, support by significant others for or against the specific behavior is far more influential than a generalized sense of social support (see Longabaugh, Wirtz, Beattie, Noel, & Stout, 1995).

A network that strongly supports frequent and excessive engagement in the behavior increases the risk of undermining self-regulation. A network filled with friends and fellow workers who use cocaine in their socializing, who value it as a mood enhancer, and who provide easy access to a supply of the substance increases the probability of abuse and dependence. The individual with such a network finds it easy to become more involved in cocaine use and to develop problems and consequences of use, especially if increasing amounts of time are spent in the network. However, it is not simply the presence or absence of the substance-abusing network that influences the choices of the individual; the individual seeks out and pays attention to some social influences and ignores others. The process of social liberation and environmental reevaluation also drive the shaping of the network as individuals select who will be the important valued others in their lives and create internal norms and comparisons (Bandura, 1986).

Societal Factors

Macroenvironment factors that influence substance use and dependence include both governmental and societal norms and policies (Connors and Tarbox, 1985). Particularly in the United States, it should come as no surprise that larger societal forces influence initiation of addictive behaviors. Our society has experimented with Prohibition of alcohol and watched prohibition create the speakeasy and a lively, illegal network of alcohol-specific support for use. Driving through the Haight-Ashbury section of San Francisco in the late 1960s, I noted that drug use was a way of life, not simply a private behavior in that community. Governmental and social influences interact with each of the stages of initiation. However, in the Action stage of initiation of addiction these influences can contribute to regular use and the transition from use to abuse and dependence.

Connors and Tarbox (1985) report that alcohol consumption is generally price-elastic, meaning that changes in price are inversely related to demand. Increases in the price of alcohol generally create a decrease in the demand for alcohol. This price-elasticity boundary seems to affect heavy as well as light drinkers. Thus, at least at a population level, cost can interfere with acceleration of use. In another example, they report that lowering the legal drinking age from 21 to 18 led to increased consumption and alcohol-related problems among the 18- to 20-year-old population (see also Holder, 1999; Whitehead & Wechsler, 1980). Controlling availability, however, has often produced mixed results. Prohibition created an alternate "bootleg" or "black market" supply system. Some regulation of accessibility seems to shift patterns of demand but not consumption. In fact, some data for Canada indicate the highest rates of drunkenness occurred in the areas with the fewest numbers of outlets for units of population (Connors & Tarbox, 1985). Government can affect consumption at a population level but needs to be careful that legislative efforts do what they are intended to do. How government and societal influences affect individual use and decisions related to increased consumption are not well examined or understood.

In summary, there are a number of interacting dimensions in the context of change that influence individuals in the Action stage of becoming addicted. Once an individual has begun to engage in an addictive behavior with any sort of regularity and entered the Action stage of acquisition, behavior-specific variables interact with a host of personal and environmental influences to promote continued engagement and loss of self-regulation. Family, societal, and social support for the behavior interacts with physiology and psychopharmacology, with the coping and reinforcement value of the behavior. Consciousness raising, self and environmental revaluation, and social liberation processes of change, in turn, shape attitudes, emotions, beliefs, and expectancies that promote unregulated use and minimize consequences and concerns.

SUMMARY

Many perspectives on the initiation of addictive behaviors have a deterministic view. They propose that once an individual with a certain physiological disposition or with a certain profile of personality or social factors engages in an addictive behavior, addiction is a foregone conclusion (Lettieri, Sayers, & Pearson, 1980). This perspective assumes that once you enter the Action stage, an automatic mechanism inevitably leads some to addiction. However, many drinkers, gamblers, and drug users with similar characteristics are able to engage regularly in these behaviors without becoming addicted. This fact undermines the foundation of any argument of inevitability. It is in the Action stage that the distinction between those who would become self-regulated users and those who move forward toward addiction becomes a concrete reality.

The Action stage of addiction is a very volatile one, with shifting patterns of use and the possible progression to abuse and ultimately dependence. However, the progression toward addiction as described in Chapter 4 is not inevitable. Addiction is best understood as the result of a matrix of various factors that represent past and present, environment and person, physiology and psychology, and personal processes of change that will ultimately determine the course of acquisition and the path to the well-maintained addiction described in Chapter 3.

Part III

QUITTING AN ADDICTION

The Journey through the Stages of Recovery

Chapter 6
_____

Precontemplation for Recovery

Cultivating Seeds for Change

*The problem of denial is really nothing more than the
conviction of addicted individuals that at the present moment
it is not in their best interest to change.*

Once individuals have established a well-maintained, dependent pattern
of engagement in the addictive behavior, they terminate the cycle of
change leading to addiction. Regular, dependent, problematic engagement in the addictive behavior becomes the status quo and persists
throughout vast expanses of a person's life. Smokers can smoke daily for
30 or more years. Drinkers can consume excessive amounts of alcohol
every week of their adult lives. Heroin "addicts" often find life without
heroin not worth living and chase the heroin high for decades. Remaining addicted becomes easier than trying to change. At the same
time, addicted individuals can be seen as entering the change process
that leads to recovery and being in the Precontemplation stage. Precontemplation for recovery appears to be a static period with little happening except an accumulation of consequences. However, in the midst
of this stasis there are seeds of change that can be cultivated and that can
move the addicted individual toward stopping or modifying the addictive behavior. This chapter will examine the characteristics of this
Precontemplation stage, the barriers that interfere with change, and the
activities that mark the transition from Precontemplation forward through
the initial stages of recovery.

DEFINING CHARACTERISTICS
OF PRECONTEMPLATION FOR RECOVERY

The defining characteristic of the Precontemplation stage is that the individual is not seriously considering modifying the addictive behavior in
the foreseeable future. In our research with adults we often employ a 6-
month time frame to measure the foreseeable future.[1] Six months is far
enough into the future to avoid the intense anxiety that more immediate
prospects for change would engender, and yet close enough in time to
detect significant decisional considerations. This definition includes individuals who are adamantly opposed to ever changing, those who put off
change indefinitely, and those who are simply putting off change for at
least the next 6 months. Individuals in Precontemplation may have tried
to change or, at least, may have seriously considered change previously
but they are not doing so now.

Many addicted individuals take a long time before beginning to
consider *seriously* whether they should either modify significantly or
change an addiction. They look like they are not ready for change. They
are *not* engaging in the cognitive/experiential or behavioral processes of
change that would shift the attitudes, intentions, or behaviors toward
change. There is little consciousness raising or self- and environmental
reevaluation going on and even less activity related to behavioral processes of change. When smokers in the Contemplation and Preparation
stages of change were compared with those in Precontemplation, Precontemplators had significantly lower levels of each of the processes of
change, with the exception of helping relationships (DiClemente et al.,
1991). In almost all studies individuals who have the lowest levels of
readiness to change and who are identified as Precontemplators experience significantly lower levels of processes of change than those in later
stages (DiClemente & Prochaska, 1998; DiClemente, Carbonari, Zweben, et al., 2001; Morgenstern, Labouvie, McCrady, Kahler, & Frey,
1997; Prochaska et al., 1991; Tejero, Trujols, Hernandez, Perez de los
Cobos, & Casas, 1997; Velasquez, Carbonari, & DiClemente, 1999).

If we examine the markers of change, a similar picture emerges.
Precontemplators have a decisional balance that is strongly tipped
against change. The pros that favor engaging in the addictive behavior
outweigh the cons. Similarly the cons for change are higher than the pros
for change (DiClemente et al., 1991; Prochaska et al., 1991; Prochaska,
Velicer, et al., 1994). With the reasons for change so outweighed by the

---

[1]In recent research with adolescents this time frame failed to yield large groups of
Contemplators who were considering use of condoms. It may be that a shorter time
frame is more appropriate with adolescents because their sense of time is developmentally different.

reasons against change it does not make sense to be contemplating or concerned about making a change.

The marker of self-efficacy is not always a helpful measure for those in Precontemplation. But temptation and a calculation of the temptation score minus the individual's efficacy score across situations can be helpful. If they are being honest, those in Precontemplation usually will endorse rather high levels of temptation to engage in the addictive behavior and lower levels of self-efficacy to abstain (DiClemente, Carbonari, et al., 1994; DiClemente et al., 1985). Those who endorse high levels of temptation and very low levels of efficacy to abstain from the addictive behavior are Precontemplators who are the most overwhelmed by their habit (DiClemente, Carbonari, Daniels, et al., 2001; DiClemente et al., 1995; DiClemente & Hughes, 1990). On the other hand, there are some Precontemplators who report high level of efficacy and believe that they could abstain if they wanted to change. They just have no desire to change at the moment.

For those in Precontemplation with a well-maintained addiction, problems in various areas of functioning are resolved in ways that support the addictive behavior. Belief systems, relationships, social systems, and basic personality characteristics become shaped to fit the addiction and to minimize problem awareness. Precontemplators are those addicted individuals who have managed the consequences and concerns that arise in the context of their lives so that they can maintain a positive decisional balance that supports continued engagement in the addiction (see Chapter 3).

Precontemplation presents significant challenges for the individual and the intervenor. "Why change?" becomes the central question. The response is complicated by a variety of issues. How intact is the self-regulation process after one becomes addicted? How do external factors interact with internal factors and what role does the context of change play? What strategies keep the Precontemplator from moving to Contemplation? What is the impact of legal and societal restrictions and prohibitions on the Precontemplator's consideration of change? How can others help? What is the best approach to reach the Precontemplator? These are some of the critical questions to be explored in this chapter to understand better this Precontemplation stage of recovery and the challenges it presents for change.

SUSTAINING OR LEAVING PRECONTEMPLATION

There appear to be several important types of activities that enable Precontemplators to neutralize any momentum that builds toward considering change. I have labeled these the "four R's" of reluctance, rebellion, resignation, and rationalization (DiClemente, 1991). At the prompting of one recent commentator, I am adding a fifth R that stands for reveling (DiClemente & Velasquez, 2002). All of these activities and experiences represent more or less effective ways of countering prompts to move toward change.

Most individuals in Precontemplation will employ several of these strategies in order to neutralize momentum for more immediate consideration of change. Reveling, rationalization, rebellion, reluctance, and resignation are often used simultaneously. There may be a single more preferred strategy for avoiding consideration of change. However, preference for one does not exclude use of one or more of the other strategies. What is important for anyone talking with a Precontemplator is to listen and to evaluate how these strategies are operating for that individual in order to understand how to best reach her or him. The following describes each of these strategies and how they interfere with consideration of change and appropriate change process activity. Then I will suggest strategies that can be used to reach out to an individual in Precontemplation who is experiencing or utilizing any or all of these five R's.

Reveling

Reveling Precontemplators are having too good a time engaging in the addictive behavior to consider change. For them the negative consequences either have not yet occurred or are less salient than the benefits. The momentum for change is virtually nonexistent, so there is little need to neutralize it. For these individuals the decisional balance is clearly tipped against change. These individuals may also be rather confident in their ability to change or control the behavior if they want to do so.

The challenge for change is to arouse concern and help the addicted individuals themselves begin to see some of the negatives of the behavior and the benefits of change. Preaching and pushing will be met with resistance. If you listen to someone who is a reveling Precontemplator, the conversation about the addictive behavior will reflect how enjoyable are the highs and how strong is the bond between the individual and the addiction. Trying to convince the individual that the behavior is not pleasurable would be met with disbelief and ridicule. It is more useful to provide objective normative feedback about the behavior and information about physical negative effects, highlighting real and potential negative consequences. This information can increase consciousness raising and self-reevaluation of negative considerations about the behavior. However, it will take a significant rise in the actual or perceived negative consequences to shift the balance. Since actual consequences may be at a low level, it may be helpful to focus on environmental reevaluation (how the behavior affects others). Efforts to engage emotional arousal (some dramatic portrayal of consequences) that fosters negative views of the addictive behavior may also begin the shift in decisional considerations. Attacking the illusory sense of elevated self-efficacy, if it exists, can also be helpful.

Reluctance

Reluctant Precontemplators are simply unwilling to consider change. They are not as much resistant as they are hesitant about the prospects of change. The current behavior has benefits and does not appear *that* bad or problematic to them. Although they are experiencing some negatives of the addiction, concerns about changing outweigh these. Change would mean disruption of the current, more comfortable and accustomed way of living. Fueling the reluctance may be thoughts like "Everyone has one bad habit" or "Whose behavior does not pose some risk or problems?" Inertia rather than energy characterize the reluctant Precontemplator.

The challenges for change are to break through the inertia and build negatives to the current behavior while building benefits for change. Considerations of change need to be energized, and hope that change is possible, beneficial, and worthwhile instilled. Consciousness raising and self-revaluation processes need to focus on these aspects and use prior experiences of successful change to offer a new personal perspective on the possibility of change. Increasing confidence in the ability to change can counter the reluctance. These individuals need to be reassured that they will be able to function without the addictive behavior and that after quitting they will be able to manage temptations to reengage in the addictive behavior. The support of individuals who have made a similar change may also engage the helping relationship process most effectively.

Rebellion

Energy is not at all lacking in the rebellious Precontemplator's approach to the problem. They are often passionately invested in their ability to make their own choices and decisions and resent anyone telling them what to do. They appear hostile and resistant to suggestions that they change. Often the rebellion appears similar to that of adolescents asserting their rights and defining themselves in opposition to societal (read parental) norms. This view of rights often hides the fact that rebellious Precontemplators are also loath to admit their physical or psychological dependence on the addictive behavior. The rebellion is a sign or mark of freedom for these individuals, who are in reality dependent on their addiction.

The challenge for change is to link autonomy and freedom with change and shift the energy devoted to rebellion into Contemplation and Preparation for change. This is clearly easier said than done. For this kind of Precontemplator the behavioral process of self-liberation seems to be important even at this early stage of change. Any modification of the addiction must be the responsibility and choice of the individual. He or she must be in charge of the change. Only then can the processes of self-reevaluation, environmental reevaluation, and consciousness raising be pursued in a personally relevant manner. Rebellion can effectively shut down concerns and considerations of change because they can be viewed as external and imposed. Motivational enhancement strategies that will be described in detail a bit later are particularly important for those Precontemplators who are most angry in their rebellion (Project MATCH Research Group, 1997b, 1998a). The process of social liberation, wherein individuals recognize and acknowledge societal restrictions and options, is least helpful for Precontemplators who feel rebellious about the addictive behavior.

Resignation

There also appear to be a subgroup of individuals in Precontemplation who feel hopeless and helpless about change. These are the resigned Precontemplators. They are either overwhelmed by all their problems including the addictive behavior(s) or they have tried to change and found it seemingly impossible. They feel unable to change and believe that they must resign themselves to being dependent on the addictive behavior. Among smokers I have called this phenomenon "the next generation solution to smoking." Plaintively and paternalistically these resigned Precontemplative smokers say that it is too late for them to stop because they smoked for 10, 20, 30, or 40 years or because they are too addicted physically and psychologically. They conclude that change is not an option for them. The only change they see as possible is stopping the next generation of smokers from starting. Most often these Precontemplators are resigned to living a life chained to their addiction. Millions of others have been able to quit smoking, but resigned Precontemplators feel that they are the exceptions and cannot change. Whether this is an excuse or a reason, these feelings of resignation allow the Precontemplator to continue to engage, either comfortably or with significant discomfort, in the addictive behavior.

The challenge for change for those who are resigned is an infusion of hope and a vision of the possibility of change. These individuals tend to have high levels of temptation and low levels of efficacy for change. Self-reevaluation needs to focus on the Precontemplator's personal concerns about change. Self-monitoring of the details of the addiction can give the resigned Precontemplator a better picture of when and why he or she engages in the behavior and offer a realistic view of the topography of the addiction. Helping relationships and environmental reevaluation that offer support by detailing the ability of similarly addicted individuals to change can increase self-efficacy. Offering data that some of the most dependent individuals have often been the most successful in some clinical trials (Project MATCH Research Group, 1998a) can help counter the hopelessness. The fact that some medications can assist in curbing temptation for a time can also offer hope for those most overwhelmed by the addiction.

Rationalizing

Finally, most Precontemplators articulate, at least to themselves, their own personal, protective rationale as to why the addictive behavior does not pose a serious problem for them. These are the rationalizing Precontemplators. They appear to have all the answers, in contrast to the resigned Precontemplator, who has none. It is easy to get into debates with this type of person. "Yes, this behavior could be a problem for others but it is not for me because. . . . " They have many reasons for believing they will avoid the negative consequences. "I am only going to smoke for a few years." "I am young and able to handle my liquor." "I won't drink like this when I have children." "I rarely go above the limit I set for myself when gambling." "I use drugs recreationally. I could never be an addict." These beliefs lead alcoholic-dependent individuals who drink massive quantities of alcohol to be convinced they are not alcoholic because they only drink beer or do not drink before noon. Similar rationales can lead individuals, dependent on cocaine or marijuana, to believe that they are virtuous because, at least, they do not do heroin.

It is important to note that the difference between reason and rationalization is often in the eye of the beholder. If the argument is *my* rationale, it is a reason. However, if *you* propose the same argument, it is a rationalization. Labeling someone as being rebellious or rationalizing fails to appreciate the Precontemplator's point of view. Labeling in any form can be a detriment to engaging and moving these Precontemplators through the stages of change because it does not address what is for them the compelling nature of their argument.

Whether rationalizing, reluctant, rebellious, resigned, or reveling, individuals in Precontemplation think and feel. What they are thinking, feeling, and saying should be taken seriously. They are not simply trying to convince us of their reasons or rationales. They themselves are the first persons they have to convince. Each strategy produces an individual convinced of and with strong conviction about the truth of their argument. Often it is not that the Precontemplator is resistant to change and then begins to employ these strategies. Rather, the resistance comes from the fact that these individuals believe personally and deeply in the various rationales and perspectives that keep them in Precontemplation.

The preceding experiences and activities of Precontemplators mute concerns and considerations and restrict change processes that would move them toward changing their behavior. Jill Walker Daniels (1998) conducted a fascinating study examining the rationalization and resignation strategies employed by smokers who were not considering quitting smoking. What she found was that the more these individuals minimized the harm related to smoking (a rationalizing activity), the less they used self-reevaluation and consciousness raising processes and the less they sought information or thought about any problems related to smoking. Those who were high in what she labeled cessation hopelessness (more resigned) were lower in self-efficacy and behavioral processes of change that could help them manage their smoking. All of the research participants in this study were not seriously considering change in the next 6 months. Even for these Precontemplators, the more they felt resigned and hopeless or engaged in harm minimization thinking, the less they were engaged in the processes of change that could lead to considerations of concern or build confidence in their potential to change.

THE TRANSITION FROM PRECONTEMPLATION TO CONTEMPLATION

The Response Ability of the Individual in Precontemplation

The previous discussion of change process activity and shifting decisional considerations places a significant amount of responsibility on the Precontemplator to do something that would promote the transition to Contemplation. Some would argue that in light of a compromised ability to self-regulate their behaviors, expecting such responsibility from Precontemplators is unrealistic. Certainly it is unrealistic to expect the addicted individual to move quickly to Action and stop the addictive behavior with minimal urging or pressure. However, it is not unrealistic to believe that he or she can begin to consider consequences and change. It is true that this consideration probably needs to be done when the individual is most sober, least intoxicated, or has the most distance from the addictive behavior. Addicted individuals are least accessible in the midst of their cocaine or gambling run, heroin rush, or eating binge. However, Precontemplators who are dependent on an addictive behavior are clearly capable of directed and self-regulated actions and thoughts. It has always amazed me to see the ingenuity and creativity demonstrated by the addicted individual in making excuses, in creating deceptions for family and friends, in procuring the desired drug and in creating the opportunity to engage in the addictive behavior. Goal-directed behavior is not impossible for addicted individuals, and neither should be some consideration of the problems and consequences of the addictive behavior. Such considerations represent movement into the Contemplation stage of change.

Traditionally, discussion of responsibility and addiction has been framed in extreme opposites. Either the addict or the addiction is responsible for the lack of change. The truth lies in the middle. Individuals do not become addicted to pharmacologically inactive substances or nonrewarding behaviors. On the other hand, potent mind- and emotion-altering drugs and behaviors do not create and maintain addictions without the participation of the individual. Nor do individuals quit and stay away from an addictive behavior without personal evaluation and effort. The process of change for addiction and recovery involves interacting external and internal forces. The individual addictions involve powerful reinforcing effects and consequences, personal choices, and environmental influences; these interact with the entire life context of the individual. Addicts are capable of the considerations needed to move forward toward recovery. When and how they can be helped to move into Contemplation, however, is complicated.

Confrontation, Consequences, and Contemplation

The Precontemplator's rejection of change has led to confrontation and external interventions, including punishment, restrictions, losses, and threats of significant losses, as the only way to "break through the denial" (Dodes & Khantzian, 1991). Imposing or coercing motivation appears the method of choice for many family members, treatment personnel, and policy makers who see Precontemplators as actively fighting consideration of change (Donovan & Rosengren, 1999; Liepman, 1993).

One strategy is to bring the person in and confront him or her about being an addict by bugging, confronting, and nagging the individual into moving toward change. These tactics are high risk because they can create a chasm between helpers and addict. If they work, they are probably most effective with those who already were considering or were more prepared to change.

There is little evidence to suggest that these punitive or aggressive confrontational approaches are effective in producing change. In fact, there is emerging evidence that confrontation produces increased resistance to change and more denial rather than a decision to change (Miller, Benefield, & Tonigan, 1993; Miller & Rollnick, 1991, 2002). Moreover, simply labeling individuals as resistant or in denial may become a way for others around the addicted individual to justify calling it quits with regard to their efforts to reform the addict. There is enormous meaning and power in a name or label. Most readers will be familiar with the phenomenon of the self-fulfilling prophecy. Saying it is so can make it so. Thus, labeling an individual's unwillingness to admit to a serious problem as resistance can actually create rebellion and denial.

Nagging can be a particularly ineffective way to move the Precontemplator, despite occasional successes. Research in partner support for smoking cessation (Cohen, & Lichtenstein, 1990; Fals-Stewart, O'Farrell, & Hooley, 2001; Prochaska, Norcross, & DiClemente, 1994) has shown that partner nagging was counterproductive and that the best way partners could help was by eliminating problematic interactions. This proved better than doing something more proactive and confrontational and better than increasing more positive helping behaviors and interactions.

There are many examples of how external pressures or control (even positive incentives like money or privileges) often produce short-term but not lasting addictive behavior change unless the individual is ready to cooperate (Curry, Wagner, & Grothaus, 1990; Higgins, 1997). Individuals jailed for drug-use offenses, even for significant periods of time, often return to use upon release. Mandated treatments produce mixed results (Anglin & Hser, 1992; Donovan & Rosengren, 1999). Curtailing supplies often creates greater demand and vigorous black markets. Clearly, external pressure is not the magic that *necessarily or automatically* motivates consideration of change or moves the Precontemplator forward in the process of change.

On the other hand, consequences hold no special magic in getting a Precontemplator to move to Contemplation, and there are numerous examples of the principle that consequences do not always teach. It has been a time-honored assumption that to move the addicted alcoholic only one of two options was available, hitting bottom or confrontation. The first was to allow the number and severity of the consequences to accumulate until these consequences reached a critical level of tolerance for that individual (hitting bottom). Only then would addicted user begin to consider change. Certainly consequences can teach. A smoker's first heart attack, the drug addict's first arrest, the gambler's first loss of a significant amount of borrowed money, the alcoholic's divorce can be instructive moments and promote consideration of change. However, consequences do not teach everyone. Often multiple consequences simply reinforce a sense of hopelessness and helplessness to change. In some cases severe consequences actually can contribute to increasing the engagement in the addictive behavior in an effort to relieve the stress or in an indirect and suicidal attempt to stop the pain. External pressure can sometimes interfere with movement out of the Precontemplation stage (Speiglman, 1997).

The challenge for family, friends, and helpers facing the multi-problem, addicted individual in Precontemplation is daunting. Family members who have a relative in Precontemplation describe the anger and frustration they experience. They feel betrayed by the empty promises that never seem to materialize into real change. They burn out on the prospect of influencing the Precontemplator. Family and friends look to therapists and treatment as having the power to make the change happen. If only they can get this person into treatment, they believe that the Precontemplator will change. "In the meantime what can we do?" they often lament. What can anyone do to get this person to change?

A few critical misconceptions lead to this sense of powerlessness. The fact is neither family members nor friends have the power to make the Precontemplator change. Treatment personnel also cannot make the person change and helpers often have even less power. Nevertheless, family members do have control over many important reinforcers and many important elements in a Precontemplator's life. Parents often complain about their lack of control over their teenage son or daughter. However, they continue to let these teens use the family car, give money for gas, provide food, clothing, and shelter without setting any limits or providing any contingencies on their behavior in order to gain these privileges. Although even "tough love" will not guarantee success, its advocates do have an important point. In their efforts to make sure that the Precontemplator does not make terrible mistakes (stealing, turning to companions that would be supportive of the addictive behavior, starving themselves to death), families often give enough financial and personal support for the Precontemplator to avoid the harshest of consequences of their addiction. In effect, these families neutralize the educational effects of negative consequences. They are short-circuiting any consciousness raising and self-reevaluation that could occur.

Families that learn the lesson of not interfering with natural consequences often can be more effective with the Precontemplator. However, the approach has benefits even if it does not provoke change. Families who set appropriate boundaries and allow the natural consequences to make an impact often feel less used and abused by the addicted individual in Precontemplation. Precontemplators will often learn to be more responsible if there are serious consequences. They may not move forward to quit the addictive behavior but they will adapt their behavior enough to avoid some of the consequences. Heavy drinkers or drug users will often avoid driving while drinking or using to prevent a second or third driving under the influence (DUI) arrest. Having to make efforts to avoid consequences also can encourage them to think more about their behavior and its consequences. Concern about consequences can lead them reevaluate the decisional considerations and move them into Contemplation.

In addition, using the term Precontemplation and labeling this state as a stage of change appears to be a more functional and less pejorative way to characterize individuals at this particular point in their engagement in and connection with the addictive behavior. If we understand the well-maintained addiction as was previously described, it is rather easy to see how these behaviors become so firmly established and resistant to change.

External pressure and environmental consequences certainly can influence individuals in Precontemplation but alone appear to be insufficient to produce movement out of Precontemplation to Contemplation. The individual must become involved. My favorite story of this kind of interaction is that of a taxi driver whom I interviewed on my way to a restaurant one evening. He was a current member of Alcoholics Anonymous (AA) and had been sober over 1 year after a lifetime of dependence on alcohol. About 3 years prior to our encounter he had been arrested for "crawling away from officers and resisting arrest." The police officer, who had previously arrested him numerous times, decided to throw the book at him. The judge was also getting exasperated and sentenced him to a year of probation with the stipulation that he must attend AA meetings for a year. He dutifully completed his sentence, going to AA meetings and then going out drinking at a bar across the street. He continued going to AA not only for the probation year but also for an entire second year while continuing to drink. Then one night at a meeting he heard a speaker with whom he felt a close kinship and he began to take the AA messages more seriously. At that meeting he went forward and requested a desire chip, the token that he was serious about quitting drinking. That was the beginning of his journey to sobriety. At the time of the taxi ride, he had achieved more than a year of sobriety, was serving as a sponsor for several other AA members, and currently was organizing several new AA meeting sites. The driving force behind his ultimate movement out of Precontemplation was becoming concerned and convinced of the need for change. In this case, being mandated to attend AA probably helped but was not enough by itself.

The more recent emphasis on motivational interviewing and the initial research on this approach also support the contention that confrontation and labeling are ineffective, at best, and harmful, at worst, in dealing with a convinced Precontemplator (Miller et al., 1993; Miller & Rollnick, 1991, 2002; Rollnick, Mason, & Butler, 1999). A more motivational approach would use empathy, understanding, and objective feedback to provide the forum where the individual with the addictive behavior can explore any slight ambivalence about change or small concerns about the problem. This opening strategy allows for a more sensitive view into the individual and his or her perception of the issues and the problem. The motivational interviewing approach is hypothesized to be a much more effective way to create and increase personal motivation and movement through the stages of change (DiClemente, 1999a; DiClemente & Velasquez, 2002; Miller & Rollnick, 1991, 2002).

Although external pressures and problems can play a role in moving a Precontemplator, it is the internal processes that are critical to moving forward in the stages of change (Simpson & Joe, 1993). It is the addicted individual who must (1) see the problem, (2) perceive the risks, (3) experience and digest the consequences, and (4) see the potential for change. So movement from Precontemplation must occur from within the individual in order to begin the process of intentional behavior change. There is certainly a role for external pressures and consequences, but we must begin to understand better how these external and environmental forces interact with the individual internal processes in order to promote movement to Contemplation more effectively.

Ultimately, processes of change such as consciousness raising that increases problem recognition, self-reevaluation that engages a personal cost–benefits analysis, and any other coping activities that create shifts in attitudes and promote accurate information processing are the critical mechanisms for moving out of Precontemplation. In addition, a seminal belief in the possibility of personal change with regard to the particular addictive behavior would assist in promoting consideration of change.

Promoting Problem Recognition and Objectivity

Problem recognition is central to resolving Precontemplation but is not a simple process. It requires that the individual identify problems and consider them as intimately connected to the specific addictive behavior rather than to other aspects of his or her lifestyle or environment. It requires the individual to evaluate as problematic the specific amount and frequency of the addictive behavior in which he or she engages. Problem recognition requires the individual to judge that a behavior producing some benefits can also be producing problematic consequences and that the problems are beginning to equal or outweigh the benefits. In order for the problem recognition process to occur, the individual must experience an emerging sense of vulnerability to the problematic consequences (Kohler, Grimley, & Reynolds, 1999). In addition, he or she must have the ability to step back and create enough space between person and behavior to allow for a more objective appraisal of the addictive behavior and its consequences.

Objectivity and honesty with the self, at least with regard to the addictive behavior, appear to make an important contribution to the movement of the Precontemplator forward toward Action. In the big book of AA, honesty with oneself is considered the critical component to beginning the road to recovery (Alcoholics Anonymous, 1952, 1976). However, objectivity with an addictive behavior is as difficult to achieve as objectivity in the midst of a passionate love affair. The two situations are very similar (Peele, 1985). Objectivity is elusive in this state of mind.

It is often easier to identify the many ineffective ways of promoting objectivity than it is to suggest effective ways. Ineffective methods fail to engage the appropriate processes of change and they often undermine the shifting of the decisional balance and the creation of a sense of hope and efficacy. A frontal attack on the behavior, listing all the negative characteristics and general negative consequences, will usually backfire because it tries to force engagement in consciousness raising and self-reevaluation. Such a presentation will probably be overinclusive and contain some consequences that the individual has never experienced; it will be relatively easy for the Precontemplator to disregard what he or she sees as hyperbole. Nagging defined as the constant repeating of one or more consequences that the Precontemplator is well defended against is particularly ineffective in promoting honesty, objectivity, and self-reevaluation. In fact, once the interaction of nagging and blowing it off becomes systematized, as happens in marriages and families, the information contained in the nagging message becomes irrelevant and very easy to dismiss almost immediately. Punishment is another rather ineffective way to promote objectivity. From the early research into reinforcement theory psychologists learned that punishment simply suppressed but did not eradicate a behavior (Craighead, Craighead, & Ilardi, 1995). Punishment often teaches the individual how to engage in the behavior in a way that avoids the punishment. Punishment most often produces crafty evasion rather than objective honesty and personal reevaluation.

Some better ways to promote more objective self-evaluation include motivational interviewing (Miller & Rollnick, 1991, 2002; Rollnick, Heather, & Bell, 1992; Rollnick, Mason, & Butler, 1999). This approach promotes an interactive stance that respects the individual engaging in the addictive behavior and attempts to begin with the perspective of the addicted individual. It promotes consciousness raising, environmental and self-reevaluation by listening, summarizing back to the individual what is heard to make sure that it is understood, and looking for any ambivalence or discrepancies between the behavior and the individual's values, beliefs, and experiences. In essence, this method leaves the responsibility for change to the individual, avoids all fighting and confrontations with the individual and promotes "rolling with resistance." Another strategy that is often included in brief interventions and seems to promote self-reevaluation is the provision of accurate and objective feedback based on a careful assessment of that individual and her or his behaviors (DiClemente, Marinilli, Singh, & Bellino, 2001). In all of these approaches the effort is to focus on the person who is in Precontemplation and discuss openly the addictive behavior and any consequences and issues related to that behavior, always beginning with the perspective of the Precontemplator. The hope is that being on the same side as the Precontemplator and understanding the Precontemplation process from the inside are better ways to promote a more accurate and personal self-assessment.

THE CONTEXT OF CHANGE

Distraction or Focus

There is an interesting and complicated interaction between the primary addiction and the life context of the addicted individual. As discussed earlier, problems in the various areas of functioning of the addicted individual can precede and follow the development of the addiction. Problems that contributed to the creation of the addiction typically become exacerbated as the individual spends more and more time engaged in the addictive behavior. Preexisting psychiatric syndromes, depression-generating belief systems and self-talk, interpersonal inadequacies, and social, employment, and family systems problems flare up and can distract the individual from seeing clearly consequences of the addiction. Moreover, new problems are created in each of these areas as a result of the addiction. These marital or relationship problems, family conflicts, and other psychiatric diagnoses complicate the considerations of change. The individual in Precontemplation can quickly shift the focus of attention from the addiction to one or more of the associated problems. Each of these problems can produce distress and disability, which are a reason for concern in their own right. However, it is important to make a distinction between additional problems as important complications for the change process and problems used to divert attention from the addiction and protect the Precontemplation status. We examine several of these complicated interactions.

Interpersonal Conflicts

Marital problems are often the identified problem that brings an addicted individual into treatment. Spouses push Precontemplators into treatment or other forms of help seeking with threats of divorce and separation (Wild, Newton-Taylor, & Alletto, 1998). Although unwilling to acknowledge the addiction as a problem that needs changing, the individual in Precontemplation may be open to discussing the marital problems. This acknowledgment can serve as a diversion as much as a useful discussion. It is precisely at this point that the question emerges as to what is figure and what is background in the process of change. Is it important to address the marital issues prior to, simultaneously with, or after trying to address the addictive behaviors? Turning down the heat on the marital conflict may provide negative reinforcement for the addiction since relief of the conflict may allow the addicted individual to believe that the problem is resolved without changing the addiction. On the other hand, if the marital conflict is fueling the dependent engagement in the addictive behavior, some resolution could give the person some breathing room that could allow for more effective consideration and concern about the addiction to arise.

Coexisting Psychiatric Problems

It gets even more complicated when there are coexisting psychiatric problems. Because many of the addictive behaviors can produce anxiety, depression, disorientation, and delusions, the problem of separating psychiatric symptoms from physiological consequences of addiction becomes very difficult (V. B. Brown, Ridgely, Pepper, Levine, & Ryglewicz, 1989; Mueser, Bellack, & Blanchard, 1992). If the depression or psychotic symptoms clearly predate the addiction, managing the psychiatric problem would seem to take priority. However, it is difficult to manage the psychiatric problem while the individual is actively engaged in using drugs or alcohol in a dependent problematic manner. This co-occurrence is problematic at every stage of change. However, it is most problematic when the addicted individual is in Precontemplation for recovery and more complicated when this individual is in Precontemplation for the psychiatric problem(s) as well as for recovery from addiction (Bellack & DiClemente, 1999; DiClemente, Carbonari, & Velasquez, 1992).

Systems Problems

Family relationships and social systems also interact with the addiction in a complicated fashion. There may have been significant problems in these systems prior to developing the well-maintained addiction. Sexual abuse, parental drug and alcohol problems, problematic employment histories, and dysfunctional social systems are often part of the backdrop of addiction (Chassin et al., 1996; Grant & Dawson, 1999; Stanton, 1997). Once again the decision of when and how to address these issues complicate the task of the Precontemplator and those who would offer help to the individual in Precontemplation. Problems that occur in these systems as a result of the addiction create additional stress and conflict and compromise helping relationships. Precontemplation can be one of the most frustrating stages of change for family, friends, and counselors in various helping systems (Prochaska, Norcross, & DiClemente, 1994).

The reality is that addicted individuals have a complex and complicated set of problems in a variety of areas of functioning that blur the focus on the addiction for addicted individuals and those around them. The context of change seems filled with issues, problems, and conflicts that can deter and distract from accomplishing the tasks needed to move from Precontemplation to Contemplation. Efficacy, decisional balance, and processes of change that are needed to move forward are undermined by the multiple problems. Although it is clear that anyone who is addicted would have a better chance of resolving problems in the context of change if they first were free of the addiction, a sequential solution—first get into recovery and then handle other problems—does not always work. Some problems must be addressed and at least attenuated before, or at the same time, so that the Precontemplator can have the physical and psychological space to begin to face the addiction. For the homeless, a safe and secure environment may be needed prior to engagement in an evaluation of decisional considerations. A truce with regard to marital conflict may need to be negotiated or some medication management given those with serious psychiatric problems before we can realistically expect any consideration of recovery. However, there is a dilemma. Providing respite and relief is a two-edged sword. It may allow the Precontemplator to regain the strength and energy needed to pursue the desired addiction. On the other hand, it can provide the safety and personal space needed to begin consideration of change and movement toward successful recovery.

There are several suggested strategies for coping with life context problems in the individual in Precontemplation for recovery that emerge from this analysis of the process of intentional behavior change.

1. First, patience and persistence are needed to address the complexity of problems that are the fabric of the addicted individual's life.

2. Some problems clearly must be attenuated prior to being able to engage effectively in the processes of change such as consciousness raising, self- and environmental reevaluation, and helping relationships. For example, any symptoms and circumstances that would make engagement in these processes impossible would need to be remediated first.

3. Harm-reduction strategies to reduce associated problems or relieve stress and distress should contain messages and strategies that can also address Precontemplation for recovery in addition to reducing harm.

4. The reality is that often multiple problems and the addiction will have to be addressed at the same time using a multicomponent and multidimensional intervention strategy. Understanding where the individual is in the process of change with regard to each of these problem areas of functioning can assist in planning and sequencing treatment (Connors, Donovan, & DiClemente, 2001; DiClemente & Prochaska, 1998; Prochaska & DiClemente, 1984).

5. Finally, it seems critical that the addiction not be relegated completely to the background, no matter what approach is used by the Precontemplator or the intervener. Allowing the addicted individual to move the addiction to the back burner reduces the potential for the increase in concerns and considerations needed to move out of Precontemplation for recovery.

Addressing Multiple Addictions

In addition to the problems in multiple areas of functioning, many addicted individuals have multiple addictions. Often when they move out of Precontemplation for one of these addictions, they remain in Precontemplation for others. Until recently few programs that treated alcohol-dependent individuals would make efforts to address nicotine addiction at the same time (Bobo & Husten, 2000; Monti, Rohsenhow, Colby, & Abrams, 1995). In fact, AA meetings have been notoriously smoke-filled events. However, the same tolerance has not been extended to alcohol dependence when it coincides with dependence on an illegal drug like cocaine. The synergy between drugs and alcohol has made it difficult for treatment providers to address one and not the other. Nevertheless, a disparity between stages with regard to the two addictions is problematic. Demanding movement out of Precontemplation for each of several addictions sets a high standard of achievement for the addicted individual and the treatment program.

Addressing multiple addictions when the individual is in more advanced stages of change for all the behaviors is much easier than addressing these addictions when the individual is in Precontemplation for one or more of them. Allowing someone to be in Precontemplation for one substance while working on changing another addiction can be a risky strategy. However, some multiply addicted individuals have successfully changed one behavior without changing all the others. Addressing some of these successively, as has been done with alcohol and nicotine in many cases, is another strategy that can be considered. Treatment providers must recognize the synergy across addictive behaviors and the complications presented in changing multiple behaviors.

CASE EXAMPLES AND OVERVIEW

In Precontemplation the person is striving to manage any consequences, problems, personal unease, or environmental pressure in a way that allows for continued engagement in the addiction. The change process is focused on avoiding consideration of change and supporting the addiction (Table 6.1). If the processes and markers of change continue to support the addiction, Precontemplators appear very difficult to influence and impervious to change. The secret is to find some seeds of discontent and cultivate them.

Peter is a 40-year-old, divorced father of two who has been using illegal drugs since college, when he began using marijuana. He became a heavy marijuana user in his late 20s and had difficulties keeping up with his job at a high-tech software development firm. He was fired from that job and became a freelance computer consultant. His wife, who married him in college and was tolerant initially of his marijuana use, became more adamant about his quitting drugs when they began to have children. Peter hid his habit and pretended to quit. The loss of his job and erratic income from his consulting work increased marital conflict, and he began to stay away from home until late at night. Fed up with his behavior and his refusal to go to counseling, his wife divorced him. Peter explained to his parents that he and his wife grew apart after college and that she changed and wanted someone who was into making money and being middle class. He would not share those values. When his parents asked him about his drug use, he exploded and told them that he was responsible for his own life and that his wife was using that for an excuse to divorce him.

Over the past 5 years Peter began to use heroin and to hang out with some individuals who were drug dealers. He worked for them in setting up computer programs that were protected and creating codes and complicated routings for e-mail communications. His access and in-

TABLE 6.1. Precontemplation for Recovery: An Overview of the Dimensions of Change

Stage task

Discovering any consequences and concerns about the problematic pattern of addictive behavior that arouse consideration of change.

Change processes at work

Cognitive/experiential processes that have been used primarily to support continued use in the face of negative consequences shift to promote awareness of and concern about the addictive behavior spurring movement out of Precontemplation.

Consciousness raising: Focus is on finding reasons and experiences that challenge views that the addictive behavior does not cause problems.

Emotional arousal: Experiences that counter reveling in the benefits of the addiction and highlight negative reactions and consequences associated with the addiction.

Self-reevaluation: Shifting discussions away from issues of independence and alternative causes of consequences (rationalizing) and onto values and considerations that create dissonance; moving from rebellion to personal realizations.

Environmental reevaluation: The person sees environment as challenging engagement in the addiction; reevaluates environmental concerns and impact of the addiction.

Social liberation: The person begins to realize shifting societal norms and how policies and laws attempt to control the behavior or provide alternatives.

Markers of change

Decisional balance: Although usually weighted strongly toward continued engagement, begins to increase the focus on negative consequences of the addiction.

Self-efficacy: Some doubts begin to surface to counter the false sense of self-control and hope begins to emerge to neutralize any sense of hopelessness about change.

Context of change

Multiple problems in various areas of functioning keep increasing but often distract the Precontemplator from focusing on the addiction and can become an alternate focus of concern or intervention.

---

volvement with drugs and his alienation from his children and family grew. His sister, Margaret, who had been close to him while growing up, did not give up and continued to call him and tell him that she was concerned for his safety. Although he believed that this alternative lifestyle was acceptable and that she was overreacting, he did have his doubts at times, particularly when she called as he was coming down off the heroin. He also was beginning to have some concerns about being around the drug dealers if there were a police raid and about being implicated in drug dealing. However, the doubts were soon erased by another dose of drugs.

Patricia was a 38-year-old, single, advertising salesperson with a large ad agency. She was living with her boyfriend of 2 years, Britt, who worked on the creative side of the agency. Patricia was a heavy drinker who could drink many of her male counterparts and customers under the table. This was a real advantage in her business but was met with a combination of admiration and disgust by them and interfered with her establishing intimate relationships with girlfriends and potential male partners. She often dated someone for several years and then broke up when they talked about marriage and family. Her parents were very frustrated with her lifestyle and continually lectured her about drinking and her failure to be married. Her father was a heavy drinker for most of his life but recently had stopped and nagged her to join AA. Patricia had always been headstrong, but did suffer from bouts of feeling depressed about life. In adolescence she had considered suicide but decided against it. When she became popular because she would go drinking with the guys in high school, she felt better about herself but always had some nagging doubts about her self-worth and her ability to really love someone.

In the past 3 months several events created additional stress and caused problems for her. Her boyfriend, who had been tolerant of her drinking and used marijuana recreationally himself, began to pressure her about their relationship, a lack of intimacy, and her unwillingness to make a commitment to him. She began staying later at the bars with her colleagues, and in the previous month was stopped while driving home and charged with driving while intoxicated. She hired a good lawyer, who assured her that he could either get the charge dismissed or get her probation. However, he did ask her to go to an alcohol treatment program to get an evaluation so he could use this in court to preempt any mandated treatment. She was scared about the legal ramifications and the possibility of a criminal record. At the same time her father became more aggressive in his efforts to get her into AA. Patricia was becoming more and more depressed and began calling in sick at work. She would sit at home and drink most of the day.

When she went to the treatment facility for an evaluation, the counselor noted many different problems. In terms of the process of change, she seemed in very different places with regard to the different problems. His analysis of the problems and her stage status with regard to these different problems is illustrated in Table 6.2. Patricia believed that her drinking was functional and an asset to her in work and relationships.

The drinking and driving was a mistake but was caused by the conflict and arguments with her boyfriend, not her being an alcoholic. She was angry at him that night and drank too much. She lived with her father when he was an alcoholic and her drinking did not compare to his. However, she was concerned about the legal issues and was willing to do what she could to resolve them. When the conversation turned to her relationships, she admitted that she was difficult to get along with and that she has problems with intimacy. She felt that these would be fixable if she found the right person to be with. At this point she was not sure if this boyfriend qualified. She alluded to issues related to her parents and their relationship but dismissed these because she had been living on her own over 15 years. She began to cry when the possibility of losing her job because of her current performance was discussed. Work was essential to her well-being, and she was very concerned that she be able to function well enough to function at work. This led to a discussion of her feelings of depression.

Patricia presents a typical, complicated pattern of problems and of her willingness to address each of these. The challenge for the counselor is how to begin to address the targeted drinking problem and, at the same time, not ignore the multiple problems in the context of change.

TABLE 6.2. A Problem by Stage of Change Analysis for Patricia

	Stage of change				
	Precontemplation	Contemplation	Preparation	Action	Maintenance
Problems					
Alcohol dependence	×				
Context of change					
1. Depressive symptoms		×			
2. Beliefs about intimacy		×			
3. Conflicts with boyfriend		×			
4. Family conflicts	×				
Legal problems				×	
Work problems			×		
5. Avoidant personality characteristics	×				

ONCE BEYOND THE RESISTANCE

If the individual in Precontemplation can begin to engage in more objective and more honest self-assessment, then he or she can begin a self-reevaluation process that can lead to the Contemplation stage of change. In order to move into Contemplation and so to begin to seriously consider change, the Precontemplator must begin to reevaluate the addictive behavior in terms of its costs and benefits. In addition, there probably needs to be some hope or expectation that change is possible and that it would bring some benefits.

There is, however, no guarantee that this self-reevaluation process will definitely lead to contemplation of change. One of the dilemmas that many therapists and family members of a person in the Precontemplation stage of change face is that the process of change is in the control of that individual. The Precontemplator can briefly take a look at these outcome expectancies and decide that what is best at this point is continuing to drink, drug, or gamble. Ultimately the decision is always up to the person engaging in the addictive behavior.

Not all of the types of treatments available for substance abusers and addicts are appropriate or efficient ways to assist the addict in Precontemplation. Some treatments, such as a 4-week inpatient treatment program, may not be an effective way to engage the Precontemplator. Program staff can spend a lot of time arguing with the clients about whether they have a problem. This can be an expensive and not very efficient way to move the Precontemplator.

If we can get the Precontemplator to come into treatment at all, it is not always clear how best to deal with him or her. Mandated treatment can produce attendance at treatment without producing movement through the stages of change, as my taxi driver illustrates. However, it can provide an incentive to consider change. Treatment programs that are more sensitive to the particular needs of the Precontemplator may have a better chance at helping to motivate movement to Contemplation. Accurate and objective personal feedback is thought to be particularly helpful for these clients in some newly developed treatment approaches like Motivational Enhancement Therapy (Miller, Zweben, DiClemente, & Rychtarik, 1992). However, the truth is that we need to learn more about effective ways to meet and move the Precontemplator toward Contemplation.

One of my graduate students recently examined the processes of influence and persuasion (Cialdini, 1992) in an effort to better understand how to reach and influence the Precontemplator. Persuasion research is often focused to how salespeople attempt to influence potential customers who are "only looking" or who are clearly ambivalent about a purchase. There are a number of these techniques and strategies that seem to be effective. The *foot in the door* strategy requires using approaches that open the door to discussion only a little. Once inside the door there can be a more elaborate sales pitch, but that cannot happen without the entry and the initial openness produced by the foot in the door. *Small steps lead to big steps* represents another influence technique that gets the individual to do something small (looking at or reading something, two minutes of a survey, making a test drive) in order to begin a process that leads to a much larger commitment. Sometimes the reverse is also true. If initially a lot is asked of an individual (a $100 pledge) and then the caller asks for only a $10 contribution, the person can evaluate the second demand as more reasonable and desire to compromise by giving this much smaller sum. All of these techniques are interesting ones to consider for use with the Precontemplator and offer some insight into learning how to persuade a Precontemplator to move to Contemplation. However, interactions with the Precontemplator cannot be a game. For long-term change to be successful the Precontemplator must buy into the process and not feel manipulated. Once a consumer has bought and used an item, it can be difficult to return it. However, the Precontemplator can always return to Precontemplation if dissatisfied with the alternatives.

Another issue is how to distribute assistance and resources needed for recovery efficiently and effectively to the Precontemplator. Although there will be some limitations on resources of necessity, the ultimate solution would be one that offers a variety of options for engaging the Precontemplator. We should be proactive in reaching out to addicted individuals in Precontemplation for recovery during specific teachable moments or windows of opportunity (Soderstram et al., 1997; Walsh et al., 1992), develop programs that can reach out to the resistant with concern and caring, and create effective engagement interventions for those who are mandated or coerced into treatment (Donovan & Rosengren, 1999). My personal fantasy would be to see more early intervention, better coordination between the courts and the treatment systems with clear delineation of responsibilities and responses to resistance and relapse, and families and helpers better trained in meeting and managing Precontemplation.

Specific approaches to target Precontemplators are being developed with research designed to measure sensitively the outcomes of various strategies. For example, there is some evidence that reaching out to smokers who are Precontemplators may be more effective than waiting for them to ask for help (Prochaska & Velicer, 1997a). In a recent matching trial of alcoholism treatment, outpatient alcoholics who were higher in state/trait anger (more rebellious) had significantly better drinking outcomes when given Motivational Enhancement Therapy (MET) than when given Cognitive-Behavioral Therapy (CBT) or 12-Step Facilitation (TSF) and low-motivated alcoholics had slightly better long-term outcomes at 1 year but not at 3 years in MET compared to CBT (Project MATCH, 1997a, 1997b). Some brief motivational interventions work well for Precontemplators (Heather, Rollnick, & Bell, 1993; Yahne & Miller, 1999). However, others may not be intensive or comprehensive enough to shift the decisional balance for the most resistant individuals (Dolan-Mullen et al., 2000; Haug, 2002; Velasquez et al., 2000). We may need to combine motivation with other types of treatments in order to maximize the potential for movement (Project Combine). The data are only preliminary in this area and much additional work is needed to understand how individuals move most effectively from Precontemplation to Contemplation and beyond.

SUMMARY

Issues and characteristics of Precontemplation for recovery have been discussed in detail in this chapter. However, much more scientific research and societal consideration of these issues are needed in order to create an atmosphere where Precontemplators are encouraged, coaxed, and prodded to consider change without interfering with the personal processes needed to initiate serious consideration of change. The optimal goal for society and the addicted Precontemplator is movement into the Contemplation stage of change.

Chapter 7

The Decision to Change

Moving from the Contemplation to the Preparation Stage of Recovery

Considering change is an exercise fraught with tension and ambivalence. Chronic Contemplation and an impulsive rush to action are the Scylla and Charybdis of considered decision making.

CONSIDERING CHANGE

Contemplation, or thinking about changing an existing addictive behavior, is a very important step in the process of successful recovery. However, addicted individuals tend to be impulsive and seek immediate gratification. They rush into an activity, failing to consider its costs and benefits. They tend not to anticipate or prepare for problems. Albert Ellis labeled the addicted individual's diminished capacity to delay gratification as "low frustration tolerance" (Ellis & Dryden, 1987). This tendency to avoid the ambiguity and frustration of decision making can interfere with the critical tasks that need to be performed in the Contemplation stage.

Addicted individuals often find it difficult to consider change long enough to make a good decision. Substance abusers interviewed during treatment intake often state that they have suddenly decided to quit. They appear convinced that they will be successful no matter what happens. There is little sense that they have considered all the actual positive aspects of the substance use or the real difficulties that changing these behaviors would entail. Most of their reasons for change involve legal or family pressures. The prognosis for such individuals should be considered guarded at best.

On the other hand, many addicted individuals get stuck in chronic Contemplation. One alcohol-dependent individual was able to deal with several related problems in therapy but he continued to drink, although seriously considering quitting. He was killed in a drinking-related accident as he was crossing a busy highway. Some other individuals, like the taxi driver from the previous chapter, move forward out of Contemplation only after a lengthy period of time spent considering change. It takes time for them to finally recognize and appreciate that the cons exceed the pros. Only then are they able to move into the Preparation and Action stages. Chronic Contemplators are not incapable of change. They are simply not convinced of the need for change despite the clear and present danger of the addiction.

Decision making is the critical outcome of the Contemplation stage and marks the beginning of the Preparation stage. Janis and Mann (1977), who originated the *decisional balance* schema for understanding decision making, warn their readers:

> Our analysis of decision-making behavior assumes that in the repertoire of every person is a proclivity to procrastinate or, if that is not possible, to invent rationalizations for ignoring the worrisome doubts that make for decisional conflict. Procrastination and rationalizing are components of the pattern of *defensive avoidance*, a means of coping with the painful stresses of decision making that can be as detrimental as the pattern of overreacting to impending threat by taking impulsive, ill-considered action in a state of panic. (p. 6)

This insightfully describes the two polar opposite approaches to decision making that are often recognized in the process of addictive behavior change. It is no wonder that this decision making process can consume so much time and energy.

Individuals will make decisions based on the expectation that the gains anticipated for a proposed course of action will exceed the expected losses associated with that particular action or behavior change. It is the tipping of the decisional balance in terms of the comparison of these two psychological vectors that is hypothesized to influence decision making and consequent action. Janis and Mann (1977) state that it is not the absolute value but the comparative value of the gains and losses that have the greatest impact on the decision. Thus a person may tolerate a less than optimal situation or behavior if the alternative is expected to yield a worse outcome.

The primary tasks of the Contemplation stage are (1) gathering decisional considerations, (2) examining them, and (3) engaging in the comparative process that would resolve decisional conflict. The goal of

Contemplation is a firm decision to change. This is needed to move effectively into the Preparation stage of change. The work of Contemplation involves an extensive, personal, and accurate evaluation of the pros and cons associated with the particular addictive behavior and the prospect of change. This evaluation occurs before addicted individuals enter treatment as well as during treatment so that the process of decision making can be examined as it occurs in the natural environment as well as during treatment. Only after understanding the tasks of Contemplation can we examine techniques and approaches that could promote decisional considerations and tip the decisional balance toward change. The same strategies that tend to keep individuals in the Precontemplation stage continue to operate in the Contemplation stage. When individuals begin to seriously consider changing the addictive behavior, often they continue to engage in rationalizations, be rebellious or reluctant, or to feel helpless and resigned to being addicted. Consequences, motivation, resistance, denial, and ambivalence continue to be important elements in promoting and hindering change in addictive behaviors throughout the process of change. This chapter will describe the critical tasks of the Contemplation stage and the types of activities and interventions needed to advance the process of intentional behavior change to the next step of preparing for action.

Understanding Contemplation

In our research, we have classified individuals who report *seriously considering* stopping the addictive behavior *in the next 6 months* to be in the Contemplation stage of change. The tasks of the Contemplator are to consider the costs and benefits of quitting in order to make a firm decision to quit or modify the behavior. Contemplators typically are engaging in consciousness raising activities. Their view of the pros and cons of the behavior can be rather balanced but often is still tipped in favor of continuing the addiction. They differ from Precontemplators in that they are beginning to engage in cognitive and experiential change process activities (DiClemente et al. 1991; Prochaska & DiClemente, 1986; Prochaska et al., 1991) and are actively and seriously considering change in the foreseeable future. Successful resolution of Precontemplation stage tasks yields an initial awareness of the problem and of the need to change. During Contemplation this awareness becomes an active consideration of the problem and a weighing of the risks and benefits of addiction or change.

The dimensions of change identified in the TTM offer a rather clear view of how this happens. The critical marker of change, decisional balance, measures the relationship between the pros and cons for change.

As the individual moves toward a decision to change there is a shift in the importance of the pros of change in relation to the cons. The cognitive/experiential processes of change fuel this shift in decisional balance. Specifically, consciousness raising activities and the feedback given by those offering a helping relationship provide information and data. This information then interacts with self-reevaluation, environmental reevaluation, and emotional arousal/dramatic relief processes, which produce new experiences and evaluations that affect decisional balance. The behavioral processes of change are not very involved at this point in the change process. Self-efficacy to quit the addiction seems to be relevant only insofar as a modest amount of it is needed so that the individual avoids becoming discouraged about the possibility of change and gives up on Contemplation. Problems and issues in the various areas of functioning that form the context of change offer important decision-making information about the consequences of the addiction. However, these problems can also distract the focus of the Contemplator from the examination of the pros and cons, contributing to the ambivalence and procrastination that interfere with resolving Contemplation stage tasks.

The Decisional Balance

Each person's decisional considerations are unique. Every reason has both a rational and an emotional dimension that appeal to the head and the heart, respectively. There can be many reasons that are intellectually convincing but have little personal emotional importance. On the other hand, a single consideration that is intellectually less convincing can have enormous emotional significance and personal value. This makes understanding anyone's decisional balance tricky, because an observer would have to gain access to the personally relevant considerations and their significance. An evaluation of the pros and cons is not simply an intellectual, rational experience. That is why both cognitive processes, like consciousness raising, and experiential processes like emotional arousal and self-revaluation, are important in shifting the decisional balance. In our research, increased engagement in the cognitive/experiential processes of change has been associated with higher endorsement of the cons of an addictive behavior (Velasquez et al., 1999).

Decisional considerations and the balance between positive and negative considerations are important markers of movement through the early stages of change (Prochaska, Velicer, et al., 1994; Velicer et al., 1985). The pros for an activity or behavior—smoking or drinking, for example—are generally high during the Precontemplation and Contemplation stages, which would militate against change (DiClemente et al., 1991; King & DiClemente, 1993; Prochaska, Velicer, et al., 1994;

Velicer et al., 1985). Conversely, the cons or negative aspects of the addictive behavior are generally low in these same early stages. Thus the *positive and negative aspects of the addictive behavior* and an individual's experience with the addictive behavior influence consideration of change. In addition, the consideration of the *gains and losses of the anticipated change* also have an influence. Many strong positive reasons for continuing an addictive behavior include consideration of potential losses and problems associated with stopping the addictive behavior (Klingemann, 1991; Miller, 1985; Miller & Rollnick, 1991). Positive and negative considerations about the behavior and the change include not only utilitarian gains and losses for self and significant others but also approval and disapproval from self and significant others (Janis & Mann, 1977).

An example of the decisional considerations for Carrie the Contemplator illustrates the scope and balance of the considerations (Table 7.1). For Carrie, the considerations that militate *against change* include the utility of her drinking in managing her anxiety in social settings and enabling her to be sexual with men she meets, her perception that she is more popular and accepted when drinking, and alcohol's ability to dull painful feelings related to family rejection. In addition, she has many reservations about how life would be without alcohol. She fears losing friends, going "crazy," and not having any social life. On the other side of the ledger are her decisional considerations that would *promote change*. These include her feelings of guilt and embarrassment when she cannot remember what happened the evening before, the recent arrest for a DWI, some friends' complaints about her drinking, and some problems at work that might be related to her being hung over. In addition, stopping drinking may help her to settle down and begin to have the children and family she has always wanted. Getting control of her drinking could also improve her relationships with her parents and her brother, who have been avoiding her. The importance and current significance of all of these considerations feed into the decisional balance about changing her drinking.

Shifting the Decisional Balance toward Change

Even when active consideration of costs and benefits begin to be weighted in favor of change, a firm decision does not always follow. Ambivalence and procrastination complicate the process. There is the very human tendency to generate a pro for every con and a con for every pro. On the one hand, smoking can cause lung cancer; on the other hand, I am young and have a few years before I need to quit. Feeding both sides of the decisional balance scale represents the ambivalence about any

TABLE 7.1. Decisional Balance Considerations of Carrie

No change	Change
Pros (Drinking)	Cons (Drinking)
• Manages anxiety • Enables sexuality • Acceptance • Dulls feelings	• Guilt • Memory loss • DWI arrest • Complaints • Work problems
Cons (Change)	Pros (Change)
• Loss of friends • Going crazy • No social life	• Children/family • Parental acceptance • Brother's acceptance

kind of change that individuals often experience, be it about job, home, or even what type of restaurant to go to for a night out. A second complication is the propensity to procrastinate when faced with a decision that is hard to make or perceived as difficult to implement. Our research has demonstrated that individuals can spend long periods of time in this Contemplation stage (Carbonari et al., 1999; Prochaska et al., 1991).

It is difficult to summon up the energy to overcome the ambivalence that fuels the procrastination. As Miller and Rollnick (1991) describe in their book *Motivational Interviewing*, feeling two ways about things is normal. Dealing with ambivalence is the critical task of increasing motivation to change. The best strategy to resolve ambivalence appears to be to bring to light all the considerations on both sides of the ambivalence. My experience indicates that individuals trying to change often attempt to restrict considerations to only one side of the ambivalence. They often will amass all the negatives of the addictive behavior in the hopes that this evidence will automatically move them to change. However, this strategy often misleads. Focusing only on the negatives gives the sense that the behavior is totally bad and completely problematic. This leaves individuals bewildered by their inability to make a firm decision to change and turn that decision into a successful long-term change. Statements like "I know that it is terrible for me but I just can't seem to quit" or "I just don't understand how I can continue to do something that is so bad for me" indicate a strategy that loads up on the cons and underestimates the pros of the addictive behavior. I confront this strategy by asking the addicted individual to elaborate on the positives of the substance abuse. If he or she says that there are few or no positives and goes on and on about the negatives, ask whether the client is completely irrational and out of touch with reality. Usually the client is surprised by this question. Then I offer my reason for asking. If addicts really believed that there were no positives to the addictive behavior and only negatives, they would be acting irrationally to continue to engage in the behavior. If there were no positives, change would not pose a problem. Most often this challenge to their exaggeration of the negatives leads to a more helpful discussion of the usefulness of the addictive behavior to the addicted individual. An accurate evaluation of what role the behavior plays in the life of the addict appears to be an important element in fostering serious consideration of change.

Bringing into the foreground the positive, helpful aspects as well as the negative consequences and risks of the addictive behavior can assist the individual to more effectively weigh the positives against the negative consequences. During Precontemplation, awareness of the problems and consequences of the addiction have been increased by engaging in consciousness raising and self-reevaluation processes of change. Reevaluation processes of change continue in the Contemplation stage. Until there is a serious and realistic assessment concluding that the negative aspects of the behavior are more important at this point in time than the positive aspects, the decisional balance will not support change.

Social cognitive theory has provided extensive descriptions of the self-regulatory mechanisms that can increase experiential processes and affect the decisional balance at this Contemplation stage of change (Bandura, 1986). Self-observation is a critical part of self-regulation, as are the personal judgments made about these observations. In fact, self-monitoring has become a standard part of almost every treatment program. Initially, self-monitoring was considered simply a means of getting an accurate baseline recording of the behavior. However, self-monitoring quickly became recognized as an intervention in itself, often reducing the target behavior before any additional intervention was implemented (Craighead et al., 1995). Getting individuals to focus on the actual behavior and become mindful of the frequency, the situation specificity, and the amount or intensity of the behavior provides information that challenges individuals' current assumptions about the behavior. As Bandura describes, this information then is put into a complex judgmental process that compares the current behavior to internal and external norms and leads to self-evaluations and self-reactions that promote decision making, whether the decision is to change or not to change.

Personal and social norms offer another avenue for intervention. Providing information or role models to support or challenge perceived norms can affect the decision-making process. For example, in the Motivational Enhancement Therapy we developed for Project MATCH, therapists provided information about the pattern of alcohol consumption reported by the client (Miller et al., 1992). Feedback to the client included a statement comparing current consumption to national norms. The statement would indicate, for example, that "your level of drinking is at the 95th percentile of drinkers in your age and gender group, which means that you drink more than 95 percent of drinkers in the United States." For many, this objective feedback challenged an assumption that their drinking was not different from most of their peers. Such information can create a reevaluation of the behavior. In fact, prior to this feedback many of these drinkers believed that they were drinking like most of their peers. Feedback is even more powerful when multiple observations support it, especially if there is a pattern to the behavior. In working with clients in therapy, feedback has been most effective when I listened long enough to see a pattern and could give multiple examples of it from the life of the client. In a similar vein, AA meetings can provide role modeling that influences these internal and external norms and engages the helping relationship process of change. When treating medical professionals who have alcohol problems, I try to get them to go to an AA meeting where doctors and nurses attend. This kind of group is more difficult for the professional to discount and more relevant for spawning direct comparisons about personal situations and drinking behaviors.

Many techniques used in the Motivational Enhancement Therapy are designed specifically to promote more complete and effective decision making. Therapists are trained to discuss the "good and not so good aspects of the drinking," reflect back to the client the ambivalence with "double-sided reflections," and listen carefully for both the positive and negative considerations (Miller & Rollnick, 1991, 2002). They asked for the client's personal evaluation of the problem and *not* simply that of spouse or family. Finally they were taught to offer frequent summaries of the decisional considerations. These were all strategies geared to promote the client's decision-making process. In all these techniques the objective is to get the client to acknowledge personal data and information to heighten realization of the social norms and personal consequences, and to raise consciousness of conflicting personal agendas that the client has but has not been actively processing.

Thus, there are a number of strategies and techniques that can be used to engage various cognitive/experiential processes of change and to promote movement through the Contemplation stage to the Preparation stage. Here again it is important to realize that there is no magic formula. Most critical is what goes on inside the individual. That process must produce a convincing shifting of the decisional balance toward making the commitment and developing the change plan. This is not

:emplators who fail to gather enough data about both
tive consequences do not have a complete picture of the
the addictive behavior. Such deficits in decision making
mmitment and eventually implementation of an Action
ion researchers consider a relapse in quitting an addic-
behavior to be a defect in the Action stage of change. However, part
of the vulnerability for relapse may lie in failure to create an adequate
decisional balance in the Contemplation stage. Firm and well-founded
decisions support action better than less-considered ones.

Helping or Hindering Contemplation and Decision Making

The Contemplation process, even when it is not chronic, takes time. The
individual, not the treatment provider or family, determines its timeta-
ble. Thus, it can be a particularly frustrating stage of change for helpers,
family, and friends. Ambivalence and procrastination are understand-
able when *I* am the one making the decision. However, these can be
maddening to me when *you* have to make a decision. The challenge for
family, friends, and helpers of the person in Contemplation can seem as
daunting as those discussed for Precontemplation. Family reactions are
also often the same as with Precontemplators: keeping quiet, not making
waves by bringing up the addictive behavior or launching angry and
blaming confrontation often fueled by years of frustration.

The strategy of not making waves tries to ensure peace in the home
and reduce any additional stress. The hope is that the individual will realize the nature and extent of the problem on his or her own. Reducing
stress might reduce the need to engage in the behavior. However, this
strategy most often neutralizes the very important and powerful social
influence of interpersonal feedback and approval that can be provided
by family and friends. A number of years ago spouses who took this
strategy were, somewhat callously, labeled "enablers" and more recently
referred to as "codependent" (Cermak, 1986). The family system in such
cases does take on a conspiratorial air when family members are trying
to passively ignore or actively hide the problem behavior. However, family members usually had tried to bring up the issue in the past and wit-
nessed or experienced very negative consequences when they did so,
with no resulting behavior change. Family members who do not make
waves are faced with the dilemma that peaceful coexistence often promotes the status quo and not change.

Feedback can be helpful to Contemplators, but when it takes the
form of frustrated and angry confrontation, there are many problems.
The most obvious is giving negative feedback when the individual is
intoxicated. The likelihood is low that any significant or memorable

information processing will occur during such an encounter. There is a phenomenon called "state dependent learning"—individuals who learn something in an intoxicated state remember it better in that intoxicated state and have problems remembering it when sober. In many angry, explosive confrontations what is learned is that when I am intoxicated, my spouse, friend, or family member explodes. So as the individual becomes more intoxicated, he or she learns to avoid going home and interacting with spouse or family member. This avoidance compounds the problem.

A second problem is that many things said in the heat of anger are often exaggerated and global. Confrontations often include personal attacks and name-calling. Family members may "pour it on" and offer a litany of the ways the addictive behavior has been problematic. This is usually done in anger and disgust. Such interactions tend to feed the self-protective mechanisms of rationalization and denial by allowing the addict to disregard patently exaggerated information. Often dire consequences such as divorce, are threatened, but family members often do not consider whether it is a thoughtful and doable consequence or whether they are committed to following through with it. The promised threat is usually not enacted. With a lack of follow-through, future threats are less likely to play a role in the addicted individual's decision-making process. This type of confrontational strategy does not usually supply usable feedback and promote decision making.

These negative and ineffective aspects of a confrontational strategy are not always easy to see. This is especially true when some reinforcing behavior change immediately follows the confrontation. However, this behavior change is usually fear driven and externally motivated. Unless the external motivation influences the internal motivation and the processes of consciousness raising and self-reevaluation, the likelihood is low that successful long-term change has been encouraged.

Both the peace-at-all-costs and the angry confrontational strategies are rather ineffective. Nevertheless, there are ways that significant others can help. Feedback from others about the personal and interpersonal consequences of the addictive behavior can make important contributions to shifting the decisional considerations of the Contemplator. However, this feedback must be heard and processed by that individual. As described in Chapter 6, significant others also have control of important reinforcers that can be used to promote personal decision making. But the reinforcing consequences must be used properly and consistently. Promising only what you are willing to do and doing all that you promise is the important advice that I would offer to family, friends, and therapists in order to ensure that words and actions are credible and powerful.

Suggested Strategies to Promote Contemplation for Change

The following are specific strategies and approaches to help promote decision making that would be helpful for family, friends, courts and treatment providers:

1. First, provide feedback when there is time and in an atmosphere that promotes openness and listening. The heat of anger, the snide or cynical comment, the critical labeling, and the passive–aggressive or openly hostile stare are actually not very effective communication strategies.

2. Demonstrate as much objectivity as possible. Be direct and concrete in your discussion. Although change of the addictive behavior would benefit you in many ways, the critical issue is how change can benefit the addicted individual. Make sure to point out that this is how the events appear to you and that the addicted individual may have a different perception. A discussion of different perceptions can be very enlightening and helpful for both parties. Listen as well as talk. In fact, spend more time listening than talking.

3. Provide feedback in the context of concern. Family and significant others need to let go of the anger and rehearse how to give the feedback with concern and love. Interventions have been created to empower family members, friends, employers, and significant others to provide effective confrontation (Liepman, 1993; Stanton, 1997), but several preparation sessions often are needed to help to defuse anger and frustration that interfere with empathy. Genuine expressions of concern for the well-being of addicted individuals enhance and encourage an exploration of their own concerns.

4. Find effective and doable consequences that reinforce your expressions of concern. The key is to discover meaningful reinforcers to withhold. Actions that reflect concern like refusing to let them drive after drinking or not allowing children or grandchildren in the car with them can be particularly meaningful. Being put on probation at work and a marital separation are other action that can reach Contemplators when these are framed in the context of concern and with an offer of support for change.

The preceding suggestions can be helpful but should not be considered guaranteed methods to move the Precontemplator or Contemplator. They probably work best for Contemplators who had already done some of the work of Contemplation. In terms of the different tasks of the various stages of change, I believe that these interventions can provide important decisional input for the addicted individual. Many of the suggested strategies are incorporated in current programs that engage families to assist in promoting change, like ARISE (Stanton, 1997), Network Therapy (Galanter, 1999), and the Community Reinforcement Approach (Higgins, 1999; Meyers & Smith, 1995).

The strategies outlined in this section have as their goal increasing the cognitive/ experiential processes of change outlined in the TTM and shifting the critical decisional balance marker of change. Whether family and friends offer consequences and concern or professionals use motivational interviewing and feedback techniques or the wisdom of the 12 Steps of AA, the addicted individual in Contemplation must become aware of and reevaluate the pros and cons of the behavior and of the change.

THE CONTEXT OF CHANGE AND CONTEMPLATION

Examining the areas of functioning, the context of change, can give a view of the additional barriers to the decision-making process. In the interpersonal area, relationship conflicts with spouse and nonusing friends often increase; family, work, and social network conflicts emerge in the family/system area; and any preexisting problems in self-esteem, identity, and character in the area of personal characteristics also seem to increase. These issues can contribute to ambivalence, distract from decisional considerations, and offer additional pros for the addictive behavior and cons for change. Because addictive behaviors actually create serious problems in many areas of the addict's life, a vicious circle develops.

In the Precontemplation stage these multiple problems are often experienced by the addict and viewed by the treatment provider as external pressures moving the addicted individual into Contemplation. However, during the Contemplation stage these problems can create stress and distress that prevents the individual from moving into Preparation and Action. Often, addicted individuals will begin to consider changing the addictive behavior but then assert that the problems with the marriage or family need to be the focus of effort. The existence of other problems can also interfere with the decision-making process, which needs time for serious thought. This is more difficult when the Contemplator is surrounded by chaos.

Chaos and environmental turmoil is one of the reasons so many treatment personnel believe that inpatient treatment is critical to recovery. Individuals surrounded by complicating problems and environments may need time away from the chaotic environment to be able to make a firm decision to change. It is often removal from the immediate environment and not necessarily medical hospitalization that is really needed. However, few programs currently offer the type of isolation and time away from the addictive behavior that is provided by the traditional, more expensive detoxification and inpatient programs. As described in Chapter 6, on Precontemplation, if this time away does not prove effective in fostering movement to Preparation and development of a plan, it may not be the best use of these intensive resources. Continued evaluation of progress is needed for all interventions (Connors et al., 2001, pp. 99–104).

As described earlier, individuals who progress to maintained dependence on the addictive behavior are ones who have integrated that behavior into their lifestyles. Individuals who use the addictive behavior as a problem-solving mechanism for life's difficulties will find the decision to stop the behavior particularly difficult. For them there is an adaptive component to the addictive behavior that increases the advantages of the behavior and makes the loss of that behavior particularly difficult to face. When the addictive behavior serves so many functions, relapse often occurs rather quickly when individuals advance to making an attempt to change.

Individuals whose primary coping mechanisms involve the addiction need to develop problem-solving and alternative coping skills even while continuing to engage in the addictive behavior. Coping skill training is usually reserved for individuals who have already made the decision to modify the behavior and are making an attempt to change. But for individuals whose coping is the addictive behavior, we may need to promote these strategies as early as Contemplation in the process of change.

Multiple problems complicate the process of change for the Contemplator. These problems need to be placed on hold for a time or partially resolved to allow the Contemplator the time and space to accomplish the tasks needed to make a considered and solid decision to change. Keeping focused on the problem of an addictive behavior while assisting with other complicating difficulties seems to offer the best strategy for moving the Contemplator to solid decision making and the Preparation stage of change.

CASE EXAMPLE AND OVERVIEW

Addicted individuals in Contemplation often go back and forth in their evaluations of the costs and the benefits of change. The cognitive/experiential processes of change need to be engaged to tip the decisional balance marker solidly in favor of change in order to accomplish the tasks, as illustrated in Table 7.2. An example of the decisional conflict and ambivalence brings to life the Contemplation stage of recovery.

Conrad is a 45-year-old veterinarian who is addicted to amphetamines and alcohol. He has used "uppers" since he was in his final year in veterinary school. He began using these substances to help with the studies and exams, but now uses them both to help him get more done and to feel good. He was married for a brief period but has been divorced for more than 10 years. He is not sure if he is gay but does frequent gay bars and engages in homosexual sex regularly. Until recently, he believed that he had the perfect life. He loved working with animals

TABLE 7.2. Contemplation for Recovery: An Overview of the Dimensions of Change

Stage task

Gathering and evaluating positive and negative considerations for change, evaluating these in a comparator process, and resolving decisional conflict in order to make a firm decision to change.

Change processes at work

Cognitive/experiential processes, particularly those promoting awareness and reevaluation of negative consequences and positives for change, promoting decision making and movement into Preparation.

Consciousness raising: Discovering negatives of the addictive behavior and positive reasons and expectancies for change.

Emotional arousal: Getting in touch with some core values that would promote change, realizing the negative reactions created by the addiction.

Self-reevaluation: Shifting views and valuing of the addictive behavior to emphasize consequences and of the potential benefits of the change.

Environmental reevaluation: The person begins to realize the impact of the addiction on others and the risks of continuing the addiction in contrast to the benefits of change.

Social liberation: The person begins to see how others in society support and encourage change of the behavior.

Markers of change

Decisional balance: Weight shifts more strongly toward change because of increasing valuing of pros and cons for change.

Self-efficacy: Growing sense that they could change the addiction.

Context of change

Multiple problems in the life Context can contribute to ambivalence, distract from decisional considerations, and can increase the need for the addiction.

and cared for them with skill. He was part of a larger practice and another partner did all the bookkeeping that was needed, so he did not have to bother with these "pesky" details. His family lived over 1,000 miles away and considered him a success but did worry about his not having a wife and family. His drug use fit in with his lifestyle, and he believed that he could control his drug use and drinking whenever he really wanted.

Recently, several events have made him reconsider his euphoric interpretation of his life. His frequent sexual partner told him that his drug use was getting in the way of their relationship and he was unsure whether he could continue going out with him. His business partner at work had begun complaining that he was not billing enough procedures to justify his pay and was not contributing adequately to the business. Conrad would disappear from the clinic for long periods of time, claiming that he had other business to do. In reality, he was off getting high. However, his most worrisome experience was the one where he went home and began seeing bugs crawling on the walls and feeling that people were out to get him.

Conrad argued both with his business and sexual partners that they were exaggerating things and promised that things would change. But his protestations made him uneasy. He was beginning to realize that he was getting high more frequently and during the day. He used to do it mostly in the evening. He also had begun using cocaine on occasion, when he could get some at one of the bars he frequented. There were some women that he found attractive in that bar, so maybe he would just get a straight sexual partner. He was not comfortable being gay but he was not really interested in women. Nonetheless, he could not imagine going to the bars and getting involved with a woman or another guy without being high. At some level, he knew that he should just quit the amphetamines. He could still drink alcohol and that could help. But the alcohol did not give him the same feelings of euphoria and energy. With the pressure at work he could not afford taking time off either to quit using or to get help. Maybe he could just cut back and hide his drug use a bit more, get the problems at work straightened out, and then think about quitting over the summer when he had some vacation time coming.

Conrad's rambling considerations of pros and cons represent the twists and turns of Contemplation, sometimes leaning toward complete change, sometimes against. A middle ground offers some solace that he is making progress and allows for delay of the "ultimate" solution. Ambivalence makes the road particularly winding. The role that speed plays in his life is significant. Relationship issues and sexual identity conflicts complicate consideration of whether and when to change. If he allows the problems of work and relationships to become more salient and can counter his fears about change more effectively, Conrad could make a decision and commit to a more complete change.

SUMMARY

The Contemplation stage begins the important work of decision making in the process of change. Evaluating the pros and cons of both the addiction and the change are at the heart of this stage. What is needed to move into the Preparation stage is a decision that is firm, proximate, and supports a commitment to follow through with the change attempt. Ambivalence, procrastination, indecision, environmental barriers, and multiple other problems can interfere with the reflection, self-reevaluation, and cognitive processing that are needed to move the individual through this Contemplation stage. Family, friends, and treatment personnel can influence this process but must do so with caution and caring.

Chapter 8

Preparing for Action

Creating a Plan

Planning and a sense of purpose and commitment are essential for effective action, although not always valued by addicted individuals.

BE PREPARED

The Preparation stage of change follows decision making and precedes significant action. Preparation stage tasks focus on securing the commitment and doing the planning needed for successful action. The advertising slogan "Just Do It" may contain an important message for routine procrastinators but it is a dangerous message for anyone attempting to change an addictive behavior. Individuals would not be diagnosed as addicted if they could *just do it* without thought or preparation. The inability to change despite serious attempts to change is one of the cardinal criteria for a diagnosis of addiction (American Psychiatric Association, 1994).

The main tasks of the Preparation stage are (1) making and strengthening a commitment adequate to support the attempt to change and (2) developing a plan for action that is sound, reasonable, and feasible for the individual to implement. Action plans lay out what is needed for this individual to successfully quit or modify the addictive behavior. This chapter highlights the need for Preparation and the challenge of building an effective plan of action.

Defining Characteristics of Preparation

The transitional nature of the Preparation stage is reflected in the dimensions of change. Alterations in attitudes and thinking begin to blend

154

with small steps toward significant action. As addicted individuals translate the work of decision making into commitment to change, they look a little like those in Contemplation as well as like those in Action stages. Engagement in the cognitive/experiential processes of change peak and begin to become less important during the Preparation stage. On the other hand, the behavioral processes of change, particularly self-liberation, increase dramatically. Self-liberation is the process of change that engages choice and commitment. It is central to successfully strengthening the commitment needed to follow through with developing the plan. Preparation also is characterized by initial use of other behavioral processes like counterconditioning and stimulus control. Planning is often accompanied by self-observation and monitoring that allow the individual to begin to avoid places and people associated with the addictive behavior and foster attempts to employ alternative coping strategies to deal with urges to take drugs, drink, or gamble. In the Preparation stage there are often small steps that are being taken or have been taken to modify the behavior, like a call for help, restructuring the environment, an attempt at self-regulation of the addictive behavior, or a recent attempt to quit the addiction. In addition, alternate reinforcing activities, such as getting involved with family, work, or school activities, can be increased so they will be available as viable substitutes for the addiction. Though they may seem anxious and hesitant, addicted individuals in the Preparation stage look ready to make an attempt to change.

As they begin to plan a strategy for conquering the addiction, people in Preparation have to evaluate how they will deal with other issues in the context of change. Multiple addictions and/or serious problems in the various areas of functioning make planning more difficult and require choices as to what to include in the change plan. Employment, family, social networks, psychopathology, psychiatric symptoms, marital relationships, and characterological problems serve as potential barriers. The possibility of assistance from others in the environment should be considered in the planning. The suggested strategy of AA to put aside all other problems and focus only on the alcohol or drug addiction until 1 year of sobriety is achieved is one way to develop a plan (Alcoholics Anonymous, 1952). However, it is not the only way, and multiple problems may need to be addressed in order to create an effective and acceptable plan.

Markers of change also reflect the transition from Contemplation to Action. The decisional balance increasingly tips toward change as commitment is strengthened. Consideration of the negative aspects of the addiction and the pros for change must be sustained in order for the planning to continue. However, self-efficacy begins to play an ever-increasing role. As individuals begin to put together a plan that they believe will work, their confidence to deal with the temptations to drink, gamble, take drugs, or smoke increases. Initial steps to manage the addiction, if successful, support personal efficacy and offer hope for success.

Commitment to Change

The first task of the Preparation stage is creating the commitment for the upcoming attempt to change. Commitment is related to decision making. However, it is not an automatic consequence of the decision-making process. Although there are many reasons why I am convinced that I "should" do something, summoning the energy, resources, and dedication needed for taking action requires another step. An additional step seems necessary even if the "should" motivating change is an internal one supported by solid decisional considerations. Commitment is a critical element of this transition.

In our research we have measured a process of change called self-liberation that attempts to capture the choice and commitment elements of change emphasized in humanistic and existential models (Prochaska & DiClemente, 1984, 1992; Prochaska & Norcross, 1999). Commitment represents the individual's readiness to place a particular change at the top of his or her personal agenda, to allocate personal time, energy, and resources to do the work needed to make the change. A miscalculation of the energy and effort needed undermines many attempts to change smoking, alcohol, and drug dependence despite good will and good decision making. Creating commitment, then, is a central task of the Preparation stage of change.

Planning for Action

Planning is the other critical dimension of Preparation. For a plan to produce significant change of an addiction it must be *acceptable, accessible, and effective*. Each of these qualities is essential. There are effective plans that are not accessible, and accessible and effective ones that are not acceptable. All three qualities are needed to engage the individual in action to break the hold of the addictive behavior. In developing their plan addicted individuals must decide how to handle the multiple and complicating problems in their lives and whether the plan is to include the help of others or formal treatment. An effective plan has concrete immediate steps for taking action.

Although individuals cannot completely prepare for what will happen in any change, planning can make the change go smoother, be less stressful, and ultimately be more successful. We understand this when it comes to making changes like moving to a new home, taking a new job, or starting a new school. Few people would make these changes without finding out something about the new location, job, or school and organizing themselves for the change. Planning is an important step in taking an action that must produce sustained change.

When it comes to addictive behaviors, individuals often refer to that elusive characteristic called "willpower" as the only thing needed for change. However, the definition is often circular and unhelpful. Successful changers have it and unsuccessful ones do not. Willpower and success are often linked together in the American ethos. However, very successful talk-show hosts, athletes, actors, comedians, and businesspersons have become addicted, suffered significant losses, and found change difficult, if not impossible (Wholey, 1984). Certainly these individuals had the willpower, dedication, and commitment to become successful. It is hard to believe that they completely lost these characteristics when it came to the addictive behavior, especially because when they finally move into recovery, many do things that take strong willpower. Changing addictive behaviors takes more than simple willpower; it takes commitment and planning specific to the individual and the behavior.

WHAT NEEDS TO BE INCLUDED IN THE PLAN

The plan to change an addictive behavior needs to be built around people's knowledge about themselves and about their habitual pattern of behavior. If drug use occurs on weekends with a certain set of friends, a plan to quit drugs while still socializing with these same friends would be difficult to implement.

Planning should also take into account the strengths and weaknesses of the individual. Individuals who lack assertiveness skills will have a difficult time in environments where there is lots of encouragement to engage in the behavior. Individuals who use the behavior to cope with feelings of frustration and anger will need to learn ways to avoid or manage these feelings. Individuals who plan to quit in the midst of other life stresses may need some special help or support. Individuals who have a spouse or partner who engages in the addictive behavior will need to find some way to neutralize this influence. The specifics of the plan may differ but the existence of a formal or informal plan appears critical for moving successfully into the Action stage.

Planning also requires some concrete details, like setting a date or taking specific steps. In studies of smokers, one important indicator of an individual's readiness to actually make an attempt to quit smoking was whether he or she had set a date for cessation (Fiore, Jorenby, & Baker, 1997). Setting a date seems to indicate that the individual has thought about the change and is developing a concrete plan of action. Whatever specific indicators of readiness are used, a plan should be based on the addicted individual's prior treatment and change experience and knowledge of the environment and resources supporting the attempt to change.

In the Motivational Enhancement Therapy developed for Project MATCH, we included a blueprint for a change plan that could be used by the therapist (Miller et al., 1992). This blueprint simply gives the categories and issues to consider when helping the client create a plan for change (Table 8.1). These include the specific change desired, the means to be used, others who are available and how they can help, what success would look like, and the problems that could pose barriers to be overcome. All of these elements form the necessary ingredients for a change plan.

Alone or with Others: Including Others in the Plan

Having someone who can empathize as well as provide encouragement and support for planning and taking action is important for many people in recovery. Sponsors have been an integral part of assisting individuals in making a commitment to the 12-Step approaches (Nowinski, 1999; Nowinski, Baker, & Carroll, 1992) and in developing the plan for sobriety based on the practices of AA. Many addicted individuals have benefited from the wisdom, commitment, and assistance of these sponsors. In my experience sponsors have been more available and integrated into the lives of the addicted individual than treatment personnel ever could be. Similarly for drug abusers, therapeutic communities and group approaches to treatment may make a great deal of sense (see Deleon, 1999; S. Brown & Yalom, 1995). However, intensive support has not always been needed for individuals to achieve successful modification of addictive behaviors. For example, it has been difficult, if not impossible, to create smoking support groups similar to those in AA. Many smoking cessation and substance abuse treatment programs report that even successful quitters do not complete all the sessions of the program, stay in close touch with sponsors, or involve others in their plan of action (DiClemente & Scott, 1997; Sobell, Cunningham, Sobell, & Tonneato, 1993). Including a support group or a mentor in a change plan should be seriously considered but is not always necessary.

The question of including others can be answered by determining what type of assistance is needed for this particular individual to implement a viable plan for action. If the addicted individual reports a significant amount of perceived support for change, then support groups or more intensive treatment programs may not be as necessary. On the

TABLE 8.1. Change Plan Worksheet

1. The changes I want to make are:

2. The most important reasons why I want to make these changes are:

3. The steps I plan to take in changing are:

4. The ways other people can help me are:

   Person   Possible ways to help

5. I will know if my plan is working if:

6. Some things that could interfere with my plan:

---

other hand, if the environment is either devoid of support for change or filled with individuals who have similar addictive behavior problems, the change plan may need to include finding others to provide helping relationships to support the change (Longabaugh et al., 1995; Longabaugh, Wirtz, Zweben, & Stout, 2001).

Another way to evaluate the need for others and particularly for support groups is to understand the individual's patterns of use and triggers for use and then to decide which of two behavioral processes are most important: stimulus control or counterconditioning. Understanding the difference between these processes can guide the decision. A brief review of these processes follows.

Stimulus control entails avoiding or removing triggers for the addictive behavior, or changing the environment in a way that helps to avoid the behavior. Examples of the stimulus control process include avoiding bars and drinking buddies, attending events where alcohol is not served, and going to self-help meetings to avoid triggers to drink. For smokers, getting up from the table immediately after eating is a stimulus control strategy.

Counterconditioning, on the other hand, involves changing the individual's response to the stimulus rather than the stimulus itself. Often addicted individuals cannot avoid triggers and must learn to cope with them. They must learn to be in situations where alcohol is being served without drinking, how to pass by an old neighborhood where they bought drugs without turning in for a hit, or how to be among smokers without smoking. Desensitization, relaxation training, distraction, and constructive self-talk are all strategies representing the counterconditioning process of change. They help the addicted individual to survive the craving or desire for the substance until that responses is extinguished.

The more an individual needs to use stimulus control instead of counterconditioning to overcome the addictive behavior, the more need there may be for a support group in the change plan. For example, alcohol-dependent individuals who have a great deal of support for drinking in their environment may need to use a great deal of stimulus control. This means avoiding most social situations and current friends in order to achieve sobriety. Since they have few nondrinking alternative environments available they need an alternative social support system to avoid cues to drink. This individual could benefit from AA attendance and the extensive support network available throughout the day and night provided by AA (Longabaugh et al., 2001). However, a gambler who has few friends who gamble and many other opportunities for amusement as well as a supportive environment would not necessarily need support groups in his or her change plan. The wisdom and knowledge of the individual who is changing the addictive behavior, who understands best the pattern of the addictive behavior and the history of previous change attempts, should be used to develop the plan.

The individual change plan has to be one that the individual will endorse and embrace for it to be implemented. Making hard and fast rules about how any addicted individual must change is as problematic as not making a plan at all. A single man announced in one aftercare group that he decided to quit cocaine and alcohol. However, he was very reluctant to give up his attendance at the bars where he would do most of his socializing, so his plan was to order nonalcoholic drinks but keep frequenting those bars. His first weekend visit to the bar was a success. He felt he had a good time without drinking. However, the second weekend it was much more difficult to sit and watch others drink without taking part. So he slipped and did have a drink, but came back to the group to discuss the problem. Some readers will immediately condemn his plan as being unrealistic from the start. However, it was his plan. It was acceptable to him and he was committed to implementing it. If I had forced him to develop another plan, it is doubtful that he would have been as committed or as open in discussing the pros and cons of his plan. Revising the plan enabled him to continue taking action to quit drinking. The path is not the same for everyone. Some addicts who drop out of treatment successfully quit their addiction. These individuals do not follow the treatment plan provided by the counselor but do follow their own change plan (Connors et al., 2001, Chapter 6). Dropout from treatment and failure to stop the addiction are not synonymous (DiClemente & Scott, 1997).

Preparation Tasks and the Context of Change

One of the significant challenges for developing a plan for change is to examine how other problems in the life context are related to the addictive behavior. When one addictive behavior is the only serious problem in an individual's life, the planning for change can proceed in a rather straightforward manner. Time and energy have to be taken from normal activities and focused on doing the activities needed to change the target behavior, be it gambling, cocaine use, or smoking. The plan can incorporate helpful aspects from other areas of life and include close family and friends as a support system for the change. In outcome studies of addictive behavior interventions, individuals who have more education, more personal and financial resources and fewer complicating problems are more successful in making the change (McLellan, Luborsky, & O'Brien, 1986). Change is still difficult for this group, but with the context of change filled with more resources they may be better able to plan and have more support for their efforts to change.

Many addicted individuals, however, have two or more addictions and multiple problems in other areas of functioning, and live in resource-impoverished environments. There may be no jobs of any substance for many of them, few alternatives for dealing with life problems, and meager resources in their current home or community environments. Without ways to resolve these complicating problems, there seems little hope of luring these addicted individuals toward change and creating a viable plan that would ensure long-term success (Smith, Subich, & Kolodner, 1995).

Staging Multiple Behaviors

Planning for these other problem areas should include consideration of where in the stages of change the individual is for the different target problems. Most individuals are in different stages of change with regard to the different problems in their lives. Some smokers are in Precontemplation about changing their marijuana use or doing something about a problematic relationship with parents. One person from my first research study stated proudly that quitting smoking had not increased his marijuana smoking, as he had feared. Clearly, he saw smoking cigarettes and smoking marijuana as very different problems and he was prepared to take action on one and not the other. Similarly, alcoholics who change their drinking behavior significantly often continue to use marijuana, and methadone-maintained clients often engage in abuse of other nonopiate drugs (Belding, Iguchi, & Lamb, 1996).

On the other hand, several successful changers with both nicotine and cocaine addictions have told me that they could not stop the use of these drugs until their change plan included some physical exercise on a regular basis. Exercise helped to fill the void created by quitting the drug use and gave them a sense of health and well-being that replaced somewhat the high of the drugs. These individuals had to take action for smoking cessation and exercise initiation simultaneously. In many cases individuals who are changing an addictive behavior will have to either begin new behaviors that are protective of the change or modify old behaviors that are now incongruent or incompatible with abstinence from the addictive behavior.

Anyone attempting to change even a single addictive behavior will need to be willing to change multiple aspects of life and environment. These "by-product changes" that occur in the context of changing a single problem behavior differ significantly from the planned, intentional change plan focused on a second and third problem behavior. A planned strategy for change would require a similar type of decision making and movement through the stages of change for each target behavior required for intentional change of any behavior. At least that is the assumption of the change model proposed here.

Multiproblem individuals, particularly those with few resources, pose a significant challenge in planning for change even if they are convinced that they should give up the addictive behavior. Although multiple problems and problematic resources create a significant barrier to changing addictive behaviors, any realistic personal change plan as well as any credible intervention strategy must not ignore the complications that interfere with decision making and the tasks of the Preparation stage of change. Incorporating multiple problems into the plan, whether or not they are addressed to any significant degree, seems most realistic. The question most often is not whether someone changing a single addictive behavior has to make multiple changes in her or his life but how many and what kinds of behaviors or problems need to be changed and in what sequence in order to develop a successful change plan for the individual.

Some of my recent research has focused on pregnant women who continue to smoke during the pregnancy. Many of these women have few resources and multiple problems beyond smoking cigarettes. Often there are conflicts with the baby's father or other partner, difficulties with parents and family, few financial resources, unstable living environments, illegal drug abuse, a history of sexual or emotional abuse, and possibly concurrent psychological distress or a psychiatric disorder. The challenge is how to move these women toward making a credible change plan for smoking that does not ignore the other very serious and real problems in their lives. It is certainly not realistic to ignore the other problems and tell them to focus only on the nicotine addiction. However, it is equally unrealistic to ignore the smoking while offering help with other problems because smoking represents the single most modifiable risk factor for premature birth and other pregnancy and postpartum problems for the baby (DiClemente, Dolan-Mullen, & Windsor, 2000). My advice for initial interviews with such women is first to identify and address the problems that are of primary interest to the women and then to incorporate a focus on health behaviors related to the pregnancy, including smoking. In actuality, smoking may be the area where these women have the most control and where they could accomplish something that would protect their baby and make them feel better about themselves while becoming more empowered to handle other problems in their lives.

Incorporating multiple problem areas or behaviors into an individual's change plan, however, can be a two-edged sword. On the positive side there can be a synergy to making multiple changes at the same time, particularly if they have some common elements, as is true with addictive behaviors. Conversion, for example, is a type of change that encompasses many areas of an individual's life and can offer multiple sources of support for changing (Miller & C'deBaca, 2001). However, such large-scale change creates negatives such as greater stress and dislocation, which can be very disorienting. Stress and disorientation can be a significant relapse precipitant for the changer. In addition, sometimes what is built as a complete change involving many different behaviors can collapse like a house of cards when relapse or problems occur in one area.

These negative aspects of an encompassing change plan are probably the reason why the 12-Step tradition and practices discourage AA members from working on other problems in their lives during the initial phase of gaining sobriety. The thinking behind this approach is that divided attention and effort can compromise the essential focus needed for achieving sobriety one day at a time. There is certainly wisdom to this strategy. Trying to fix marital problems, to solve family relation problems, or to begin a new career demands serious concentration and effort and can cause significant stress.

However, a "one size fits all" change plan that focuses exclusively on a single addictive behavior or even on a constellation of drug and alcohol behaviors is not always the best strategy for developing a change plan. One of my clients was discouraged by AA peers from going back to school and learning a new set of technical skills because she was too young in recovery from her poly-drug dependence. However, for this individual it was important and, I think, critical to include changing her problematic educational status (a dropout from school because of drug involvement). It is true that the stress of taking courses was significant and created additional problems. However, for this individual handling these issues became an important diversion from drugs and created an alternative area of focus and functioning that was incompatible with using drugs (counterconditioning).

Personal Plans and Treatment Programs

For most addictive behaviors there are a variety of treatment programs of differing intensity and orientation (McCrady & Epstein, 1999; Tucker, Donovan, & Marlatt, 1999). Should they choose a program or an approach for their change plan? How are individuals to choose from this bewildering array? Should they do it on their own or seek professional, formal assistance? I suggest that it is the personal plan rather than the treatment program that may be the critical dimension for changing any of the addictive behaviors. Each problem, whether cocaine or nicotine dependence, gambling or eating disorders, has some unique features that need to be addressed in the plan. However, development of a realistic plan with the commitment both to follow through on that plan and to revise the plan as needed are critical elements for successful behavior change. The more the plan engages appropriate processes of change, shifts critical markers of change, and is comprehensive and realistic in addressing the context of change, the better, more effective it should be. However, I have seen some strange change plans that seemed to effectively engage this process work for certain individuals. In any case, personal plans and treatment plans should focus on the process of change and use a similar series of steps to address the addictive behavior and the life context (Table 8.2).

The effectiveness of the change plan can only be judged in the Action stage of change when the plan is implemented. That is the reason why the plan has to be one that can be changed if it is not working. The plan is not the end point of the process of change. Taking action to make the change is the real bottom line for moving out of the Preparation stage and into Action.

CASE EXAMPLES AND OVERVIEW

Preparation stage tasks empower the addicted individual to implement the decision to change in a manner that offers hope for success. Commitment and specific strategies to be used in taking action are the main focus (Table 8.3). There is a shift from cognitive/experiential processes to behavioral processes of change, and the markers of change shift in emphasis from decisional balance to self-efficacy and temptation. Contextual problems begin to play an important role as they can significantly influence the potential for change and complicate a change plan. Case examples can only begin to approximate the complexity.

Paula Prepared, a 33-year-old homemaker, decided that this time she was really going to quit smoking. In addition to stopping smoking during her two pregnancies and resuming as soon as she finished breastfeeding, she had made several prior attempts to quit. Once when she was 22, she quit for 6 months but returned when she started seeing the man she eventually married, who also was a smoker. When she turned 30, she tried again but lasted only 1 month. Recently she found out that a

---

TABLE 8.2. Planning for Change Using the Change Dimensions of the TTM

1. Identify stage of change for target problem.
2. Identify processes of change needed to address tasks of that stage.
3. Identify problems in the context of change and how they interact with change of the target problem.
4. Evaluate stage of change for context problems and when they can be most appropriately addressed.
5. Develop a plan to address target and other problems that includes:
   • Strategies to promote key processes
   • Focus on the critical markers of change
   • When and how to address other problems

TABLE 8.3. Preparation for Recovery: An Overview of the Dimensions of Change

Stage task

Creating and strengthening commitment needed to support action and developing an accessible, acceptable, and effective plan for change.

Change processes at work

Cognitive/experiential processes peak and begin to become less important. Behavioral processes of change, particularly self-liberation and initial use of stimulus control and counterconditioning, become important in creating the commitment and plan.

Reinforcement: Small steps toward change are successful and reinforce the commitment; alternative reinforcements begin to be viewed as valuable.

Counterconditioning: People and places that trigger the behavior are identified, as well as alternative coping strategies to cope with the urges.

Stimulus control: Self-observations and monitoring uncover and begin to avoid the presence of triggers in the person's life.

Self-liberation: The person makes choices about what elements and strategies to include in the plan and commits to implementing the plan.

Helping relationships: The person seeks out others who can encourage and support changing the addictive behavior.

Markers of change

Decisional balance: Continues to be weighted strongly toward change, supporting both the decision to change and the commitment.

Self-efficacy: Confidence in the various elements of the plan as well as in the ability to change the addiction increases.

Context of change

Multiple addictions and problems in the life context complicate the change plan; sequencing when and how to deal with contextual problems offers significant challenges; understanding the stage of change for additional problems can offer some direction.

---

teacher she admired had lung cancer. Her health concerns and her awareness that her children were now getting to an age when they may begin smoking convinced her that she must quit for good.

Paula talked to her physician about quitting and whether a new medication, Zyban, could help her to be successful. After discussing the pros and cons, she decided to use a nicotine gum as an aid to reduce her smoking from the pack and a half a day that she currently smoked. The nicotine gum would help her deal with nicotine withdrawal. She would lower the dose of the gum gradually over 6 weeks as suggested by her doctor until she would just quit altogether. She set the date for quitting and purchased the gum at the pharmacy. She also knew that her husband's smoking would be a problem for her. She talked with him and told him how important this was for her. At first, he tried to talk her out of quitting right now but then agreed to smoke outside the house and to try not to smoke when she was around. Paula also knew that the children's hectic schedule produced stress and made quitting more difficult, so she timed the quit date to be after they finished the school year.

Paula was well prepared and had a plan that seemed reasonable and effective. There were a few wild cards in the mix. Paula's father had recently been diagnosed with a serious heart condition and was undergoing treatment. If he became seriously ill, she would have to travel from Baltimore to Philadelphia where he lived, to help her mother. She was an only child. This stressor could significantly impact her plan.

Fred Furious presented another picture of preparing to quit smoking altogether. The recent increase in the cigarette tax made him very angry and upset. He was convinced that he needed to quit just so he would not give his money to a state government that was punishing him for smoking. He also thought that turning 50 and growing concerns about health were good reasons to finally quit smoking. There would be other benefits. His wife and kids would finally stop nagging him about his smoking and he would no longer have to go into that obnoxious, smoke-filled enclosure reserved for smokers at O'Hare Airport when he traveled.

Fred spent a couple of days mulling over his decision and planned to quit smoking this weekend. He had tried nicotine gum before and just went back to smoking, so this time he would quit cold turkey. The weekend would give him some time to get over the first days without cigarettes. He would smoke his last cigarette on Friday and then destroy the rest. This time he would really make it stick and not relapse like before.

Fred's plan seemed solid but did not take into account that he was scheduled to play golf with his business associates who were smokers on Sunday and that he was going out for dinner on Saturday evening with a couple whose wife smoked. This was also a high stress time at work and he had several important presentations in the next couple of weeks. He would certainly face significant challenges to his quitting smoking early in his attempt to quit.

Paula and Fred offer contrasting plans and different levels of detail and preparation. Although each of them could falter and stumble as they implemented their plan, Paula appears to be anticipating potential threats to action better and to have a more detailed contingency plan. Both seem committed to quitting. Fred's anger can be a potent force if it can be sustained and directed at supporting the change. Contextual problems with parental illness and business stressors make the prediction of successful action more difficult because planning seldom covers all contingencies in the life context.

SUMMARY

Although planning may be difficult for individuals who are impulsive and addicted, as are most substance abusers, commitment to a plan of action is essential in order to implement the decision of the Contemplation stage. The plan should be a personal one that is chosen by the individual and can include self-help resources as well as formal treatment programs. One critically important issue that must be addressed by the plan is how to manage other life problems while implementing the change plan for the target addictive behavior. Multiple problems in other areas of functioning complicate planning and steal resources needed to follow through on the action plan. Once the plan is in place and the commitment secured to begin to take action, the individual can move forward into the Action stage of change.

Chapter 9

Taking Action
to Change an Addiction

*Leaving an addiction is one of the hardest things I have
ever done.*

BEGINNING BEHAVIOR CHANGE

The Action stage of change requires a concentration of energy and attention in order to interrupt the habitual pattern of addictive behavior. During Action, addicted individuals begin to break the physiological, psychological, and social ties that bind them to the addictive behavior. They separate themselves from the old pattern and begin to create a new one. This stage requires commitment and active use of the behavioral processes of change. The work of Contemplation and Preparation has laid the foundation for this active behavior change by providing the specifics of the plan and the commitment to act on it.

There is a significant discontinuity between the tasks of the first three stages, which focused on changing cognitions, attitudes, and experiences, and those of the Action and Maintenance stages. Being ready to stop smoking is one thing; actually going through the physical withdrawal and psychological loss is quite another. There is a qualitative and quantitative difference in the activities and attitudes needed in Action from those needed before.

Defining Characteristics of Action

The four main tasks of Action are (1) breaking free of the addiction by utilizing behavioral change processes and the strategies of the plan, (2) commitment, (3) revising the plan in the face of difficulties, and

(4) managing temptations and slips that can provoke relapse. The goal is to establish a new pattern of behavior. All of the behavioral processes of change are needed to initiate and sustain the separation from the addiction. Commitment (self-liberation) must be sustained. Counterconditioning, stimulus control, and reinforcement management must be employed to break the bonds of the addiction. Helping relationships are particularly important for support during this attempt to live life without the addiction.

Self-efficacy is the marker of change that is most critical at this juncture in the process of change. Confidence in one's ability to stop the addiction, built vicariously during the Preparation stage, is tested in the Action phase. Successful separation from the addiction increases efficacy to cope with a variety of situations without reengaging in the addiction. Successful coping with temptations to use reduces the level of temptation as well as increases self-confidence to abstain. However, if temptation remains high and coping is inadequate, then Action is jeopardized.

Slips—brief episodes of use—are events that interfere with successful Action. Yet slips also create an opportunity to problem solve defects in the current Action plan. Most Action attempts do not end in successfully maintained change. A full relapse back into the addictive behavior pattern recycles the individual to earlier stages of change. The tasks of those earlier stages must be redone or accomplished more fully if the person is to move back again into the Action stage. Recycling successfully through the Action stage on successive cycles enables the addicted individual to move into the Maintenance stage of change. This chapter describes the specifics of behavior change needed during this Action stage to continue on the road to recovery.

Breaking Free

The important task of the Action stage of change is to break away from the addictive behavior and to create new patterns of behavior. Action begins on the first day of the attempt to quit or modify the addictive behavior. Action continues through each day of the week and each week of the month until the ties to the addictive behavior are less binding and the task of breaking free requires less intense effort and focus. It usually takes 3–6 months to firmly establish a way of living and coping with day-to-day life without the addictive behavior. Well-maintained addictions are integrated into the lifestyle and coping repertoire of the individual. Breaking free means cutting the ties to the addiction across the broad range of life situations.

Leaving an addiction has been likened to leaving an intense love relationship (Peele, 1985). Familiarity and conditioning combined with potent physiological effects make the loss of the addictive behavior particularly poignant and difficult. In the initial phase of Action, each of the connections between lifestyle activities and the behavior must be severed. For example, with addicted smokers cigarettes are connected with eating a meal, talking on the phone, taking a break, getting up in the morning, and so on. As we saw in Chapter 3, each activity has set the stage and provided the cue to smoke. These cues are classically conditioned, like the ringing of the bell to signal salivation for Pavlov's dogs, and serve as signals that powerful reinforcers are coming. It takes time and energy to sever these connections, and a certain nostalgia may remain that encourages the individual to renew the connection with the addiction.

Abstinence and Slips on the Road to Recovery

Taking action requires significant modification of the addictive behavior. In most cases this will require abstaining from the behavior for at least some period of time. The role of abstaining from the behavior often has been misunderstood. Abstinence can serve as both a short-term *and* a long-term goal of recovery and plays an important and unique role during the Action stage of change. Once addictions have developed into well-maintained problematic patterns of behavior, they have escaped self-regulatory control. The addictive behaviors are not well regulated and do not respond to consequences (see Chapter 3). Once individuals are addicted, reinstating self-regulation is a very difficult and problematic Action strategy. Smokers who have for a period of time cut down on the number of cigarettes smoked often find themselves smoking more in order to maintain a level of nicotine in their system or because the behavior returns to normative levels of nicotine ingestion. Dieting has been a very unsuccessful enterprise for many overweight individuals; most gain back the entire weight lost on the diet (Brownell et al., 1986). Alcohol-dependent individuals often report that returning to some kind of social drinking is difficult because of their tendency to overdrink (DiClemente et al., 1995; Marlatt & Gordon, 1985; Vaillant, 1995).

The longitudinal data demonstrate, however, that while difficult, the return to self-regulation is not an impossible goal. My belief is that the best, if not the only, way to achieve a return to self-regulation is through a learning process that includes at minimum a sustained period of abstinence during the Action stage of change. In fact, self-regulation requires the ability *not* to engage in the behavior across all situations so that self-control is reestablished. Therefore, abstinence in the Action stage is an important goal whether the long-term goal is complete abstinence or significant modification of the addictive behavior (responsible gambling, drinking, medicinal drug use).

Total abstinence during Action may be the goal but it is not always the reality. Slips are brief reengagements in the addictive behavior that indicate that the commitment or plans are defective. Slips represent an opportunity to evaluate the difficulty and the temptations that are encountered and to revise the plan accordingly. The emphasis on total and complete abstinence as the only acceptable outcome for addiction has obscured the fact that many individuals experience a slip during the Action stage, learn to remedy the defects in the plan, and go onto successful recovery. Slips are often part of the process of taking effective action and should be understood as part of the learning process. However, once slips become more often or more extensive, they become part of a relapse and represent a substantive return to the addiction, as discussed later in this chapter.

The Right Road

There is disagreement about how to get through the first days and weeks of the Action stage. Some insist, particularly for the severely dependent, that it be done in an inpatient setting to protect the person from any physiological dangers and to shelter from those daily cues to return. There are numerous detoxification programs that require an inpatient stay, even for smoking cessation (Hurt et al., 1992). However, others believe that simply monitoring the detoxification process with or without the use of cross-tolerant drugs in an outpatient setting works as well as the more expensive inpatient detoxification (Miller & Hester, 1986). In smoking there is the controversy of whether to quit "cold turkey" versus "cutting down" on the number of cigarettes gradually. Many believe that cold turkey is the only way to ensure success because reduction in numbers of cigarettes can undermine motivation to abstain (Orleans & Slade, 1993). However, as we saw in the Preparation stage, many successful quitters begin to cut down on the numbers of cigarettes smoked as they get ready to quit (DiClemente et al., 1991). In addition, some individuals have to avoid all cues in the early phase of stopping while others prefer to quit without disrupting their natural environment.

Is there a single, most effective way to get through this early stage of Action? Probably not. The list of Action strategies that have been used to break an addiction includes acupuncture, electrical shock and other aversive conditioning techniques, hypnosis, behavioral coping skills, 12-Step approaches, anticraving medications and natural remedies, therapeutic communities, inpatient 28-day programs, single-session primary care interventions, community reinforcement approaches, fear-inducing motivational techniques, and sensory deprivation (McCrady & Epstein, 1999; Miller & Heather, 1998; Miller & Hester, 1986; Tucker et al., 1999). All have been used as Action options by many individuals to achieve successful cessation or modification of addictive behaviors. This has led some investigators to claim that it does not matter what you do as long as you do something to break the habit. This is clearly an over-statement because there are documented instances where some techniques have been demonstrated to be ineffective (Miller & Hester, 1986). However, we are only just beginning to understand how very different techniques and therapies can produce similar results for some of the population affected by addictive behaviors (Babor & Del Boca, 2002; Carbonari & DiClemente, 2000; Longabaugh & Wirtz, 2001; Project MATCH, 1997a). Despite the many different strategies there does appear to be, nevertheless, a common path through a set of change processes that are needed to negotiate the Action stage.

A COMMON PATH FOR ACTION

As individuals move from Preparation into Action, they need to decrease experiential change processes and increase behavioral process of change (DiClemente & Prochaska, 1985; Perz et al., 1996; Prochaska et al., 1991). Over and over again our research has demonstrated a significant relationship between the behavioral processes of change and taking action to modify or quit an addictive behavior. Individuals in the Action stage of change usually endorse more behavioral process activity than do those who are in earlier stages of change (DiClemente et al., 1991; Fitzgerald & Prochaska, 1989; O'Connor et al, 1996; Stotts et al., 1996).

This should not be surprising since addictions have a large behavioral component. As we saw in Chapter 3, addictions are appetitive behaviors (Orford, 1985). The behavioral processes of conditioning, stimulus generalization, and reinforcement help to lock in the routine pattern of activities labeled addictive. In order to break the habit it is necessary to make use of the same behavioral processes of change. The forms that the processes now take are counterconditioning, stimulus control, reinforcement management, and helping relationships, in addition to self-liberation or commitment. They represent some of the most powerful principles of learning that psychologists and behavioral scientists have uncovered. Successful action requires counterconditioning activities that include finding alternatives to the addictive behavior, especially in high-risk situations. Stimulus control activities do some managing or avoiding of the cues or triggers for the behavior. Reinforcement management activities involve creating a more addiction-free environment, reinforcing and rewarding oneself, and having others help to reinforce the change. Self-liberation activities strengthen the commitment to action. Strategies for prompting, organizing, and instigating these activities differ greatly, as can the reasons given for their success. However, the research indicates over and over that successful change has these change processes in common (DiClemente & Prochaska, 1998; Goldfried, 1980; Prochaska et al., 1992).

What does this mean for the resolution of the controversies about the setting (inpatient vs. outpatient) and methods (cold turkey vs. cutting down) for taking action to change addictive behaviors? According to the TTM, the critical issue is whether the setting or methods of the treatment have been successful in engaging these behavioral processes of change in the addicted individual. In addition, substantial commitment is needed to implement these behavioral activities. This need for commitment is probably why common wisdom attributes successful change to willpower. It is easy for a successful changer to say, "Well, I just did it with the force of my will [or character]." It is also easy to attribute success to this program or that technique after the change has been successful. In both cases individuals seem to forget other previous quit attempts when they may have had equal amounts of commitment, a solid program, and effective techniques, but a flawed personal plan of action. Settings, methods, techniques, and commitment are important but incomplete explanations for successful action. Individuals must be prepared to take action and engage in the behavioral processes of change in order to change the environment, find other ways to cope, and actively avoid high-risk situations.

Treatment Compliance, Commitment, and Behavioral Processes in Action

The inadequacy of commitment to explain the entire process of successful change of addictive behaviors is also evident in the treatment literature on compliance. The correlation between compliance and successful change is a solid but modest one. All treatment programs require some commitment to attend or follow through with the program. There is usually a positive correlation between posttreatment success and compliance with procedures. Compliers do better than noncompliers in achieving successful change of addictive behaviors (DiClemente & Scott, 1997; Donovan & Rosengren, 1999; Mattson et al., 1998). Compliance can be seen as a measure of commitment and often serves as a marker for success. However, compliance is not equivalent to success (Wickizer et al., 1994; Wierzbicki & Pekarik, 1993). Some clients come to therapy religiously but fail to take effective action. For these individuals the commitment to attend either is not equivalent to the commitment to change, or the commitment to attend is not connected to the commitment to implement the behavioral processes needed to change. Some possible reasons for this lack of concordance are that unsuccessful compliers have not made the solid decision to change, do not have the skills to implement the behavioral change processes, or have environments that overwhelm the implementation of the change processes.

Other clients drop out of treatment but successfully change their addictive behavior. In fact, I was surprised to see data from a number of studies showing that dropouts to treatment are not necessarily failures to change. In a recent paper, Carl Scott and I described the relationship between compliance and readiness to change as orthogonal, representing two separate and not necessarily highly correlated dimensions (DiClemente & Scott, 1997). Addicted individuals can rate as high on both dimensions, low on both dimensions, or high on one and low on the other. Understanding the complexity of the relationship between compliance, commitment, and change can help make sense of what clinicians often see in the treatment of those with addictive behaviors (DiClemente, 1999b).

The key to successful action is committed use of the proper processes of change to break the bonds of addiction. Getting addicted individuals to go to treatment is only a first step and, from a process of change perspective, probably represents less than half the battle to overcome addictive behaviors. Every clinician knows that presence on a treatment inpatient unit or at an outpatient treatment program is not a sure sign of motivation to change and that completion of the 28-day or 12-week program is not equivalent to successful action on discharge. Commitment to and compliance with a treatment program or method are not equivalent to successful addictive behavior change.

A Process Profile for Successful Action

The addiction field needs indicators beyond commitment, willpower, and type of treatment to judge success during the Action stage of change. Currently we are examining a multicomponent set of constructs that constitute the TTM's view of action (Carbonari & DiClemente, 2000). Looking at the data from over 900 outpatients and 700 aftercare patients in Project MATCH, we examined predictors of drinking during the 1-year posttreatment period. We divided up the patients into those who were completely abstinent, those who had some drinking but did not engage in heavy drinking, and those who had returned to substantial, heavier drinking. When these groups were compared on TTM variables, including measures of stage and processes of change as well as evaluations of temptation to drink and efficacy to abstain from drinking, clear differences emerged. We then looked at the scores of these three groups separately for outpatient and aftercare patients (Figures 9.1 and 9.2). Those who were most successful in taking action in the 12 months after treatment had at the end of treatment significantly higher scores on the Action subscale and lower scores on the struggling with Maintenance subscales of the University of Rhode Island Change Assessment (URICA), greater use of behavioral processes of change, lower temptation to drink, and higher self-efficacy to abstain than those who were the least successful. Interestingly, those who achieved a moderate level of success in changing their drinking in the year after treatment had scores on these variables that were between the most and least successful patients.

Although outpatient and aftercare patients differed in severity of problem and amount of treatment given prior to the MATCH treatments, the end of treatment composite profile on these variables were remarkable similar. Patients with more than three of these indicators in the right direction above or below the mean of the entire group had significantly greater odds of being in the most successful group. Patients with less than three of the five success indicators in the right direction had significantly greater odds of being in the heavier drinking outcome group. These findings offer the hope of providing a process-oriented measure of activities and attitudes that will be a sensitive indicator of successful action (Carbonari & DiClemente, 2000). It is clear that measures reflect-

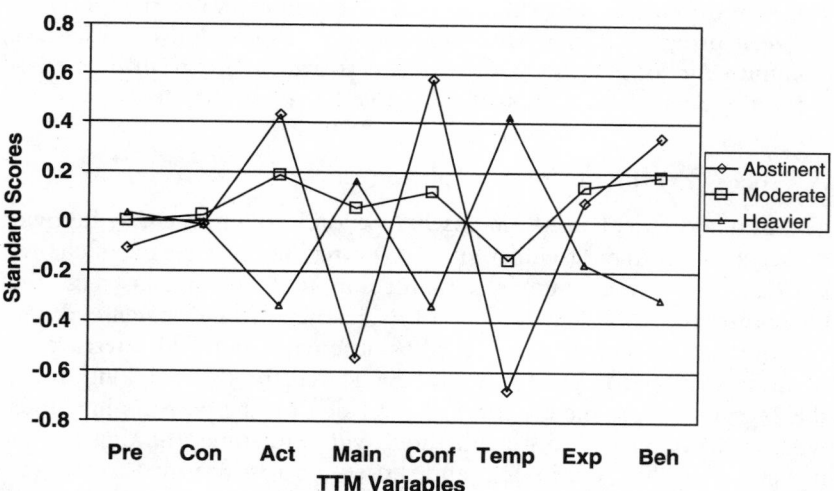

FIGURE 9.1. TTM profile of successful action for outpatients in Project MATCH. Pre, Precontemplation; Con, Contemplation; Act, Action; Main, Maintenance; Conf, Confidence; Temp, Temptation; Exp, Experiential processes of change; Beh, Behavioral processes of change. From Carbonari and DiClemente (2000). Copyright 2000 by the American Psychological Association. Reprinted by permission.

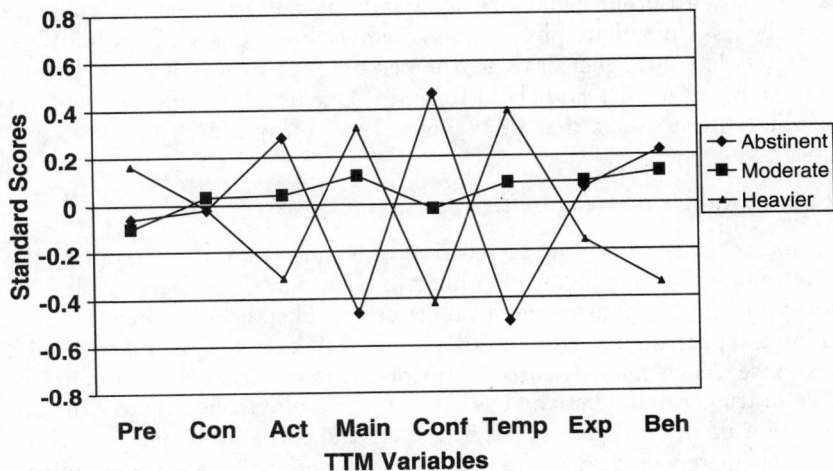

FIGURE 9.2. TTM profile of successful action for aftercare patients in Project MATCH. From Carbonari and DiClemente (2000). Copyright 2000 by the American Psychological Association. Reprinted by permission.

ing the process of change can be most helpful in predicting outcomes for those entering the Action stage of recovery.

STRATEGIES FOR INTERVENTION

Breaking the most immediate and most visceral of the ties that bind the individual to the addictive behavior is the primary task at the start of action. Solid commitment and a good plan can make this initial phase a bit easier. However, actually breaking the dependent pattern of behavior is a difficult, uncomfortable, and stressful experience. Physiology and habit play a significant role. Breaking any habitual addictive behavior requires the individual to suffer disruption to the physiological and psychological systems that depend on the behavior. Smokers who experience the anxious and, at times, disorienting withdrawal effects or find themselves with nothing to do with their hands must endure these effects until they get through the first few days when the drug nicotine is being flushed out of the system. With some drugs like alcohol and heroin the physical withdrawal effects can be painful and dangerous, including extreme physical disruption and pain (heroin withdrawal) or being significantly out of touch with reality (the delirium tremens—DTs—of alcohol withdrawal). With other behaviors like gambling and eating disorders there may be less immediate physical involvement but a gnawing sense of loss that acts like a magnet drawing the person back to the addictive behavior. As many former addicts have said, "Leaving the addiction was one of the hardest things that I have ever done in my life."

Behavioral Processes of Change

Breaking the conditioning connection is as important as interrupting the physiological or biochemical connection. In fact, there are clear behavioral links to the pharmacological effects of substances of abuse. Conditioning represents the creation of a learned linkage between a cue and a response. As we have discussed in prior chapters, cues play an important role in triggering addictive behaviors. Successful change requires the unlearning of the linkages between the cues and the addictive behaviors. One client reported that after achieving some abstinence from cocaine, he had to be particularly careful as he drove around the freeway at a particular exit. This was the exit for his drug purchases. Several times he noticed himself pulling over to exit as he drove around, and once he found himself off the freeway before he caught himself. The cocaine and freeway exit connection was a strong one. It took a long time to neutralize or extinguish this connection.

Breaking the connections between the cues and the behaviors requires either changing the cue (stimulus control) or changing the response (counterconditioning). In either case it requires that the individual take some concrete steps. Individuals who do neither are forced to rely completely on willpower to resist recurring urges. Paradoxically, urges often strengthen when the individual concentrates so strongly on resistance to a present cue. Refusing to engage in the behavior helps break the conditioned connection with the cue, but it is not necessarily the most efficient way to do so. Just saying no does not always decrease the intensity of the cue or the strength of the craving. Several individuals preferred to quit smoking while carrying an unopened pack of cigarettes with them. They reported that the presence of the cigarettes reduced the feeling of being deprived of cigarettes, but it also kept the habit alive to some degree. In almost all cases this strategy was used for only a short time. Then they disposed of the cigarettes—a more typical stimulus control strategy.

Part of the power of the addictive behaviors is that they have such strong, immediate, and consistent reinforcement effects compared to many of life's alternatives. Thus it should not come as a surprise that changing these behaviors requires some reinforcement or contingency management. These strategies can range from counting the money the smoker is saving every day that she does not smoke to getting AA tokens or chips for various milestones on the path of recovery. Reinforcement is a powerful strategy in successfully changing the addictive behaviors.

Reinforcers not only provide relief for negative states, but they also offer the direct rewards of positive new behaviors. Furthermore, reinforcement effects create a synergy with counterconditioning strategies. When individuals in the Action stage use alternative behaviors (deep breathing instead of smoking) or engage in incompatible behaviors (jogging instead of smoking), they often find these other behaviors have their own rewards and so are reinforcing in their own right. Individuals who have not found alternative activities that can provide some measure of relief, pleasure, or satisfaction are at significant risk for returning to the addictive behavior. Finding new sources of reinforcement is particularly important in the late Action and Maintenance stages of change.

Important sources of reinforcement for human beings are the presence and support of significant others. The process that we call helping relationships identifies the contribution of having someone whom the individual can talk with and share the struggles involved in moving through the stages of addictive behavior change. It is in the Action stage, however, that these relationships can provide reinforcers for the change. Several of my clients have reported that they have had images or remembered words from our sessions that encouraged them or supported them through a particularly difficult temptation to use. Clients who report greater satisfaction from intimate relationships while sober or who have a personal cheering section that accentuates the positives of the change seem to have a better prognosis for successful change. In fact, more than one client has expressed disappointment in the fact that the praise and rewards for sobriety did not last nearly as long as the nagging and complaining about the addictive behavior. It seems that those who live with addicts are better at complaining about what they do not like than they are at reinforcing and praising positive changes in the lives of these addicts. However, there is peril in not praising. Change that is taken for granted by significant others can be more easily reversed.

Action and Environmental Reinforcement

Successful change requires the addicted individual to manage the interpersonal and social environment in order to achieve and sustain successful action. This is particularly important in the early period of the Action stage, when the attempt to change is new and the individual's most vulnerable to slipping back into the addictive behavior. Breaking the personal connections to the addictive behavior is more difficult if the individual continues to be surrounded by people and places that promote engagement in the addictive behavior. In fact, it is for just such a person that the need or rationale for inpatient or residential treatment is most compelling (Longabaugh et al., 1998). Residential programs have been promoted as a way of ensuring that the individual gets a priming dose of sobriety or behavior change and an escape from the stress and pressures of the normal environment (DeLeon, 1999). In Project MATCH, individuals who successfully completed an inpatient or residential program and then went into the MATCH aftercare did very well in terms of percentage of days abstinent during the posttreatment period and had outcomes that were better than the outpatient subjects (Project MATCH, 1997a). These better outcomes occurred even though the aftercare subjects had more serious initial alcohol problems and consequences related to their alcohol consumption than the outpatients.

One way to understand this result is that these individuals, who entered a residential program, had achieved a priming dose of abstinence that gave them an advantage. This advantage was then reinforced by the aftercare MATCH treatments as these subjects returned to the natural environment. This residential program period of abstinence combined with support on discharge was associated with significant changes in drinking throughout the 1 year following aftercare treatment (Project MATCH, 1997a). It is not clear from this study what types of individuals actually need an inpatient or day hospital program in order to take successful action because subjects were not randomly assigned to inpatient or outpatient treatment in this study. Moreover, many of the individuals who entered the inpatient program had prior treatment for alcohol problems, so the effects of recycling were not taken into account. However, there are recent studies indicating that individuals with greater alcohol involvement do better in inpatient treatment and have better psychosocial outcomes (Rychtarik et al., 2000).

It is important to note that in the Project MATCH study, the reported use at the end of treatment of behavioral processes of change was predictive of successful drinking outcomes (Carbonari & DiClemente, 2000). Even during the second week of treatment, subjects who reported greater use of behavioral processes had higher percentage of days abstinent posttreatment (DiClemente, Carbonari, Zweben, et al., 2001). Many of the participants discharged from the inpatient condition returned to the environments where they used to drink. Behavioral process would be expected to assist them to modify the cues, responses or reinforcers in the environment that would assist in promoting abstinence. One way or another individuals who are going to engage in action to change addictive behaviors will need to address the role of the environment.

The environment represents both places and people; both are powerful influences on the addictive behavior. Action is most difficult when the addicted individual continues to be surrounded by others who are engaging in addictive behaviors. For pregnant women who stop smoking for the pregnancy the best predictor of postpartum relapse is the presence of a smoking spouse (Mullen, Richardson, Quinn, & Ershoff, 1997). For pregnant women who fail to quit smoking during pregnancy, a smoking partner is an important correlate (DiClemente, Dolan-Mullen, & Windsor, 2000; McBride et al., 1999). Family members who are also abusing alcohol or drugs represent an important predictor of relapse in almost all studies (Marlatt & Gordon, 1985; Merikangas et al., 1992). In short, it is difficult to overcome spending time with individuals who provide access and model the problematic behavior. Sustaining action in the face of these obstacles to change requires solid commitment. It also requires effective cognitive and behavioral coping skills to counter the influence that people and places can have on the individual. Seeking alternative support systems can also be helpful. One of the intriguing findings for the Project MATCH outpatient participants was that long-term outcomes at 3 years for those with alcohol-saturated environments were better if they were treated in the 12-Step Facilitation program and used the support of AA groups (Longabaugh et al., 2001; Project MATCH, 1998a)

RELAPSE AND THE ROLE OF RECYCLING

Relapse is most often defined as a return to the problematic behavior, the opposite of successful action. When I first entered the field of addictive behaviors, relapse was considered unique to the addictions and very discouraging for researchers and treatment personnel. The infamous relapse curves demonstrated by Hunt, Barnett, and Branch (1971) seemed to indicate that long-term successful change (total abstinence) in heroin use, cigarette smoking, and alcohol dependence was an elusive goal. The lack of sobriety in long-term abstinence rates of only 20–30% was sobering. This led some to claim that addicted individuals did not change and that addictions were the most recalcitrant behaviors known to behavioral science. That was before we began to realize that most intentional human behavior change included a relapse phenomenon. Researchers began to point out that compliance to medical regimens and adherence to positive behavior changes like regular physical exercise had relapse rates similar to those for addictive behaviors (McClellan, Grissom, Zanis, & Brill, 1997).

Relapse has different meanings depending on whether the desired outcome is total abstinence or allows some engagement in the behavior.

Although not recommended by most current treatment philosophies, many individuals consider themselves in recovery if they engage in minimal drinking or occasional drug use without returning to any problematic use (Fletcher, 2001; Vailliant, 1995). In these cases treatment personnel would consider the individual as relapsed. Long-term follow-up studies of individuals who have quit drinking or using drugs indicates that total continuous abstinence is not always the norm as individuals move through the Action and Maintenance stages (Cisler & Zweben, 1999). Slips and infrequent periodic use in highly variable patterns seem to be common even among individuals who are able to sustain the change and never return to any problematic engagement in the addictive behavior (Cisler & Zweben 1999; Simpson, Joe, & Lehman, 1986; Vaillant, 1995). This is an area where additional longitudinal research is needed to understand which patterns of maintenance provide for successful sustained change. Sustained total abstinence represents the clearest but not the only picture of successful maintenance (Fletcher, 2001; Project MATCH, 1997a, 1997b; Simpson & Sells, 1982).

No matter how it is defined, relapse is an integral part of human intentional behavior change. Human behavior change requires a learning paradigm, and we do not learn ordinarily without trial and error. In fact, one-trial learning is a rather rare event and is most often associated with traumatic learning. A child who burns herself touching a stove may learn quickly not to touch a stove. A serious case of food poisoning may stop someone from ever eating a particular food again. However, most learning is like learning to ride a bicycle: often falling over in our first trials, then gaining small successes and some confidence about our abilities. Successive approximations are the way we learn most new behaviors or change old ones. It is clearly the way that most addicted individuals find their way to recovery.

Relapse versus Slip

Individuals in the Action stage of change often encounter situations, stresses and temptations that significantly tax coping efforts and action plans. They often give into a temptation and engage in the addictive behavior on an occasion. Those who regard abstinence as a single piece of fabric that once torn is forever ruined see this single event of reengagement in the addictive behavior as catastrophic relapse. Behavioral scientists, like Marlatt and his colleagues, have attempted to make a distinction between a "slip or lapse" and a "relapse or collapse" (Marlatt & Gordon, 1985). The slip is a single occasion or two of use. The relapse represents a significant return to the problematic pattern of use or engagement in the behavior. From this perspective slips provide the occasion for learning in order to avoid the relapse. The goal continues to be prevention of relapse. Relapse represents a failure for this change attempt and something to be avoided. However, it should not be equated with total failure and the inability to change.

Both slips and relapses provide important occasions for learning and should be seen as part of the ongoing process of change. Of course, if an individual can learn from a slip, make a midcourse correction in his or her planning, and continue successful action, this is a good outcome and can enhance the individual's ability to achieve the change goals. However, if the individual does not make the correction and slips begin to accumulate, the problematic pattern of engagement or use can be reinstituted. In this case the personal plan and/or the abilities to take appropriate action appear inadequate and flawed. This too should be an occasion for reflection and learning about what went wrong in order to make a better plan for change in the future.

Relapse—the return to the problematic pattern of behavior—requires a recycling through earlier stages of change in order to get ready for a return to action. Recycling is at the heart of this stage model of the process of change. The vast majority of individuals do not successfully achieve change of an addictive behavior on a first attempt. Successful changers report multiple attempts that were unsuccessful. Most addicted individuals report making attempts over a long period of time before being successful (DiClemente & Prochaska, 1998). Recycling through the stages of change in some sort of spiral fashion seems to be at the heart of long-term successful change (Prochaska et al., 1992). Relapse is the event that commences the recycling process. It provides feedback about flaws in the current plan for changing the addictive behavior. Relapse offers an opportunity to learn how to develop the next plan to avoid the pitfalls of the failed attempt.

Relapse Prevention

Over the past 15–20 years, the focus of most addiction research and treatment has been on the prevention of relapse. Alan Marlatt and colleagues developed a model of the relapse process and offered numerous ways to short-circuit and prevent relapse (Marlatt & Gordon, 1985). Since then, there have been many attempts to develop relapse prevention programs in the hope of creating more durable change attempts (Quigley & Marlatt, 1996). A review of the literature (Connors, Longabaugh, & Miller, 1996; Donovan, 1996) indicates that these programs have had some modest success but have not provided the technology or strategies to avoid all relapse. For some addicts these programs help to prevent a slip from becoming a relapse and enable entry into the Maintenance stage of change. For others the data indicate that these programs postpone or delay relapse, giving these individuals more sustained change and a better chance that the next attempt to change would be more successful. However, for many individuals it is difficult, if not impossible, to prevent relapse completely, even with the most sophisticated relapse prevention programs (Quigley & Marlatt, 1999). Maintained recovery is not an impossible goal for individuals who relapse. To achieve it, relapsers have important lessons to learn about their pros and cons for change, the power of the addictive behavior, or the influence of stress and the social environment. In addition, relapsers must reassess their skills and abilities and review their use of the behavioral processes of change.

Recycling

If relapse is an integral part of the basic change process and all relapses are impossible to prevent, then we need to focus less solely on preventing relapse and more on promoting recycling. In other words, we need to focus on relapse as providing critical learning events. The research data on recycling come from longitudinal research on the process and outcomes associated with addictive behavior change. In one research project we examined the probability of an individual in a stage at one time point moving to another stage 6 months later. We found that the majority (60%) of smokers in Precontemplation and Contemplation were at the same stage at both time points (Carbonari et al., 1999). But the majority of individuals in Preparation who made one previous quit attempt in a 6-month period were likely to make more than one quit attempt (60%) and found themselves in various stages of change 6 months later. A significant number of those in Action (abstinent anywhere from 1 day to 6 months) at the first time point had successfully moved into maintenance (46%). However, many other smokers who were in Action at the first time point had recycled and moved back into Contemplation or Preparation 6 months later. A small but significant number of individuals in Action had moved all the way back to the Precontemplation stage and were not seriously considering any attempt to quit smoking in the next 6 months.

Individuals differ as to where they end up after a failed quit attempt with some, usually the majority, going back to considering or preparing for the next attempt (Prochaska & DiClemente, 1984). Others may give up at least temporarily after having failed to sustain the action attempt. Large numbers of relapsers seem to need some time to regroup and renew commitment before making the next attempt. In our minimal intervention studies I noted that many individuals made an attempt to quit smoking soon after entering the study and getting the manuals or other self-help materials. However, in the subsequent follow-ups at 3 months, 6 months, or 1 year, the numbers of new attempts among these individuals were low. These individuals appeared to need a refractory period before they were ready for a new attempt to take action. A certain amount of time may be needed before they can recycle back through the early stages all the way to the Action stage.

This spiral movement over time and the process of recycling through the stages until the individual achieves successful recovery provide a generally optimistic framework for addictive behavior change (DiClemente et al., 1992; Prochaska et al., 1992). However, it does not suggest that recycling to success occurs in swift succession over a brief period of time. The process of change can take place over extensive periods of time, particularly if success depends completely on trial and error learning, as often occurs in the natural environment (Carbonari et al., 1999). This type of learning can be rather inefficient without some guidance or coaching. The purpose of treatments, self-help, and other types of interventions is to make the learning more efficient. If they are helpful, interventions reduce the time spent in the process of change and in the number of relapses and recycles needed to successfully move through the stages of change. The hope is that by understanding better this process of change we can facilitate movement and recycling through the stages and reduce the time needed to achieve successfully established and maintained change.

TAKING ACTION AND THE LIFE CONTEXT

Resources and problems in other areas of functioning can enhance or undermine initial Action strategies and plans. Contextual problems can hinder implementation of a plan. Family conflicts, addiction-saturated social systems, and psychological and emotional problems can reduce commitment, interfere with coping activities, create stresses that compound difficulties, and offer environments that make abstinence extremely difficult. Conversely, supports and resources that can help to resolve daily hassles, offer material and emotional assistance, and relieve some problems provide a life context that promotes change.

Successful action also provides a new perspective on problems in other areas of the individual's life. Problems that seemed trivial in light of the serious problems caused by the addiction look different in the light of abstinence. Once change of the addiction has begun, change of other problems becomes more feasible, and often more necessary, in order to sustain the change. Anger and aggressive behaviors become more accessible to change once the addiction is removed from the equation.

Spousal conflicts can be addressed more effectively after there is a period of abstinence from drinking and drug use. Certainly there is a question of timing. When to tackle an associated problem will be discussed in depth in the next chapter. In Action the primary focus must be on changing the addiction.

CASE EXAMPLE AND OVERVIEW

The Action stage is filled with behavioral processes of change, shifts in self-efficacy, successful distancing from the addiction, and coping with the loss of the addiction (see Table 9.1). The decision to change must be strong enough to sustain action. Positive experiences that come from abstaining from the addiction ideally would support this decision. Activities that engage the behavioral processes of change require energy and focus. Social environments can offer support both for returning to the addiction and for abstinence. Choosing where to spend time is critical. Personal success enhances confidence in one's ability to abstain across a growing number of situations and cues. Temptation begins to recede as confidence grows across situations.

Anthony Action is a 45-year-old appliance repairman who has been using marijuana for the past 20 years. He is married and has two children, a boy, 15, and a girl, 12. He and his wife used to smoke together at concerts and on the weekends to relax. He also was into motorcycles and would smoke with some of this group of friends. About 4 years ago his wife quit using marijuana. She was concerned about the children and any potential negative effects of parental drug use on them. Although they concealed their use from the children, she believed that her son realized that they used when he was around 11 and found some funny-looking cigarettes. He had a course in school on drugs where they showed them various types of drugs. When he asked, she told him that she and his dad used to smoke and that these were from an earlier time. She quit then and made Anthony promise never to have any marijuana in the house. Since that time, Anthony would smoke with friends and before coming home from work. However, over the past 2 years he was becoming increasingly concerned about his son. He knew that young Tony smoked cigarettes and drank alcohol. He had been in trouble in school several times for smoking. Anthony felt like a hypocrite lecturing his son while continuing to smoke marijuana. In addition, he felt that the marijuana was having a negative effect on his work and his relationship with his wife.

Recently, Anthony decided that he would quit and 3 weeks ago did so. This was much more difficult than he thought it would be. His initial

TABLE 9.1. Taking Action: An Overview of the Dimensions of Change

Stage task

Implementing and revising the change plan; maintaining commitment to change in the face of difficulties; managing temptations and slips that provoke relapse.

Change processes at work

Behavioral processes of change, particularly stimulus control, counterconditioning and reinforcement management, are needed to create change. Self-liberation sustains commitment and helping relationships support change.

Reinforcement: Extrinsic and intrinsic rewards reinforce the change and commitment; alternative reinforcements begin to replace the addiction.

Counterconditioning: Alternative coping strategies are used to deal with emotions, people, and places that trigger the addictive behavior.

Stimulus control: Avoidance of cues and triggers early in Action increases probability of abstinence; minimizing contact with others who engage in the behavior.

Self-liberation: Sustaining commitment to abstinence and the change plan and to revising the plan.

Helping relationships: The person turns to others for encouragement and support for abstinence and for changing the addictive behavior.

Markers of change

Decisional balance: Pros for change may increase as abstinence is experienced as positive; balance continues to be weighted toward change.

Self-efficacy: Confidence in the ability to abstain increases as success in behavior change occurs and extends over time; slips challenge and successful coping increases efficacy; temptations to use decrease in intensity and frequency.

Context of change

Multiple addictions and problems in the life context often interfere with success and provoke relapse; energy and attention can be focused on other problems as the period of abstinence extends over time.

---

plan was to avoid his smoking buddies and spend more time at home, where he did not smoke. But he was more irritable than he expected and was getting into conflicts with both his son and daughter, who were not used to him being home. He also was surprised at how angry he would become. Obviously the marijuana had made him mellow and covered his anger. At first, he thought it was just withdrawal from the drug that was making him so angry and anxious. However, he began remembering that before he began to smoke, he used to be more anxious about being with people and more frustrated with others. He had had some loud arguments with his father over his lack of ambition and his choice of spouse. The family relationships were still strained but there was little contact, so it did not seem to be a problem anymore.

Anthony made it through the first 3 weeks without smoking but was still feeling shaky. He was beginning to leave the house to spend time with friends because of the conflicts at home. He was very tempted, particularly around his two smoking buddies, who were shocked to learn that he was trying to quit. They respected his wishes but were not going to not smoke in front of him. Anthony knew that he had to make some choices about whether to hang around them since he was very tempted when he was in their company and smelled the smoke. Several times he had second thoughts and wondered if quitting was really necessary. One night he almost asked his buddy to give him a toke but thought better of it because he believes that if he starts back, it will be difficult to stop again. He has begun to talk with his wife more about how she did it while he continued to smoke.

Several events that are coming up in the next few weeks will be particularly difficult. There is a family reunion with his parents and siblings to celebrate his parents' 50th wedding anniversary. His dad will likely ask how he is doing in his job and possibly make some comparisons with his younger brother, who is a very successful realtor. Another upcoming event is the annual Fourth of July rally of the motorcycle club. Anthony typically spent several days before and after the event with his friends smoking and drinking. Although he was feeling pretty confident in being able to abstain from marijuana in most situations, he was not sure what would happen in these two. He did not want to blow up with his father and would feel bad about not participating in the rally because it was the highlight of the year for him and his friends.

It is not clear how Anthony will do in the next few weeks. He has made a significant attempt to change. His efficacy and his commitment seem a bit shaky. It would not be surprising to learn that he had a slip one night with his friends if he does not use either stimulus control or counterconditioning. Managing his emotions will be another critical issue, as will finding alternative reinforcers in his social and family network. When and whether he will address his anger and frustration with his father and his feelings about not being very successful are interesting questions for which there is no current answer.

SUMMARY

As its name implies, the Action stage of change is filled with important action plans and strategies that break the connections between the individual and the addictive behavior. With the successful implementation of the Action strategies, addicted individuals begin to create the needed distance from the addictive behavior that allows recovery to begin. It is a tenuous time because the power of the addiction is strong. Only a committed, planned, comprehensive effort can break the multidimensional connections in the areas of physiology, cognition, affect, behavior, and environment that constitute an addiction. However, it is the initial successful action begun during the Action stage of change that lays the foundation of permanent change. Turning that foundation into a solid, sustained recovery is the task of the next stage of change.

Chapter 10

The Long Haul
Well-Maintained Recovery

Sustaining recovery involves developing new, strong, and healthy habits as well as repairing the damage done by the addiction.

THE FUNCTION OF MAINTENANCE

The challenge of human behavior change is to make change permanent. In the Maintenance stage of change, not engaging in an addictive behavior becomes established as a personal norm for the formerly addicted individual. Individuals negotiate their way successfully through the Maintenance stage by (1) actively countering any threats and temptations, (2) checking and renewing commitment, (3) making sure that the decisional balance remains negative for reengaging in the addictive behavior, and 4) establishing a protective environment and a satisfying lifestyle. In the Action stage the task is often simply to refrain from the addictive behavior. However, the absence of the addictive behavior is not sufficient to successfully maintain the change and become an ex-addict. In order to sustain recovery, new behaviors and reinforcing experiences must become part of a new way of living in the world.

As individuals successfully maintain the change, they increasingly use less and less energy and active coping. They develop a solid sense of self-efficacy—of confidence in their ability to avoid the problematic behavior and manage any remaining cues to reengage. Once successful Maintainers have achieved sustained change, they can best be seen as having terminated the cycle of change (Prochaska, Norcross, & DiClemente, 1994). Termination indicates the successful conclusion of the process of stopping the addictive behavior and the end of the cycling through the stages of change (DiClemente & Prochaska, 1998; Prochaska et al., 1991). Formerly addicted individuals are always vulnerable to reinitiation. However, once they have left the cycle of change and are focused on other challenges of life, over time they begin to look more and more like their nonaddicted peers (DiClemente, 1994; Moos et al., 1990). Successfully maintained change is considered by society to be the desired outcome for the cessation or modification of any addictive behavior.

There is a critical difference between well-begun action and the sustaining of that action over a long period of time. An addiction is by definition a behavior that resists feedback about consequences and efforts to change. Moreover, there is a tendency for the addictive behavior to regain its position of dominance even after periods of abstinence.

Why is maintenance of this change so difficult and so important? Once intrinsically rewarding addictive behaviors escape self-regulation, bringing them back under control is exceedingly difficult. Smokers and drinkers often experience this dilemma. They achieve some measure of abstinence, then they begin to believe that they can control the behavior. The thinking often goes like this: "Boy, if I could just smoke two or three cigarettes a day [five a day, ten a week, etc.]." Or "If I could have a drink or two every once in a while, I would be in great shape healthwise and not have to quit this habit completely." "After all, there is a part of smoking [drinking] that I really enjoy." However, maintaining this level of control over smoking or drinking is very difficult for someone who has been dependent on nicotine, alcohol, or other mind-altering drugs. Most often the number of cigarettes or drinks increases a little at a time, and before they realize it these smokers and drinkers are back to smoking a pack or more a day or drinking dependently. This is because addictive behaviors become entwined with the basic coping mechanisms of the individual. Often the addictive behavior becomes a major coping mechanism for how the individual handles bad or unpleasant things that happen, interacts with others, feels good, and, at its most extreme, feels normal. Maintaining recovery means establishing or reestablishing basic coping mechanisms that do not include the addictive behavior. Maintenance usually requires that individuals who have been dependent build a new pattern of behavior that excludes all or, at minimum, any significant engagement in the addictive behavior.

The Maintenance stage takes a significant amount of effort over a substantial period of time. If the Action stage takes about 6 months, the Maintenance stage takes years. However, it is more than time that demarcates the Maintenance stage and makes it the final step in the cycle of change (Prochaska et al., 1992). Maintenance is defined by the critical tasks that need to be accomplished to enable the addict to leave the addiction behind and look forward to a new life free of it. The tasks of the

Maintenance stage of recovery are, first, to sustain change for an extended period of time over a wide range of situations and, second, to avoid slips and relapse into the old pattern. Individuals move into the Maintenance stage once they have achieved short-term success in the Action stage of change and have begun to establish a pattern that excludes the addictive behavior. Discovering alternative activities and experiences can provide some measure of comfort and coping formerly provided by the addictive behavior (Higgins, 1997; Vuchinich, 1999). The next challenge is to manage the less frequent cues and triggers to reengage in the behavior. Building a satisfying and well-modulated lifestyle that offers alternatives to the addictive behavior accomplishes this most effectively. Once this successful alternate lifestyle is in place, there is less need or temptation to reengage in the addictive behavior.

A sociologist colleague has written a book on the process of leaving a profession, marriage, or other role, of reestablishing an identity separate from the prior identity, and of successfully becoming an "ex" as in an ex-wife, -husband, -priest, -nun, -executive, and so on (Ebaugh, 1988). The process that we are outlining as comprising the important tasks to be accomplished in this Maintenance stage of change is similar. Successfully becoming an ex requires a shift in one's perception of oneself. All of us know of individuals who, although divorced, have never been able to get beyond being someone's ex-spouse. This self-perception gets in the way of building new relationships, a new life, and a regained sense of wholeness. An unsuccessful ex always has something missing in his or her view of the self. The successful transition and the pitfalls to being an ex as described by Ebaugh are similar to those experiences and activities that are needed to maintain addictive behavior change and become an ex-addict. As long as a large portion of the individual's life seems missing, there will be a longing for the addictive behavior. Such a person is not able to successfully move forward and will continue to struggle with Maintenance of the change. The danger of a return is ever-present.

Although behavioral theorists, B. F. Skinner in particular, often talked about the role of new positive reinforcers to change problematic patterns of behavior, there is renewed interest in this topic with addictive behaviors. Behavioral economics is the study of the competing reinforcements that shape behavior in the lives of individuals using an economics perspective (Vuchinich, 1999). In recovery, for example, the new lifestyle created to replace the addiction should offer rewards that are potentially as meaningful and fulfilling as those problematically offered by the addictive behavior in order for the personal economics to work. Satisfying alternate reinforcers decrease the value of the addictive behavior. Without these alternatives the addiction continues to hold its value and fascination for those addicted, even though they are not currently engaging in the addictive behavior. Taking away an addiction leaves a void that must be filled by alternative satisfying reinforcers for the economics of recovery to work. Only then can individuals exit from the cycle of change.

Whether an individual will be unable to successfully exit the cycle of change and will need to remain in recovery forever depends on how that individual handles leaving the addictive behavior. The dictum "once addicted, always an addict" seems less an issue of a label (recovering vs. recovered) than understanding the process of becoming an ex.

Defining Characteristics and Dimensions of Change: Maintenance and Termination

The period of time spent in Maintenance varies dramatically. After about 3–6 months in the Action stage, individuals who have successfully remained in recovery move into the Maintenance stage and face the tasks described earlier. How long they remain in this stage depends on how well and completely they accomplish these tasks. How hard they have to work at remaining in recovery is an important indicator. Individuals who have to continually monitor addiction cues and triggers, who long for the addictive behavior, who fail to find adequate alternate reinforcers, and who have been unsuccessful in extricating themselves from an addiction-infested environment remain in Maintenance and must continue to use behavioral and cognitive/experiential processes of change.

In some research we have used an arbitrary time frame of 2 years in Maintenance to indicate the exit from the Maintenance stage (Carbonari et al., 1999; Prochaska et al., 1991) and to define termination similar to the way time frames are used to define successful cancer treatment (5-year survival). However, this has been done out of necessity. The more satisfying way to define termination is an individualized assessment of the critical dimensions of change outlined earlier (DiClemente & Prochaska, 1998). The markers of self-efficacy, temptation, and the behavioral processes of change are good indicators to use in this assessment. Individuals who experience little or no temptation to engage in the behavior and are very confident (self-efficacious) in their ability to manage or abstain from the behavior across a variety of tempting situations have successfully completed the Maintenance stage and can exit the cycle of change. The other important indicator is related to the processes of change. Change process activity devoted to modifying the addictive behavior declines during the Maintenance stage of change. As self-efficacy increases, change processes decrease in frequency and intensity of use. Termination represents the point where there is little or no activity devoted to this process of change (DiClemente & Prochaska, 1998; DiClemente et al., 1985; Prochaska & DiClemente, 1984; Prochaska et al., 1992).

Although efficacy, temptation, and behavioral processes of change are the most important indicators, other dimensions of change are also involved. The decisional balance remains tipped in favor of change, but often endorsement of both the pros and cons diminish in importance (Velicer et al., 1985). The negatives of the addiction and the positives of change continue to outweigh opposite considerations. However, once addicted individuals achieve substantial recovery and successfully become an ex there is little consideration of pros and cons except for occasional reminiscing. In fact it is a danger sign of potential relapse or reinitiation of the addiction if the positive aspects of the addiction are still valued rather highly or become somewhat idealized in retrospect.

Cognitive/experiential processes of change decline during the Action and Maintenance stages of change consistent with the shift in focus from attitude change and decision making to behavioral change. It is a striking and rather consistent finding in our research that some coping activities appear mismatched to Action and Maintenance stages and can precipitate relapse. Smokers who report engaging in higher levels of cognitive/experiential types of coping activity (consciousness raising, self-reevaluation, environmental reevaluation) during the Action and Maintenance stages of change have a greater probability of relapsing compared with recovering peers who engage less in these processes (DiClemente & Prochaska, 1985; Perz et al., 1996). In particular, during Action and Maintenance the use of self-reevaluation (being upset with oneself about the problem and thinking negatively about oneself and the problem) has proven to be problematic. Individuals who remain engaged in berating themselves about the past behavior, who are preoccupied with the addictive behavior, or who may be constantly generating guilt and negative feelings about the addictive behavior are not as successful in maintaining change (Perz et al., 1996).

MECHANISMS INFLUENCING
MAINTENANCE OF RECOVERY

Once an individual has negotiated successfully the first 6 months of the Action stage of change, he or she has encountered all the most frequently occurring cues and triggers to engage in the addictive behavior. The individual has experienced 6 months of weekends, 6 months of Mondays and Fridays, which incidentally number only 24 or 25 of each. These numbers are in sharp contrast to the many years of days and weekends spent engaged in the addictive behavior. However, after 6 months or so, some stability is achieved for those who have avoided relapse and sustained change. It is this initial stability that marks the transition from the Action stage to the Maintenance stage. In Maintenance the addicted individual will encounter cues and triggers that are less frequent or that have been encountered before but not at such a level of intensity. If an alcoholic, for example, takes action in March, the first 6 months will take him through the summer but not a Christmas with family members who are heavy drinkers. Two of my first research interviews were with women who had successfully quit smoking for 4–6 months only to have relapsed in emergency rooms, one with a husband with a suspected heart attack and another with a grandchild who was injured. Less frequent events and intense stressors are two critical types of triggers that must be negotiated successfully to sustain change and manage the Maintenance stage of recovery.

To successfully cope with these challenges to the Maintenance of sobriety and recovery, the addicted individual will need to engage behavioral change processes together with some cognitive change processes in order to sustain the change. One reason that individuals fall back and reengage in the addictive behavior is precisely the naive belief that the change process is brief and over quickly. These naive changers think that after a brief period of successful change they "have it made" and do not have to do anything in order to maintain the change. Maintenance tasks take a long period of time.

Maintainers need to continue actively sustaining the change. However, the focus of the coping activities shifts. Successful Maintainers use a wide-angle lens and focus more on the larger picture and less on the need to struggle day to day with triggers to reengage. This shift in coping may be as subtle as refocusing on new activities or as dramatic as changing whole areas of life, like getting an education or job training. As individuals move farther and farther into the Maintenance stage, change process activities most directly related to changing the addictive behavior become less and less salient. During maintenance not engaging in the addictive behavior becomes more habitual and the norm. The tugs and pulls to return become less frequent and intense. Life becomes livable and, most times, more satisfying without the addictive behavior.

Maintaining Commitment and Decisional Balance

In the process of creating a new lifestyle and an identity free of the addictive behavior, several specific cognitive and environmental factors need to be addressed. Marlatt and Gordon (1985), in their groundbreaking work on relapse prevention, identified a number of thinking patterns that are problematic for long-term recovery. To a certain degree behavioral relapse (reengaging in the behavior) may be secondary to a cognitive relapse process (thinking about the behavior) during the Maintenance stage. In the Action stage a slip and a return to the addictive behavior often can occur before the individual really spends any time considering it. In Maintenance there are subtle cognitive activities that undermine the process of change prior to any behavioral return to the addictive behavior. Marlatt and Gordon (1985) have identified two of these problematic cognitions as the "abstinence violation effect" and "apparently irrelevant decisions."

The abstinence violation effect is well known to anyone who has been addicted. It is a belief in abstinence as a fragile state that is completely violated by any engagement, intentional or not, in the addictive behavior. Abstinence once breached, even inadvertently, is forever broken. A single breach can therefore grant permission to return to the entire pattern of behavior (Shiffman et al., 1997). With this belief a lapse can turn quickly into a relapse. As Marlatt and Gordon describe it, violators can quickly go from a lapse to a complete collapse.

There is something to be said for rigid beliefs about abstinence. Even if it does, at times, promote a return to the addictive behavior, a rigid belief about abstinence does have a supporting rationale born of the experience of many addicted individuals. One of the dangers of successfully maintained change is that it can breed overconfidence and cockiness. "I have learned my lesson, I will never do that behavior *to excess* again"; "I have been able to control this behavior for 8, 10, 12 months so *I must be able to control it now*"; "*One drink* cannot hurt me." These quotes represent thoughts that have contributed to the first reengagement and the ultimate return to the problematic pattern of the addictive behavior. In order to protect individuals from the potential for relapse, many addicts and treatment personnel suggest that abstinence should be treated as a fragile and single fabric that cannot be torn and mended. Both overconfidence and the abstinence violation belief are problematic patterns of thinking and illustrate the dilemma of the Maintainer: how to negotiate the very narrow passage between being confident but not too confident and being able to cope with a lapse without giving oneself permission to relapse. There is a delicate balance that must be achieved in order to successfully complete the tasks of the Maintenance stage and move forward to possible termination from the cycle of change.

"Apparently irrelevant decisions" represent shifts in thinking and in decisional considerations that promote a return to the addictive behavior. The shifts include the slow erosion of the commitment to change and a subtle increase in the positive valence of the addictive behavior. After the passage of time or intervening events, the commitment to change can be undermined. A former, overlearned pattern of behavior will have some continuing influence for a long time. In fact, for most people it will always be easier to return to the addictive behavior than to stay in Maintenance during the initial period of this stage. A process of entropy can occur, where the forces that push toward a return to the addictive behavior sometimes get stronger. Entropy wears down commitment to continue change in the same way that gravity makes continual orbiting around the earth difficult.

A related mechanism undermining Maintenance is the shifting of positive and negative expectancies. The human tendency to remember the positive and forget the negative plays a role in the Maintenance stage of change. The farther away the former pattern of addictive behavior, the less problematic that behavior often appears. Increasingly, only the more positive aspects of the behavior are remembered. This kind of reidealizing of the behavior rekindles desire and reduces resistance to the ever-present cues to reengage in the behavior.

Countering these subtle shifts in commitment and thinking are important tasks of the Maintenance stage of change involving the self-liberation, consciousness raising, and environmental reevaluation processes of change. When thinking about the former addictive behavior, the Maintainer should actively recall the negative aspects and problems created by that behavior. However, our research does make it clear that individuals in Maintenance should not dwell too much on how bad the behavior has been or on self-recrimination because these thoughts could contribute to relapse. Periodically checking on commitment is another good idea. During the course of Maintenance the commitment to healthier alternative behaviors ideally becomes stronger and stronger. A commitment to a positive alternative is a better option and a more protective long-term strategy than simply a commitment to stay away from the behavior. However, if this positive commitment is taking a long time to develop or there is a waning of commitment to "all this healthy stuff," renewing the commitment *not* to engage in the problematic addictive behavior is a needed option.

For some individuals in the Maintenance stage continued vigilance is not necessary because thoughts about the former behavior have faded. Not having to think at all about the past is a good indication that these individuals have moved forward toward sustained change. In our research, individuals who are in Maintenance and have moved away from any thoughts about the addictive behavior often will complain, only half jokingly, that the only time they think about cigarettes, for example, is when we ask them all these questions in our surveys.

Although it is important to be vigilant about waning commitment or reidealizing the abandoned behavior, each Maintainer must find the strategies and alternatives that work best for him or her. The principles are the same, but the personal strategies can be different. Use of the processes of change needs to be titrated to the experience of the individuals as they progress through Maintenance and encounter the twists and turns of life after addiction. This argues for helping individuals evaluate themselves and their vulnerability as they negotiate the rather narrow passage through the Maintenance stage of recovery.

Creating a Solid Sense of Self-Efficacy

In much of our research, a critical mediator of Maintenance is the development of a solid sense of self-efficacy to abstain from or manage the addictive behavior (DiClemente, Carbonari, Daniels, et al., 2001; DiClemente et al., 1985; Project MATCH Research Group, 1997b). As individuals successfully sustain the behavior change, they develop a growing sense of confidence to perform the behaviors needed across a variety of situations (S. A. Brown, Carrello, Vik, & Porter, 1998; Shiffman, 1982).

It is precisely in the Action and Maintenance stages that the mediational role of self-efficacy appears to be most important (DiClemente et al., 1995). In the earlier stages of change, when individuals are in Precontemplation, Contemplation, and Preparation, efficacy estimates are often influenced by hopeful expectations or feelings of despair rather than by an accurate evaluation of one's ability to abstain or stop the addictive behavior. Once the individual has achieved some measure of success, he or she is able to more accurately evaluate how difficult the task is and how much effort and energy are needed to sustain and maintain the new behavior. Early in the Action stage, efficacy to abstain from drinking, smoking, or gambling is variable. An individual's confidence often depends on the type or intensity of the cue presented. For example, a person can be rather confident in his or her ability to not drink in social situations but not at all confident about abstaining when angry or frustrated. Confidence grows with successful coping in the various settings and situations where the behavior was predominant. As individuals move through Action, use the various behavior processes of change, and successfully cope with the most frequent situations and triggers, they develop more confidence in their ability to resist temptations.

In the Maintenance stage this confidence or self-efficacy becomes consolidated. Temptations to engage in the behavior become less frequent and intense as the individual creates a different lifestyle. During Maintenance the more the individual continues to struggle with temptations and finds it difficult to sustain the change, the lower the self-efficacy to abstain and the less motivation there is to continue the change. Thus, increasing efficacy and decreasing temptation become markers of successful Maintenance. Remaining tempted with a lower sense of self-efficacy to abstain indicates that the individual is not progressing well through the Maintenance stage and continues to be vulnerable to relapse (Carbonari & DiClemente, 2000).

A solid sense of self-efficacy to abstain from or manage the former addictive behavior is a good predictor of future successful maintenance and a marker of successful movement through the Maintenance stage of change (Project MATCH, 1998a). It is difficult to sustain artificially inflated or cocky self-confidence for long periods of time. "Fake it until you make it" works only for so long. It is difficult to simply bluff your way through the Maintenance stage.

Developing efficacy over time differs for individuals. Some become confident early in the Action stage, with this confidence simply growing to the maximum with the passage of time. Others experience a more variable growth pattern where efficacy plateaus for a period of time and then grows in the face of certain challenges. For some others the experience is one of struggling with temptation and trying to maintain sufficient efficacy to cope successfully with these temptations over a sustained period of time.

Managing the Interpersonal Environment

A final important influence in the Maintenance stage is that of the interpersonal environment surrounding the Maintainer. Individuals who have been most effective in maintaining cessation usually change the environment to minimize cues that rekindle thinking, craving, or longing. Protected in this way, these individuals also have a better chance of surviving any slips or lapses when their thinking begins to wander or their commitment erode.

An environment that supports the change can be a wonderful asset to the individuals struggling to maintain a change of an addictive behavior. Understanding employers, reinforcing and supportive spouses, inspiring sponsors, caring family, and accepting peers help the person leave the past behind and create a new and alternative life pattern. These reinforcing effects support and consolidate the change. Unfortunately, the damage done during the time of engaging in the addictive behavior and a prior pattern of relapsing and recycling may have compromised the supportive environment available to most Maintainers. Often there are only a few supportive individuals left in the social network by the time the addicted individual finally achieves a good measure of maintained change. Sometimes only colleagues from AA or Narcotics Anonymous (NA) and a particularly resilient and persevering parent are available and able to provide this support. Maintenance is more difficult without the helping relationships and reinforcement management processes of change that are so critical to recovery. But it is not entirely impossible.

A more difficult challenge is the presence in the immediate environment of people, places, and activities that support the addictive behavior (Longabaugh et al., 1995). Maintainers with an environment supportive of the addictive behavior are the most vulnerable to lessening of commitment and cognitive shifts toward a more positive view of the addictive behavior. If an individual in such an environment makes it through the Action stage, he or she must have acquired some good coping skills. Many individuals with addictive-behavior-infested environments relapse during the Action stage. During Action most of the more successful changers will have modified the environment in order to succeed. However, there are many Maintainers who have elements in their environment that continue to be encouraging or supportive of the addictive behavior, be it a friend and former drinking buddy, a family member who continues to gamble, a spouse who continues to smoke, or colleagues who continue to use drugs. Managing to maintain commitment and retain a negative decisional balance in the face of the modeling, availability, and possible encouragement of others requires courage, strength, and active coping. Somehow individuals with less supportive environments must separate their actions from those of others and create an internal buffer to protect the change because a more complete external or environmental buffer is not possible. How Maintainers cope with environmental pressures to return to the addictive behavior is an intriguing subject that has received far too little scientific scrutiny (Longabaugh, Wirtz, Zweben, & Stout, 1998; McCrady & Miller, 1993).

EXITS FROM MAINTENANCE: RECOVERY, RELAPSE, AND RECYCLING

There are two ways to exit from the Maintenance stage of change. Successful negotiation of the tasks of Maintenance leads to sustained recovery and exit from cycle of change. But if the individual is not successful in establishing an alternative lifestyle, slips and relapse are real possibilities. Relapse represents the less successful way to exit from the Maintenance stage; the individual needs to recycle through certain stages once again in order to learn how to achieve successful maintenance of recovery.

Recovery

Termination of change has been referred to as a final end state in the TTM. There are a number of reasons why it is better to consider termination from the cycle of change than to envision Maintenance as a permanent condition that accompanies successful change of an addictive behavior. For those individuals who have successfully consolidated the change into a new and satisfying life with very little potential for a return to the problematic behavior, the change cycle has ended. Their energy needs to be focused on other areas of life. The change has become habitual and it would take considerable effort to go back to the former addictive behavior. Maintained recovery is the norm in this individual's thinking and behavior. The entire gestalt of life now supports a new lifestyle committed to not engaging in the addictive behavior. But it is not impossible for someone to return to an addictive behavior after being in termination. One workshop participant disclosed that she returned to smoking after 8 years of abstinence and feeling that she terminated the cycle of change. However, this return should not be called a relapse. Once having terminated the cycle of change, a return to the addictive behavior should be considered reinitiation rather than relapse. This reinitiation would proceed in a similar fashion to the process to be outlined in the stages of addiction. In fact, upon reflection this smoker admitted that she had reconsidered smoking and made a decision to return after those 8 years of abstinence. The ex-smoker, -drinker, or -drug user who has terminated the cycle of change can always return to the former behavior and reinitiate more quickly and more efficiently than a neophyte.

All of these considerations have led me to reevaluate the idea of perpetual Maintenance as promulgated by many treatment and recovery philosophies such as AA. In the AA tradition the alcoholic is told that he or she is always only one drink away from being a drunk and is always in recovery and never recovered. This is done in order to emphasize the dangers of relapse and the struggle against overconfidence. This AA perspective is certainly one that supports the fact that long-term maintenance is needed for successful recovery from an addictive behavior. However, continuing a focus on drinking behavior, even though the focus is on avoiding drinking, may have the unwanted consequence of keeping the habit alive in some paradoxical manner.

Relapse

Relapse is less frequent in the Maintenance stage than in Action but still occurs. Several researchers have noted that relapse continues to be a

problem that affects 10–15% of Maintainers over the course of the ensuing year or two after quitting and initiating a period of abstinence
(Carbonari et al., 1999; Moos et al., 1990; Vaillant, 1995). Relapsing
after spending a significant period of time in Action and Maintenance
stages is a mixed blessing.

The ability to maintain abstinence for long periods of time is a positive indicator for change and bodes well for ultimately being able to sustain recovery and terminate the cycle of change (Abrams, Herzog,
Emmons, & Linnan, 2000; Carbonari et al., 1999; Farkas et al., 1996;
Prochaska et al., 1991). In fact, several studies have argued that a composite of addiction (dependence) and change variables that includes the
longest previous quit attempt can be a more effective predictor of successful smoking cessation than stage of change (Abrams et al., 2000;
Farkas et al., 1996). However, these studies demonstrate an inadequate
understanding of the recycling process. Increasing time in the Maintenance stage demonstrates that the individual has learned to make the
changes and create alternatives that support recovery. However, since
the individual returned to the addiction, there are some defects and inadequacies in the change plan that need to be remedied. The learning principle of successive approximations would support the potential for these
individuals to be more successful maintaining change the next time they
recycle through the stages and take action. Comparing measures that reflect recycling through the stages against the smokers stage status at the
beginning of an arbitrary period of time defined by a research study
seems counterproductive. Successful periods of abstinence can provide a
firm foundation for recycling and more effective and efficient movement
toward recovery.

On the other hand, a relapse after a period of significant success can
be particularly disheartening. Often these individuals become discouraged about the possibility of conquering the addiction. Some even return
to the Precontemplation stage of change (Carbonari et al., 1999). They
need to be convinced that they have the skills to do it again if they can
muster the courage and conviction to recycle through the stages.

Recycling

Recycling from the Maintenance stage of change may be more efficient
and effective than recycling early in the Action stage. The best estimates
of the number of addicted individuals who relapse come from longitudinal studies of smokers. In one study stage status was examined at time
points 6 months apart over 30 months. In this study, during a 6-month
period approximately 15% of those who had achieved at least 6 months
of maintained abstinence from smoking relapsed back to smoking

(Carbonari et al., 1999). A few (2%) moved all the way back to the Precontemplation stage for recovery with no serious consideration of quitting again in the next 6 months. Most, however, were in the Preparation (6%) or Action (7%) stages of change. Instead of being discouraged about change, these relapsers were in the midst of planning or taking action to quit smoking. Those who have maintained recovery for at least 6 months have gained a significant amount of confidence in their ability to manage many of the triggers to engage in the addiction. They know how to use the behavioral processes of change effectively enough to produce some stable change. They have sustained a negative decisional consideration long enough to support the decision and continuing commitment to stop the addiction for a substantial period of time. In summary, they have learned a lot about how to change the addiction.

Recycling through the stages of change is about learning from the relapse. Recyclers must figure out what went wrong so late in the process of recovery and find a remedy. Was there a problem with erosion of commitment and decisional considerations, or simply an event or trigger in the external environment that was unanticipated and powerful? Or was the reason for the relapse in the context of change? The latter is often the case. Problems in other areas of life functioning (marital, psychiatric, employment, etc.) create difficulties or distress that overwhelm behavioral coping or undermine efficacy needed to sustain the change. Whatever the origin, the recycling process must reestablish the decisional balance and reevaluate and create another change plan in order to transition forward once more though the stages of recovery.

MAINTAINING RECOVERY AND MANAGING OTHER LIFE PROBLEMS

Once the individual has gained some distance from the addictive behavior and no longer has to struggle on a day to day basis simply to stay sober, he or she is free to work on other problems that may have preceded or resulted from the addictive behavior. Poor academic achievement, problematic relationships, and little vocational direction or training can contribute to the onset of an addiction. Once-addicted individuals accrue multiple consequences, so that their lives are filled with the residual debris, for example, legal problems, angry and disappointed children, poor work skills, and the like. It is in the Maintenance stage that these problems begin to be addressed and managed.

As mentioned earlier, individuals who are successful over time in resolving or at least successfully managing problems in other areas of functioning come to look more and more like their peers who did not become addicted (DiClemente, 1994; Moos et al., 1990). Solutions to employment, relationship and meaning of life problems increase the distance from the addictive behavior and assist the individual to create a new lifestyle that is protective. Changing the addictive behavior reverberates in multiple areas of the individual's life in a way similar to that of becoming addicted.

As the formerly addicted individual successfully remains in recovery, it becomes easier to see what problems are caused by the addiction and what are separate problems. Maintained recovery allows the individual to focus on problems in the life context that need attention. This is particularly true for psychiatric problems faced by dually diagnosed individuals. Those suffering from manic–depression, major depression, or schizophrenia will need significant assistance. Individuals whose drug abuse interfered with academic achievement and the development of valuable work skills will need remediation so they can build a new life distant from the addiction. Those with impaired social and interpersonal skills will need to learn or repair them in order to build a network of support that will sustain change. The Maintenance stage is often very busy with addressing problems in areas of functioning.

The process used to recover from an addiction is the same process used to address any life problems (Prochaska & DiClemente, 1984; Werch & DiClemente, 1994). The specific behaviors that need change will differ but the process of intentional behavior change is the same. Addicts in recovery will have to move through similar stages of change for problems in other areas of functioning. They will have to acknowledge the problem and need for change, create a decisional balance that supports change, make a viable plan for change, and follow through with the actions needed to change the new target behavior. Then they will have to work to sustain that change over time. Experience with the process may make changing other behaviors a bit easier. The successful Maintainer has negotiated the stages for the addiction. However, failure to recognize the need to transition through the same stages and successfully complete similar tasks can fuel an inefficient search for a separate process for each problem. Learning how to change an addiction offers valuable tools and experiences to deal with one's entire life context.

CASE EXAMPLES AND OVERVIEW

This stage is marked by significant shifts in self-efficacy, successful distancing from the addiction, and creation of a new life filled with new alternative reinforcers (see Table 10.1). Becoming an ex-addict requires continued vigilance and effort until the individual can exit the cycle of change. Personal success in managing the addiction and in creating a new lifestyle enhance efficacy to abstain. The gap between the levels of temptation to engage in the addiction and confidence to abstain continues to increase until they peak and support exiting from the process. Life-context problems continue to improve and are managed in ways that support recovery.

TABLE 10.1. Maintaining Recovery: An Overview of the Dimensions of Change

---

Stage task

Sustaining change over time and over a wide range of situations; avoiding slips and relapse; creating a new life filled with alternative rewarding activities and coping mechanisms.

Change processes at work

Behavioral processes of change, particularly reinforcement management and counterconditioning create competing rewards and increased efficacy for recovery. Some experiential processes are needed to protect against problematic thinking patterns. Processes needed to deal with life context problems become more salient.

Reinforcement: Alternate behaviors produce rewards that reinforce recovery, replace the addiction, and create the new lifestyle.

Counterconditioning: Alternative coping strategies are used to deal with emotions, people, and places that trigger the addictive behavior and become the norm for dealing with life.

Helping relationships: Social networks supportive of abstinence replace addiction-encouraging ones.

Consciousness raising and self-reevaluation: Recognizing and reevaluating thinking that could support reidealization of the addiction, the abstinence violation effect, and/or apparently irrelevant decisions.

Markers of change

Decisional balance: Balance continues to favor recovery; concerns about pros and cons decrease in intensity as new lifestyle takes hold; protect against reemerging addiction pros.

Self-efficacy: Confidence to abstain grows and temptations decrease. Efficacy becomes a critical indicator of success.

Context of change

Other problems in the life context begin to be seen more clearly once the struggle with the addiction eases and to emerge as a focus for change either because they threaten recovery or are needed to create a new life sufficiently rewarding to sustain recovery.

Margaret Main is a 40-year-old single mother, who had become a heroin addict in her late 20s. During the 12 years when she was using, she experienced a number of severe consequences, including losing custody of her two children, arrests for prostitution, severe bouts of venereal disease that ultimately required a hysterectomy, and other serious health problems. She has been clean for the past 18 months and still goes to outpatient groups at the treatment center where she spent 3 months in residential treatment and then went to a halfway house where she currently lives. For the past year she has been working as a computer technician. The treatment program she attended had an innovative work preparation component. It helped women who had graduated from high school to learn basic computer technology and to be hired by a high-tech company supported by a federal grant. Margaret was hired full-time after the training and is now earning a decent salary and is looking for her own apartment. She has distanced herself from her former heroin-using friends and has begun attending church. She has also reestablished connections with her family and regularly visits her children who live with her mother. She has also begun to work on her issues of mistrust and anger with her father and other men in her life.

Margaret is well on her way to recovery. Her growing confidence will be protective and her newfound profession should offer satisfaction and support for building her new life. Her move to her own apartment will test her recovery. She has begun to date a coworker who has had a drinking problem but is also in recovery. Her therapist is concerned about this relationship because her partner has some history of violence toward women. Margaret, however, is not as concerned because she believes that he has changed and he has always treated her with respect. He also seems to be very accepting of her children, which is very important for Margaret. There are still some hurdles to overcome and some areas where there are clear and present dangers to her sobriety. Using a variety of behavioral processes of change, Margaret continues to build a life that excludes the former addiction. She is discussing issues and becoming aware of potential problems before they take her unprepared, as happened in previous attempts to get clean. Every once in a while she gets one of her old feelings that used to lead immediately to drug seeking. These feelings are becoming less and less frequent, and she knows that they will go away in a rather short time. She has a quiet confidence that this time she will make it.

Margaret's story is in sharp contrast to her housemate, Rita Relap. Rita went through the same residential program and has been in the halfway house for 6 months. She has been in recovery for 9 months but has had two slips, one right after she came to the halfway house and another about 3 weeks ago. Rita did not qualify for the computer technician program and has obtained a job working for a janitorial firm that has a large contract to clean the local schools. Rita is 35 and has no children. She was married to a high school sweetheart for 5 years, but when he left her life went downhill and she developed a serious cocaine addiction. Rita misses the excitement and highs that the cocaine provided to her life. She has been diagnosed with dysthymia, a low-grade constant depression, and is getting some antidepressants for this condition. However, she has been gaining weight and feels like she is becoming less attractive. Rita has one close friend at the halfway house and does attend some NA meetings, but is pretty much a loner. At work she is becoming friends with a man who is younger but straight and somewhat demanding.

Although Rita is in the Maintenance stage of recovery from her cocaine addiction, her prognosis is poor for remaining in Maintenance and terminating the cycle of change. Temptations are still strong. Slips indicate some weakness in her plan for sobriety and continued access to the cocaine. Complications from her psychiatric disorder and her current relationship undermine her positive feelings about recovery and thus her efficacy to abstain. The treatment staff has been discussing all these issues with her but have noted that Rita seems discouraged and down. Although recovery and continued Maintenance are possible, additional positive reinforcers for sobriety, a more extensive support system, and significant additional work on her life-context problems would be needed to make it happen.

SUMMARY

The focus of the Maintenance stage of change is driven by the need for generalization of learning across situations and time. Learning how to avoid the addictive behavior, however, represents only part of the process. The learning needed for successful recovery from an addiction requires learning new behaviors and modification of many other behaviors in order to sustain the change long-term. Maintenance goes beyond a concentration on a single addictive behavior and extends into larger areas of the individual's life. The TTM uses the same stage perspective and dimensions of change to conceptualize the process of change for these multiple problems and includes the interaction of these multiple problems and their solutions within the tasks of the Maintenance stage of recovery. Successful negotiation of the tasks of the Maintenance stage leads to the termination of the process of change for recovery from addiction. Termination indicates the end of the cycle of change and is marked by dramatic decreases in temptation and behavioral processes of change and significant increases in self-efficacy to abstain from the addiction. Termination allows addicted individuals to invest their entire energy and attention on creating the alternate lifestyle needed to become a successful ex-addict and ensure sustained recovery.

Part IV

DESIGNING INTERVENTIONS TO MATCH THE PROCESS OF CHANGE

Chapter 11

Prevention

Interfering with the Process
of Becoming Addicted

*Becoming addicted involves transitions across multiple stages
of change and shifts in processes and markers of change
interacting with various aspects of the context of change. The
process of intentional behavior change that is common across
addictive behaviors offers a template for creating sensitive
credible and targeted prevention programs.*

PREVENTION ACTIVITIES: TARGETS AND GOALS

Prevention in the arena of the addictions has multiple meanings and interpretations. For some it means stopping an already existing problem, such as regular cigarette smoking, in order to prevent future illness. For others prevention signifies eliminating any experimentation with addictive behaviors. Still others consider prevention the process of instilling attitudes that prevent thinking about engagement in any health-threatening addictive behavior. The stages of becoming addicted described in Part II offer a way to segment the process. Together with the other change dimensions of the TTM they can sharpen the focus of prevention efforts.

TYPES OF PREVENTION

The traditional view of prevention was developed in the context of medical diseases. It consisted of a tripartite division of prevention based on the goals and targets of intervention efforts: primary, secondary and tertiary prevention. These types of interventions more recently have been relabeled according to the type of population targeted by the intervention (population-based, at-risk, and currently affected). A discussion of these three types of prevention can set the stage for understanding how to integrate prevention efforts with our process of change perspective.

Population-based prevention, once referred to as primary prevention, has as its goal the protection of individuals who have no signs or symptoms of the disease. These individuals, as a group, usually have minimal direct exposure or vulnerability to that particular disease at the present time. Population-based prevention looks at entire groups of individuals regardless of whether any risk factors are present and attempts to inoculate the population against the disease. Some good examples of such programs would be fluoridation of the water supply to prevent tooth decay or vaccinations of all infants or children to prevent polio or smallpox. In many of these cases, even though the likelihood of contracting the illness is small, prevention efforts are deemed worthwhile because the disease is so devastating. For addictive behaviors, primary prevention attempts to educate or inoculate the total population against experimentation, engagement, use, and/or abuse.

Interventions targeting *populations at risk*, or secondary prevention, concentrate on individuals with one or more risk factors for developing a disease, who may have been exposed to the disease, or who may have initial or prodromal signs of the illness. The goal of prevention for those at risk is to protect these individuals from developing the condition or to provide an early intervention before the problem can develop fully in order to produce the best possible prognosis. Examples of this type of at-risk prevention include offering tetanus shots to individuals who have been bitten by a potentially rabid animal, immunization programs for individuals exposed to particular viruses (TB shots for those who work in medical settings), and screening for particularly vulnerable individuals (mammography for women over 50 or with a family history of breast cancer and colorectal cancer screening for older males). Prevention for those at risk for addiction would target individuals with specific risk factors to try to stop them from engaging in the addictive behavior or, at minimum, from developing abuse or dependence.

Prevention with *afflicted populations*, tertiary prevention, is characterized by interventions that prevent deterioration or provide harm reduction. Critics claim that these interventions are misnamed prevention because they focus on individuals who already have the illness or disease. However, the prevention goal in these interventions is to provide as much of a "cure" as possible for those already afflicted with an illness or, at minimum, lessen the impact of the condition on other physical systems. For example, most common cold remedies are designed to relieve common symptoms while the cold virus runs its course and is defeated by the body's immune system. Treatment for symptom relief can be conceived of as prevention because it does prevent some of the more debilitating effects of the illness and allows the person to function better at work or home. Usually interventions implemented earlier in the course of the illness result in a greater probability of preventing associated problems. Prevention with afflicted populations inhibits progressive deterioration and debilitation and is essentially a harm reduction strategy to be used when the problem has already emerged.

With people already afflicted with an addiction, prevention includes interventions and treatments to abbreviate the time spent in maintained addiction or to reduce severity of consequences to self and society. Treatments that lead to recovery can prevent additional damage or deterioration and provide hope to counter fatalism and hopelessness. Research has demonstrated that deterioration of medical conditions can be facilitated by patient pessimism about recovery (Becker & Maiman, 1975). Additional advantages to battling an illness, whether treatment-facilitated or not, is that the struggle provides the individual with some protection against further incidents of the illness by strengthening natural immunities (Clark et al., 1999).

The Need for a Modification in Perspective

This tripartite view of types of prevention has been applied with mixed success to psychological and behavioral problems (Trull & Phares, 2001). Potential difficulties arise when applying this prevention framework to behavioral problems that are not completely biologically based disease processes. Medical diseases often have a clearly defined presence or absence, with predictable precursors and a predictable course. For instance, laboratory tests can indicate whether a certain virus is present; deterioration can be clearly distinguished from no change; and recovery is often definable and recognizable. However, even with medical diseases clarity of condition, course, and recovery is not always possible. It is certainly obscured when the problem or illness involves behavioral components and a less predictable course (e.g., diabetes, hypertension, addictions, chronic pain).

Whenever intentional behaviors are an important component of an illness or problem, intentional behavior change becomes an essential part of the prevention process. Problems involving changes in behaviors, such as diet, drinking, a medication regimen, drug use, or exercise, require individuals to adhere to prescribed regimens and make lifestyle modifications. When it comes to health-threatening behaviors, prevention must include changing both attitudes and behaviors in order to achieve the desired goals. However, evaluation of success in these programs is problematic because the course of the "illness" is variable and the definition of optimal outcome not always very clear.

With addictions the behavioral end point is often more apparent. Not using heroin or cocaine is measurable, as is the number of cigarettes smoked. However, measures that use absence of a behavior as a prevention outcome can be problematic. For example, a program that encourages youth to "just say no" to heroin and cocaine could measure nonuse as a positive outcome. However, youth, particularly those at younger ages, who are not thinking about these drugs and have no access to them have little reason to learn how to say no. For addictions and other health-threatening behaviors the distinction between use versus nonuse offers a dichotomous outcome that is problematic for evaluating different types of prevention activities, particularly those directed at entire populations or at-risk populations.

A PROCESS PERSPECTIVE ON PREVENTION

Application of the TTM of intentional behavior change to the initiation of addiction can address many of the conceptual and practical problems that plague prevention efforts with health-threatening behaviors (Raczynski & DiClemente, 1999). Addictive behavior prevention programs usually have as their ultimate common goal prevention of regular abusive and/or dependent engagement in the addictive behavior. However, this goal focuses on the end point of the process of becoming addicted, identified as the Maintenance stage of addiction. The stages of change identify important earlier transitions in the process that can increase the specificity of prevention efforts. The process of becoming addicted progresses through a series of stages that catalogue a growing commitment to use, a diminishing of self-control, and a growing biopsychosocial dependence on the addictive behavior, as it becomes an integral part of the individual's lifestyle. In particular, the stages, processes, markers and context of change provide a framework for a more precise application of all three types of prevention activities.

Specifying Targets for Prevention Programs

In each of the previous chapters I have highlighted the key processes of change that are involved in moving forward through the transitions toward addiction. These processes can provide targets for prevention efforts. Critical processes of change can be activated in ways that interfere with the transitions forward through the stages of an addiction. For example, if an individual is in the Contemplation stage, seriously considering using cocaine and ready to experiment with that substance, the objective of a prevention intervention would be to influence the self-reevaluation and environmental reevaluation processes as well as consciousness raising. Consciousness raising activities should be engaged in order to heighten awareness of the dangers of use and realities of peer use on the one hand and to decrease positive outcome expectancies on the other. Reevaluation processes should be activated so that heightened awareness and personal values interact to increase negative considerations and decrease positives for any cocaine use. If interventions fail to engage these processes, they will be ineffective in halting this Contemplator's progression forward through the stages of cocaine addiction.

As individuals move into the Preparation and Action stages and begin to experience the reinforcing effects of the substance and of peer support for use, interventions must interfere with the conditioning process and offer alternative reinforcers using the reinforcement management process to create rewarding environmental support for nonuse. Processes of change offer a series of mechanisms that can influence the process of initiation. The goal of prevention interventions would be to effectively engage these processes of change, targeting the critical biopsychosocial factors discussed in Chapter 4. This would reduce the probability of movement forward in the stages of acquisition and addiction. Evaluation of prevention activities should examine first whether the intervention was successful in engaging the appropriate processes and then whether they prevented the transition from one stage to the next.

The stages and processes of change identify key elements on the road to addiction that are specific to the targeted addictive behavior. The context of change categorizes areas of associated risk and protective factors that can influence the acquisition process for many different addictive behaviors. However, these factors must be evaluated in light of the stage of change for each addictive behavior. Developing problems in various areas of an individual's life can promote or discourage movement through the stages for one or more addictive behaviors. For instance, depressive symptoms, divorce, family problems, interpersonal difficulties, and school failures contribute to a complex probability matrix that makes it easier for an individual to move from one stage to the next in the process of becoming addicted. Prevention activities directed at improving problems in these contextual areas of functioning can interfere with the development of the addiction directly or indirectly by making the transition from one stage to the next more difficult. The impact of risk and protective factors, however, differs depending on the stage transition in question. There is an interaction of these factors with different parts of the process of change involved in becoming addicted.

This interaction between stage transition and other factors may explain why different studies have found conflicting results about the role of risk and protective factors at different points in the process of initiation (Glantz & Pickens, 1992). Factors that are important in the transition from Precontemplation to Contemplation are different from those that are important in the transition from Preparation to Action. Moreover, many studies have found interactions between risk and protective factors (Jessor et al., 1995; Newcomb et al., 1993). The complex relationship of these factors with the processes of acquisition and addiction indicates that the same factor can act as a protective factor at one stage transition and a risk factor in another. A strict, religious upbringing, for example, can protect Precontemplators from becoming Contemplators. However, once these individuals move into the Contemplation and Preparation stages, this rigid belief system can act as a risk factor and accelerate the movement to Action and problematic patterns of use. Stewart and Brown (1993) have found a reciprocal relationship between family functioning and adolescent substance abuse. This reciprocity between family dynamics and the substance abuse problem operates in one way as the individual develops the substance abuse problem, and in another way after the adolescent stops the addictive behavior and achieves abstinence. Lori Chassin and her colleagues (1990, 1996) have found that similar factors can be both protective and risk factors in the process of initiation.

As is illustrated in Figure 11.1, a stage by addictive behavior matrix can offer a view of where an individual is in the stages of addiction for each type of addictive behavior. Allen is a 17-year-old high school senior in an inner city school. He began smoking regularly at 15 and now smokes 5–10 cigarettes a day. Although he experimented with marijuana on and off since 15 and has an older brother who uses marijuana regularly, Allen began using marijuana regularly last year as he got into listening to music while stoned. He adamantly states that he uses only "soft drugs" and that he has no interest in heroin and cocaine. Those drugs can get you into real trouble, according to Allen. He has used amphetamines once and is not sure he likes the effect. Six months ago one of his friends introduced him to ketamine, a drug with hallucinogenic properties. Although he did not like the effect at first, he did it while listening to music and it seemed a better experience. He does not seek out this drug and has only used it a couple of times. However, he is open to using ketamine if someone offers it and he does not have any marijuana. Allen drinks alcohol on occasion and has overdone it several times in the

Type of Behavior	Stage of Initiation				
	PC	C	PA	A	M
Alcohol				x	
Nicotine					x
Marijuana					x
Heroin	x				
Cocaine	x				
Amphetamines		x			
LSD			x		
Gambling	x				
Eating Disorder	x				

FIGURE 11.1. A stage-based prevention matrix: An example of Allen.

past 6 months when he was out partying with his friends. Although he prefers marijuana, alcohol is the more popular drug among his larger peer group, so he joins in as needed. The past couple of times he drank a lot of beer and has had some real hangovers, when he did not remember what they were doing the night before. He also drank excessively with his girlfriend when they were together and having sex. Allen does not have any eating patterns that are problematic, with the exception of his overindulgence in sweets when he is using marijuana. He is not interested in gambling and believes that people waste their money when they bet.

Figure 11.2 offers a matrix of stage by context of change that can identify what types of problems and resources in the various areas of functioning may be playing a role in the stage transitions that are occurring and already taken place in Allen's case. As is obvious from his stage profile on the various addictive behaviors, it would be difficult to identify overall risk and protective factors that operated in the same way for each addictive behavior and every transition. Whatever aspects of his life that were protective in terms of heroin and cocaine were not operative with regard to nicotine and marijuana. There is a set of contextual factors that serve as risk and/or protective factors for Allen. However, they need to be analyzed separately for each behavior and for the relevant transitions.

In the life situation arena, Allen is not achieving in high school and has little interest in school or college. His parents are divorced and he lives with his mom who works long hours and provides little supervision for her sons. These factors seem to have accelerated the transitions from

Context of Change	Stages of Change			
	PC → C	C → PA	PA → A	A → M
Specific Behavioral & Situational Issues				Multiple addictions
Beliefs & Expectancies	Soft vs. hard drugs		Sex & alcohol	
Interpersonal			Girlfriend/ intimacy	
Social Systems (Family, Employment, Social)		Brother & peers	Peers	
Enduring Personal Characteristics				

FIGURE 11.2. Complicating problems and stage transitions for Allen.

Preparation to Action and Action to Maintenance for alcohol, nicotine, and marijuana. Music seems to be an important pleasure in his life but is intimately connected with use of substances of abuse. His earlier movement through the stages for nicotine addiction makes him more vulnerable for moving through the stages for other substances.

In the area of beliefs and expectancies his dichotomous view of "hard versus soft drugs" is protective in preventing movement out of Precontemplation for heroin and cocaine but clearly a promoting factor in the transition through Action and Maintenance for nicotine and marijuana. His alcohol expectancy connecting drinking and sexual encounters facilitated his movement from Preparation to Action and would contribute to the transition from Action to Maintenance if not altered.

With regard to the interpersonal and systemic areas of functioning there are clear indications of involvement as well. In the interpersonal area it is not clear how he relates to his girlfriend and whether there are any complicating issues. However, the alcohol and sex connection does indicate that there may be problems with intimacy that could foster continued use of drugs to mask these issues. On the other hand, systemic issues play a role in many of the transitions. His absent father and lack of family support for avoiding addictive behaviors make it easier to consider and engage in risk-taking behaviors. His brother's marijuana use compounds problems and certainly fostered the movement to and through Action for his marijuana addiction. His social system and peers also appear to be involved in multiple problematic behaviors and seem to support his use, making his movement into Preparation for ketamine easier and fostering the transition to maintained marijuana use. How-

ever, these same peers seem to be similar in their views of heroin and cocaine, which prevents the transition from Precontemplation for those
substances.

Although there may be some deeper emotional problems or characteristics that could also play a role in the transitions for the different addictive behaviors, these are not clear at present. Issues of identity and
self-esteem probably contribute to his overdependence on peers. Marijuana's effect in helping him avoid facing himself and any self-concept
problems could play a role in moving toward addiction, particularly
with marijuana.

These matrices provide a comprehensive but complex picture of target areas for prevention. However, greater precision in outlining connections and targeting transitions offers significant advantages for guiding
prevention efforts. Although we speak of preventing addictions, for Allen it is a bit late for prevention in the case of nicotine and marijuana.
With these maintained addictions, recovery interventions are needed at
this point. However, in other areas we need to prevent the late stage and
dangerous transitions for alcohol and ketamine and support primary
prevention for heroin or cocaine use, gambling, and eating disorders.
Even in less complicated cases, individuals often differ as to where they
are in their transitions through the stages for various addictive behaviors. Contextual factors interact with each of the behaviors, but not always in a uniform manner. Although the complexity of this view of stage
transition by contextual arena is a bit daunting, the matrix seems to reflect the actual complexity of the process of becoming addicted (Scheier,
Botvin, & Griffin, 2001).

There is another important benefit of using the TTM to understand
addiction and assist in the application of prevention strategies. Numerous problems occur in prevention and treatment because there is not a
clear understanding of the process of change. Treating everyone who
uses as being in Action misrepresents the process of change involved in
becoming addicted. There are some scary examples of this misclassi-
fication problem. Adolescents with very low levels of use and sometimes
with only a history of experimentation have been placed in extended
stay, residential, or hospital-based treatment programs (DiClemente,
1999a). This represents an inappropriate use of a treatment intervention
for a problem that needs a prevention approach. On the other hand,
many educators attempt to use primary prevention strategies like generic
education for students who have already developed dependent, regular
use of a substance. Education about experimentation for individuals
well into the Action and Maintenance stages of addiction represent well-
intentioned efforts that are too late and too little.

For many years researchers and clinicians conceptualized almost all interventions targeting adolescent smoking as a prevention activity. For example, only recently have they come to realize that adolescents are actually in the Maintenance stage of nicotine addiction (smoking regularly and dependently for more than 6 months). Individuals in the Maintenance stage of addiction need cessation activities and treatment to move them through the stages of recovery, and not prevention programming that is population-based or even directed to the at-risk subgroups (Choi, Ahluwalia, & Nazir, 2002). Because adolescents were dissimilar to confirmed smokers typically seen in smoking cessation programs who had smoked for 20 or 30 years, the erroneous assumption was that adolescents needed prevention and not treatment. A process of change perspective sharpens the focus and offers clearer distinctions between stages of acquisition and addiction and stages of recovery and between prevention and treatment.

Confusion created by the lack of differentiation between the addiction and recovery change process is widespread in the field of addictive behaviors. This confusion contributes to the lack of effectiveness of some of our prevention efforts and the high cost of some of our treatment endeavors (Ennett, Tabler, Ringwolt, & Fliwelling, 1994). More importantly, this confusion creates serious misunderstandings among individuals who engage in the addictive behavior as well as among family members, community leaders, and others. Application of the stages of change in conjunction with the identification of processes of change and understanding the influence of contextual areas of functioning on stage transitions can clarify and organize different types of prevention activities. Moreover, distinguishing between stages of addiction and stages of recovery can establish important boundaries between prevention and treatment activities.

Clearing Up Confusion about Types of Prevention

Using the framework of the TTM we can examine the tripartite prevention perspective in a new light and discuss the goals and efforts that would characterize each of the types of prevention.

Population-based prevention activities should be directed at individuals in the Precontemplation and Contemplation stages of becoming addicted. *At-risk prevention* activities should target those individuals who are in the Preparation and initial Action stages of addiction. When the focus of the intervention is on those in the Action stage who already engage in the behavior (drink or gamble) and the goal is to promote responsible and controlled use, prevention addresses an at-risk population and tries to facilitate a transition to maintained, self-regulated use. However, individuals in Precontemplation or Contemplation who have excessive risk and/or minimal protective factors also could be singled out and targeted with at-risk prevention programming.

If the program targets problem drinkers, as do many early intervention programs, prevention is reaching *already afflicted individuals* in the Action stage for becoming addicted. Individuals already well into the Action stage of change should be considered already afflicted and need programs that could prevent movement to a maintained addiction. However, once individuals have reached the Maintenance stage of addiction, programming should shift to using the stages of recovery. Interventions would be needed to meet these individuals wherever they are in the process of recovery from an addiction. Diversity of targeting and programming is enhanced by using the process perspective and focusing on preventing transitions forward through the stages of addiction or, once addicted, promoting movement through the stages of recovery.

PREVENTING TRANSITIONS THROUGH THE STAGES OF ADDICTION

Population Prevention for Precontemplation to Contemplation Transitions

The transitions identified by the stages of change provide an interesting new way to envision and direct prevention interventions. The goal of population-based prevention of addictive behavior is largely to keep individuals in Precontemplation and to prevent forays beyond the Contemplation stage. If any movement into Contemplation occurs, the goal is to keep any consideration or experimentation with the behavior from developing a positive evaluation and decision to engage. The ultimate goal of any program that encourages Contemplation or consideration of the addictive behavior is to move individuals back to Precontemplation.

Targeting decisional considerations and risk factors that would lead to serious consideration of the addictive behavior prevents movement from Precontemplation to Contemplation and beyond. Individuals in Precontemplation for any engagement in the behavior could be kept there, or Contemplators could be assisted to develop decisional balance considerations that would be tilted firmly against adoption in order to keep them from progressing toward Preparation. Ultimately, this decisional balance would protect the individuals from moving out of Contemplation and be instrumental in moving them back into the Precontemplation stage, where they would have no serious consideration of engaging in the behavior.

Keeping individuals and populations in the early stages for adoption is not as easy as it seems. To a greater or lesser extent most people in our society will be introduced to a variety of addictive behaviors. Keeping young children ignorant of the lure of alcohol, drugs, nicotine, and other types of addictive behaviors is not easy and may not be possible in our current society. However, that does not mean that all youngsters will automatically move into the Contemplation stage for engagement and addiction. Many children will stay in Precontemplation for most addictive behaviors throughout their childhood and adolescence. Ultimately they become adults in that same stage of Precontemplation for these behaviors.

A critical question is how much, if anything, should be done for those in Precontemplation for initiation, especially when they are children and young adults. Precontemplators already are not thinking about or considering engaging in the addictive behavior in the foreseeable future. They could just be left alone. However, the problem with a benign neglect prevention strategy is that these naive Precontemplators would be ignorant about the behavior. Whenever confronted by an event or situation that introduces them to or influences them to try the addictive behavior, naive Precontemplators have few protective reasons or resources to support them. What happens when young Precontemplators for smoking cigarettes see billboard and other advertisements about the wonderful benefits of smoking certain brands of cigarettes? If they are not armed with some realistic, negative considerations of this behavior, they may be more vulnerable to the influence of the advertising. Doing nothing and hoping children continue to be ignorant of all addictive behaviors seems a high-risk strategy, particularly when the behavior is highly visible or promoted in the immediate environment or society.

However, inundating youth with information about all the dangers of every addiction early in their childhood also seems to be a risky strategy. Primary prevention programs that target very young children and give them too much information about the addictive behavior may actually end up promoting progression toward initiation of the behavior. For example, some well- intentioned programs propose to teach all first and second graders about the dangers of drugs in general and detailed risks associated with specific drugs. In many neighborhoods and schools, these children will not have any significant exposure to drugs for several more years. What the drug prevention program proposes to do is to provide information that will protect the child in the future. However, they may actually be introducing the child to consider the addictive behavior well before the natural environment would. Even though the message is a negative one, the reality is that these children are being given specific, detailed information that could make them more knowledgeable and possibly more open to experimentation. Providing too much specific information or knowledge and offering this information too early in the life experience of the individual may backfire as a primary prevention strategy, especially for young children, who are in Precontemplation. On the other hand, if a child could be exposed to the addictive behavior as early as first or second grade, this type of program may help to inoculate these youth with accurate information and realistic attitudes. However, a prevention program focused on these children would not be broadly population-based; rather it is a secondary prevention program because it targets at-risk youth.

Primary population-based prevention programs always tread a narrow line between under- and overexposure. They must provide the general population with attitudes, experiences, and skills to remain committed to not progressing through the stages of initiating an addictive behavior. At the same time, prevention intervention messages and information need to be developmentally appropriate, generationally and culturally sensitive, tailored to the specific addictive behavior, and credible.

Population prevention programs must be designed to match the developmental status of the target populations. Attempts to develop fine-grained discriminations in the attitudes and beliefs of very young children are simply misguided. The messages have to be simplistic, clear, and rather dichotomous. Children understand black and white, and not shades of gray, at early ages. Simplistic messages can ultimately backfire, however, as children become more mature and their thinking becomes more differentiated. Messages must be developmentally appropriate and also must adapt as the child grows in sophistication in order for prevention to keep pace with the internal thinking processes. Thus, no simple prevention message could keep children of all ages in Precontemplation for engaging in an addictive behavior.

We must remember that what is negatively valued in one generation often becomes valued in the next. In my relatively short lifetime, crewcuts and head shaving have been viewed as punishment, a mark of military service, a sign of radical right-wing movements, and simply an acceptable hairstyle. The ying and yang of social behaviors make prevention of specific behaviors and styles of living rather tricky, particularly if the messages are perceived as one generation telling another generation what to do and how to live.

The narrow line between preventing and promoting an addictive behavior is particularly tricky for drug use, cigarette smoking, smokeless tobacco use, gambling, and eating disorders. Each of these has carried both negative and positive valences at different points in the history of the generations. Positive views as well as the prevalence of these behaviors have risen and fallen over the past 100 years here in the United States and around the world. At a societal level a moderately negative view of the behavior may be the best protection against the creation of addictions. Such a moderately negative view could discourage interest in initiation without stirring rebellion and make the move from Precontemplation to Contemplation less probable.

Of course, the messages and the approach need to vary depending on whether complete abstinence or responsible engagement is the goal. The approach of population-based prevention for alcohol consumption should differ from that used for heroin use. If the behavior is legal and one that the majority of the population will ultimately engage in, like drinking beverages containing alcohol or gambling, primary prevention should emphasize the when, where, and how of legal, responsible, self-regulated use. Prevention programs targeting alcohol should promote attitudes and behaviors that would keep alcohol a beverage among other equally acceptable and desirable beverages and offer some specific guidelines for use that would be clearly contrasted with abuse and dependence. For heroin use, on the other hand, population prevention should attempt to dissuade experimentation or use and probably not focus on the distinction between use and abuse, as would be done with alcohol or gambling.

The decision of how to handle each potentially addictive behavior involves cultural and societal considerations. Interventionists need first to understand the current culture and attitudes toward a particular addictive behavior in order to be culturally sensitive. Then they can develop programs that would fit into that perspective so that they can counter problematic societal attitudes and create protective ones. The place of the addictive behavior in a particular society also influences population prevention. Smoking has a different place and role in various countries and cultures. Whether men and women smoke is largely culturally determined. Some Central American countries have legalized marijuana use but frown on dysfunctional use (Page, Fletcher, & True, 1988). In the United States legal gambling has gone from being a limited behavior confined to specific locations (e.g., racetracks and casinos) to a behavior that is as close as your local food mart and a major source of revenue for state budgets. Obviously, primary prevention messages have to recognize the realities of the behavior in the society if the messages are to be at all credible.

Credibility is actually another important issue in population-based prevention programs. Messages that are not solidly based on accurate information and current knowledge can be discarded rather easily when an individual encounters information from peers that contradicts and invalidates the prevention message. This is even more important with at risk prevention. However, credibility is critical for population-based prevention programming as well. Messages that exaggerate the potential dangers of a behavior (e.g., cocaine will kill you on the first use, or cigarettes always lead to using other, illegal drugs) can easily be discounted once any exceptions are encountered either among peers, adults, or role model media figures. In fact, during the teen years, adolescents become very critical of parental messages. Self- and environmental reevaluation are constantly processing messages from authority figures. It is developmentally appropriate for them to challenge these messages and to argue the opposite. Messages that are too global or exaggerated are particularly vulnerable to this onslaught. Even well-founded information has a difficult time in this environment but has a better chance of surviving the adolescent self- and environmental reevaluation.

At-Risk Prevention for the Transitions from Contemplation to Preparation to Action

Prevention activities that target at-risk populations typically focus on individuals transitioning from Contemplation to Preparation as well as on individuals in Preparation and Action stages of initiation (see figure 11.3). Anyone who progresses forward out of the contemplation stage can be considered at risk for initiation of addiction. Such movement signifies that the individual's positive considerations of the addictive behavior outweigh negative considerations. Continued experimentation and gradual movement toward more regular use are the hallmarks of Preparation. Regular use and the loss of self-regulation are signs that the individual is in the Action stage. Secondary at-risk prevention programs can help individuals at any of these junctures. But the specifics of those programs will differ depending on the specific stage. Thus a broad range of activities can be considered, including those that target individuals who may use little but have positive attitudes toward use and those who have serious risk factors for initiation. At-risk programs may also target beginning problem drinkers to prevent them from losing control of their drinking and developing alcohol abuse or dependence (Baer, Kivlahan, Blume, McKnight, & Marlatt, 2001).

The breadth of at-risk prevention can be challenging and confusing. It can focus on attitudes and beliefs about the behavior, the behavior itself, or risk and protective factors. Examples of each of these may be helpful. Some at-risk prevention programs focus on children who are in neighborhoods filled with illegal drug use and provide media testimonials by popular athletes or entertainers about the dangers and risks of using crack cocaine. Dramatic portrayals of these dangers (overdose, death) are used to raise awareness and shift evaluations of the behavior, thus promoting a personal self-reevaluation that would protect the child against experimentation and use. In this case the clear target is the changing of attitudes and expectancies related to the substance that

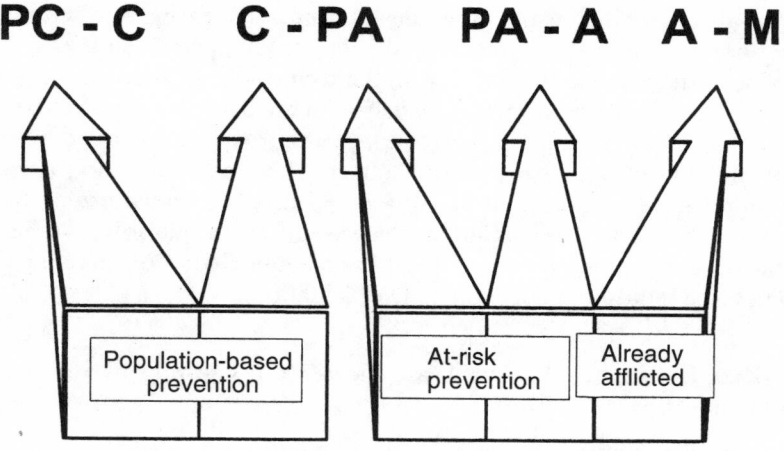

FIGURE 11.3. Types of prevention and stage of addiction transitions.

would keep at-risk children in Precontemplation. In contrast, zero tolerance programs focus on the behavior itself and primarily on those individuals in Contemplation and Preparation stages. These programs attempt to provide rather severe consequences for any engagement in the
behavior in an effort to increase the cost of any experimentation. Other
programs use a different approach: They focus on risk factors by offering special tutoring at school to improve academic achievement or to
teach stress management and coping skills. These programs concentrate
on providing protective factors to decrease vulnerability to influences
that would move individuals from Contemplation to Preparation or Action. Other programs provide jobs or gainful employment, offer alternative activities that would keep youth off the street corners, and provide
family counseling for the children of parents with drug or alcohol problems. All of these programs focus on subpopulations of high-risk youths
who are at different critical stages of change in the process of becoming
addicted.

It is often easy to identify high-risk youths from personal profile or
environmental risk. However, the broader and the more impersonal the
criteria that are used to define the population at risk, the greater the
probability that those caught in the net will include some youths who
are actually in Precontemplation or who have already developed strong
personal decisional considerations against initiation. At-risk prevention
programs need to be conscious of the potential heterogeneity of the indi-

viduals they target in order to provide sensitive and credible messages. Just because a group of youths come from a high-risk crime area, for example, it is wrong to assume that all or even a majority has experimented frequently or that they currently use drugs regularly. Prevention programs that do not have a thorough knowledge of their target population end up addressing assumptions and prejudices about that population and not the reality. When this happens, messages and approaches can be irrelevant or insensitive, if not dangerous and damaging. For this reason it is critically important to assess the stages of initiation in the targeted population before employing at-risk prevention activities.

The matrix in Figure 11.2 can be particularly useful in developing secondary prevention programs. As shown, the three critical transitions for at-risk prevention are the movements from Contemplation to Preparation, from Preparation to Action, and from Action to Maintenance. Preventing these transitions to addiction is the key task of secondary prevention. However, each transition requires different prevention strategies and different goals. For example, increasing experimentation, a growing social network supporting engagement in the addictive behavior, and an increasingly positive attitude about the behavior mark the transition from Contemplation to Preparation. Interventions designed to prevent this transition should concentrate on how to decrease experimentation, counter any positive experimentation experiences, and attempt to increase the social network with individuals who are able to support nonuse (Werch, Pappas, Carlson, & DiClemente, 1998). All these interventions attempt to engage the relevant processes of change. At this transition the relevant processes are self- and environmental reevaluation related to this specific addictive behavior, the creation of helping relationships, consciousness raising, and supporting an individual's commitment (self-liberation) not to engage in the behavior. These types of interventions concentrate on the addictive behavior itself. However, the context is also important. Achievements and success in other areas of life, or a lack of problems in these areas, can assist in preventing the transition from Contemplation to Preparation. Depending on the assessment of the context of change for a particular individual or group of individuals, additional interventions could be developed. Boys from broken homes where there is no male figure (family/social system) and who are having difficulty in peer relationships (interpersonal) may be at greater risk for this transition from Contemplation to Preparation. A big brother or male mentor program with an interpersonal skills training component would be valuable in targeting this transition for this group.

If the targeted transition is from Preparation to Action, other goals and strategies are important. In this transition individuals move from experimentation to more regular use and begin to develop a pattern of use and a narrowing of other activities. Although frequently the behavior continues to be under self-regulatory control, there are more incidences of impaired control. Consequences may also begin to occur, but generally at low levels of severity. At-risk prevention activities at this point should heighten any negative experiences with early use, emphasize the seriousness of both experienced and potential consequences of use, and attempt to foster broad engagement in other activities to prevent narrowing of focus (Monti, Colby, & O'Leary, 2001).

In addition, complicating problems in the context of change may be related to this transition from Preparation to Action. For example, individuals who begin to engage in bulimic behavior more regularly may have issues related to individuation (Selvini-Palazzoli, 1974) and trouble separating from their families of origin. In addition, they may have a growing distortion of self-image and beliefs about weight and weight gain. Interventions that would be most helpful for these individuals are those that promote individuation, like an adolescent Outward Bound experience where they are challenged to learn and perform on their own, separate from family—that can provide accurate feedback related to physical abilities and image. These experiences can engage the cognitive/experiential processes of self-reevaluation and environmental reevaluation as well as social liberation that could discourage progression from Preparation to Action. Providing interventions that focus on the specific stage transition for the addictive behavior as well as complicating problems in the context of change creates more intensive prevention for this vulnerable subgroup in the process of developing severe bulimic behavior.

Harm Reduction and At-Risk Prevention in the Action to Maintenance Transition

At-risk prevention in the transition from Action to Maintenance must take into account that the target population no longer consists of naive experimenters but of more seasoned regular users who believe in their self-regulatory capability to control the behavior. Moreover, the social networks of those in Action often are filled with peers engaging regularly in the behavior. This is no time for vague warnings or general education about the negatives of the behavior. It is especially important at this point to focus on the experiences of the individual and to capitalize on any ambivalence and negative considerations that are present.

Offering these individuals data-based personal feedback may be critical (DiClemente, Marinilli, Singh, & Bellino, 2000; Kreuter, Strecher,

& Glassman, 1999). Particularly, offering information about any current negative consequences or initial signs of potential dangers could be especially helpful. Miller and his colleagues at the University of New Mexico have demonstrated in several studies that a "drinker checkup program" reduced substantially the consumption levels of problem drinkers for up to 1 or more years (Miller, Sovereign, & Krege, 1988; Yahne & Miller, 1999). This checkup provided an extensive, objective assessment of the drinking patterns and consequences to individuals with concerns about their drinking. The program targeted problem drinkers who were not dependent but often were problematic users or abusers of alcohol. This at-risk program is an excellent example of one directed at the transition from Action to Maintenance stages of initiation.

The transition from Action to Maintenance is particularly influenced by problems in the context of change. The more extensive the problems are in areas of functioning, the greater the probability that there will be a loss of self-regulatory control (McLellan et al., 1986). Loss of control can occur because the individual does not have the energy to use his or her self-control over the addictive behavior after dealing with the other problems. At other times multiple problems both contribute to and result from the erosion of self-control over the addictive behavior.

Interventions that identify and target problems in various contextual areas can be particularly helpful in supporting self-control and preventing the transition from Action to Maintenance. However, it is important to maintain dual focus on both the addictive behavior and the other problems in order to effectively prevent addiction. Efforts that concentrate on resolving problems in the interpersonal or family contextual areas while ignoring the drinking, eating, drug use, or gambling behavior can allow the individual to avoid examining the behavior. Ignoring the addictive behavior can feed the erroneous belief that other problems, and not the addictive behavior, are the entire cause of current distress. This can actually increase the probability of transitioning from Action to Maintenance by supporting the maladaptive feedback mechanisms subverting accurate self-reevaluation. This maladaptive feedback is already developing in the individual during the Action stage of change.

At-risk prevention can encompass a confusingly broad range of activities. But specific stage transitions along with the processes and markers most appropriate at these transitions offer a precise way to pinpoint the risk and define a direction for prevention activities. The interaction of context with these transitions enables programs to incorporate risk and protective factors as they relate to the particular stage transition of the individuals targeted for prevention efforts.

Paying Attention to the Heterogeneity in the Process of Change

Program planners and developers who utilize this stage model for at-risk prevention will need to understand the stage status of the individuals that they are addressing with their program. Prevention is a rather new and developing science (Coombs & Zeidonis, 1995). Some prevention advocates rather naively believe that they can simply develop a single program and apply it to large numbers of individuals. Youth who are the typical targets of prevention efforts are not only in different schools, at different ages, of different ethnicities, and in different environments but also at different points in the stages of engagement and addiction. Programs that do not recognize or address heterogeneity in all these areas will not have the credibility, power, or influence to prevent progression toward addiction at all the different points of transition.

As more and more prevention programs are evaluated for both short- and long-term effects, many are found not to have been clearly effective in preventing acquisition of the addictive behaviors (Clayton, Cattarello, & Johnstone, 1996; Lynam et al., 1999). A number of other programs have demonstrated an ability to delay engagement but not prevent it completely (Botvin, Baker, Dusenbury, Botvin, & Diaz, 1995; Pentz, 1999; Tobler, 1986). Outcome evaluations such as these should also be supplemented with process analyses to better understand the mechanisms of prevention or its failure in the context of the process of change (Longabaugh & Wirtz, 2001; Pentz, 1999).

Analyzing prevention activities in the light of stage transitions and problem areas they address can provide important information with which to evaluate current programs and plan future ones. In addition, identifying which processes of change are being targeted in each prevention program could assist in dissecting programs and examining their inner workings.

Interestingly, changes in process activities during the stages of adopting a new behavior appear to parallel process activity found in the cessation of addictive behaviors (Glanz et al., 1994; Hudmon et al., 1997; Marcus et al., 1992; Pallonen et al., 1998; Perz et al., 1996; Prochaska et al., 1991; Suris, Trapp, DiClemente, & Cousins, 1998). Specific processes are most relevant for different types of prevention. For population-based prevention, cognitive/experiential processes are most prominent because attitudes and decisional considerations are the primary focus of the interventions. As the initiation process moves through the Preparation, Action, and Maintenance stages, behavioral processes like reinforcement management, conditioning, stimulus control, and helping relationships become more prominent. Contrary to the cessation process, however, it seems that the cognitive/experiential processes remain important throughout the stages of addiction and that the behavioral ones grow in importance as the progression involves more and more behavioral aspects of the addiction (Lee & DiClemente, 2000). This seems to be true in the initiation of health protection behaviors as well as in the initiation of addictions (Werch, 2001; Werch, Carlson, Pappas, Dunn, & Williams, 1997).

PREVENTION AND MAINTAINED ADDICTION

Treatment for the Addicted

Individuals who have reached the Maintenance stage of addiction have well-defined patterns of the behavior and have a dependent, problematic, and well-established physiological and psychological connection to the addictive behavior. Up to this point in the change process, prevention interventions attempt to interfere with and prevent the individual reaching this Maintenance stage of addiction. However, once the person is addicted, efforts must shift to treatment or harm reduction. These efforts are best included in the tertiary prevention category, a focus on the already afflicted. From the stages of change perspective this represents a shift from the stages of addiction to the stages of recovery.

In other words, as people move through the Maintenance stage for addiction and terminate the process of becoming addicted they become Precontemplators for cessation. Interventions then should be directed at helping addicted individuals begin to move through the stages of change for cessation and recovery. Part 2 of this volume described the process of movement through these stages of recovery. Interventions and strategies designed to facilitate movement through the stages of recovery are the focus of the next chapter and therefore are not discussed here. However, one additional intervention, harm reduction, should be included under the heading of prevention rather than treatment.

Harm Reduction

Harm reduction is a strategy that focuses on preventing risks associated with addiction and not necessarily on stopping the addiction. Harm reduction can also be a component of population-based or at-risk prevention activities. For example, efforts to get parents to provide rides for their drinking adolescents focus primarily on harm reduction and only indirectly on drinking. These programs target teens in the Preparation and Action stages of change predominantly. However, most harm reduction efforts concentrate on individuals who have moved into the Maintenance stage of addiction and are in Precontemplation for cessation. Methadone maintenance programs, for example, are often aimed not at cessation but simply offering the possibility of stable employment and reduction in criminal activity. Needle exchange programs currently being used to reduce the risk of HIV transmission among addicted individuals are also preventive, harm reduction programs. These types of interventions are classified as prevention because they attempt to prevent additional problems or deterioration in individuals who already have the illness or problem.

Harm reduction strategies have generated controversy when applied to addictive behaviors. Those opposed to harm reduction believe that these strategies promote addiction and restrict recovery activities. Harm reduction proponents see this criticism as naive and point to the fact that successful cessation is difficult and takes a long time (Marlatt & Tapert, 1993). Not providing interventions that can improve the health and well-being of the addict until they have achieved successful cessation would be cruel and unethical in their view.

The issues on both sides of this controversy can be clarified and addressed using the TTM perspective. Harm reduction strategies with individuals in Preparation and Action stages of addiction should include prevention activities designed to weight the decisional balance against further use or move them toward self-regulation. Otherwise, harm reduction could reduce negative consequences at a time when they may be needed to signal trouble, provide feedback, and create shifts in the decisional considerations away from addiction. Thus, simply allowing adolescents to continue to drink to excess and providing transportation so they will be protected from harm could promote stage transitions into Action and/or Maintenance of addiction. This should not be made into an argument against this type of program, however. The danger of a fatal car crash that would injure a number of individuals is serious and independent of someone becoming addicted. However, individuals using this safety net on multiple occasions demonstrate that they are moving through Preparation or Action toward the Maintenance stage of addiction. For such individuals additional prevention efforts must be taken if there is any hope of stopping the process of becoming addicted. If this type of harm reduction program (you drink, we drive) is implemented by parents who have their eyes closed and are willing to protect their child at all costs while ignoring the developing alcohol problems, then it could be considered problematic. However, parents are using this type of program responsibly if they are willing to evaluate where the adolescent is in the process of becoming addicted and take appropriate actions to interfere with that process. In fact, "don't drink and drive" programs can be beneficial not only in reducing injuries and death but in preventing movement forward toward addiction, when used skillfully.

The problem is a bit different with individuals who have well-maintained addictions and are in Precontemplation for recovery. These individuals are addicted and currently unwilling to take steps to change the problematic behavior in any significant way. Providing harm reducing alternatives to these addicted individuals is better than simply allowing them to amass consequences until they reach their own personal "bottom." Bottoming out is based on the premise that individuals must suffer a certain number of consequences in order to gain sufficient motivation to change. However, there is little empirical evidence for this premise. Many individuals who become addicted stay that way for long periods of time. Consequences are only part of the equation that makes for change.

Methadone maintenance and needle exchange programs for heroin addicts, for example, are important harm reduction interventions. However, they have the potential to do more than reduce harm. Providers with needle exchange or methadone programs gain access to individuals in Precontemplation for recovery that would otherwise be impossible for traditional treatment personnel. Once there is the contact, there is a possibility for offering additional interventions and promoting movement through the stages of recovery. This opportunity makes harm reduction interventions beneficial not only for reducing associated risks but also for promoting recovery. Moreover, just as problems in various areas of life functioning promote movement through the stages of addiction, assisting addicted individuals in resolving current or preventing potential problems in these multiple areas can promote movement through the stages of recovery. Harm reduction efforts are worthwhile and valuable if they are cognizant of the stages for both addiction and recovery, recognize their potential impact on the processes and markers of change, and take advantage of the contact to promote addiction prevention or recovery-related interventions. Harm reduction implemented in ways that interfere with the process of recovery or promote progression toward addiction would be irresponsible and problematic.

PREVENTION POLICY AND PROGRAMMING

Myths and Reality

Policymakers view prevention as the elegant solution to the drug problem because stopping addictions before they start seems the most logical and compelling way to eradicate drug abuse and other addictions. However, prevention policy and programming often embrace several myths that have been discussed in other chapters and are summarized here.

- *Myth 1*. Becoming addicted is an all-or-none phenomenon. This could be called the *on/off myth*. In the usually fragmented way we think about addictions, this myth is applied primarily to illegal drug abuse and sometimes to cigarettes, alcohol use, or gambling behavior. Preventing any engagement in the addictive behavior becomes the goal of those who subscribe to this myth. Therefore, any lifetime engagement marks the failure of prevention efforts. As we have seen in previous chapters, the reality of addiction involves a process of change and is not well represented as an all-or-none experience.
- *Myth 2*. Creating a completely negative view of the addictive behavior at individual and societal levels is the best way to protect individuals, no matter what their age, from considering and engaging in it. Prevention policy and programming that follows this myth emphasizes the negative aspects of the behaviors from early childhood. Parents and educators are encouraged to train the children in these negative and hostile attitudes whenever they have an opportunity. Proponents of the myth believe that prevention requires ongoing extremely negative messages delivered in the best Madison Avenue, marketing style. Counter-advertising is designed to counter positive messages and keep a negative "spin" on the addictive behavior among the population. However, negative marketing can backfire and is particularly dangerous during the adolescent stage of human development. All negative messages about the addictive behavior do not contribute necessarily to prevention of the addiction.
- *Myth 3*. Schools are the best place to reach and teach children in order to prevent drug abuse and other addictions. Prevention proponents with this view see schools as the main prevention venue. Information and education delivered in the schools become the primary prevention strategies. At times these strategies are integrated into the curriculum but most often they are delivered by some organization that is not a part of the school, like law enforcement or treatment specialists. However, prevention programming in schools is unlikely to succeed if it is not integrated into curriculum, is unaware of the process of becoming addicted, fails to address family and peer influences, and lacks developmentally appropriate messages. Moreover, often schools do not reach the most vulnerable kids at the most vulnerable periods in their lives.
- *Myth 4*. Prevention of any single addictive behavior is either completely linked to or totally independent of other addictive behaviors. Examples of such dichotomous thinking abound: Cigarette smoking is the gateway to all illegal drug use (there is a correlation but it is not clearly

causal); alcohol is completely unrelated to illegal drug use; medications are not drugs; drug abusers will use any drug available; college drinking is completely unrelated to later alcohol abuse or dependence. Under the influence of this myth prevention efforts become targeted either to all or to only one addictive behavior. The reality is that there are connections among various addictive behaviors and that the trajectory through the stages of addiction for each is unique but often interrelated.

One or more of these myths can usually be found in the conceptual background of many prevention efforts, creating confusion and complicating policies and programming. Those programs that are sponsored by agencies or community groups with limited or narrow concerns about one or more addictive behaviors are most vulnerable to the myths. Unfortunately, these myths are part of the current belief systems of many legislative and policymaking bodies as well. The reality is contrary to the myths. Initiation of each addictive behavior involves a process and path that is NOT best characterized as an on–off phenomenon. Negative messages can heighten awareness, sensitize, create a positive rebound, and provide fuel for rebellion. Schools often do not reach the population of children most vulnerable to the initiation of drug and other addictive behaviors. The interaction of use and abuse among various addictive substances and behaviors is complex. Dispelling myths and focusing on the process that underlies the initiation of single and multiple addictive behaviors can increase the specificity, effectiveness, and coherence of prevention policies and programs.

Societal Policymaking and the Need for a Stage-Based Etiology of Addiction

Those who wish to prevent and reduce addictions in society should begin with an in-depth understanding of the specifics of the addictive behavior and of the target population. Staging has been done rather successfully for recovery with populations of current smokers. We have some good estimates of the percentage of smokers in the various stages of cessation and recovery for different populations of smokers in California, Australia, the Netherlands, and other locations (Keller, Nigg, Jakle, Baum, & Basler, 1999; Schmid & Gmel, 1999; Velicer et al., 1995). This information can be extremely helpful in designing strategies for community interventions for cessation of smoking. Researchers are just beginning to do the same for the stages of acquisition and addiction in order to guide prevention efforts (Hudmon et al., 1997; Pallonen et al., 1998). What is needed is a stage-based epidemiology that can inform and guide policymaking and programming.

Surveys often obtain information only about use. They identify how many individuals, between certain ages or in certain grades at school, used a particular drug in the past month or in the past year. This type of epidemiological data often generates more heat than light and offers too little information to guide prevention efforts. However, to really understand where youth are in the acquisition of addictive behaviors, we need evaluations of behavior-specific outcome expectancies and intentions to use, as well as current and historical patterns of use. Then we can track populations as they increase or decrease movement toward the initiation of various addictive behaviors. Although such data is not available currently, I predict that positive expectations for drug or alcohol use increase before experimentation and repeated use increase. Using the occurrence of drug use as the early warning sign for intervention is problematic. By the time any subgroup is engaged in repeated use, a number of these individuals are well on their way to abuse or addiction. Prevention efforts at that point are like trying to stop a car after it has begun rolling down a hill, gathering momentum. Prevention interventions, policies, and activities should be addressed to individuals in earlier stages in order to head off movement into the Action and Maintenance stages of addiction. Matching intervention efforts with current stage-status of populations can be one of the most important contributions of the addiction and change model proposed here. Matching requires that we have an in-depth understanding of the transitions from each stage to the next, the developmental stage of the target population, and the social environment.

Policy makers concerned about the initiation of addictions need a more comprehensive and complex view of the problem. Societal messages about the benefits and risks of various drugs are omnipresent and subtle. They range from billboard messages promoting cigarettes and alcohol to the touting of legal wonder drugs. It is naive to believe that the only influences on heroin or cocaine use are messages specific to these two drugs. The entire societal and personal context influences initiation (see Figure 11.4). A comprehensive process of change perspective offers a unique way to examine these complex problems and it offers multiple tasks and targets to guide prevention policy and interventions.

SUMMARY

The description of the process of change and the paths of addiction and recovery offer a detailed, pragmatic, process view of addiction that can assist prevention specialists and policymakers. Programs and policies that correspond to the process of change and address individuals at dif-

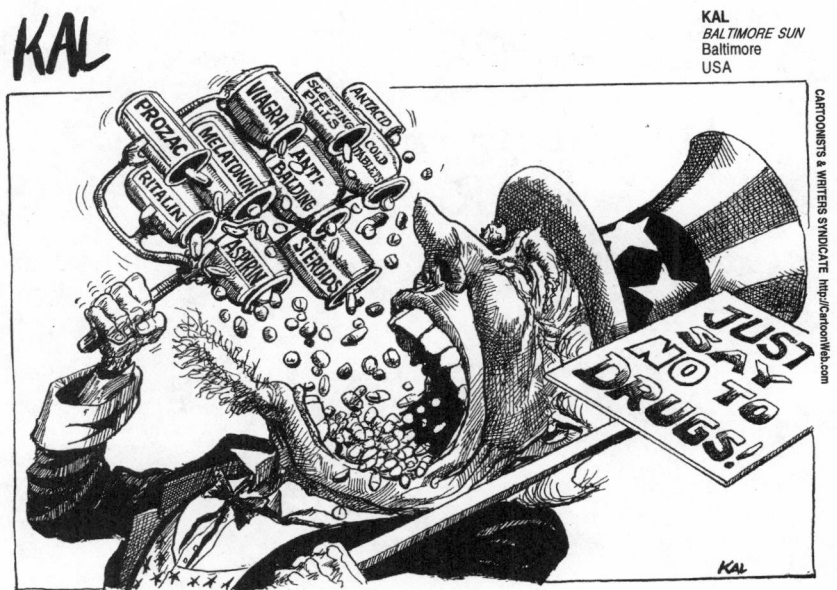

FIGURE 11.4. Mixed messages and the prevention of addiction. Reprinted by permission of Kevin Kallaugher (KAL), Cartoonists & Writers Syndicate/cartoonweb.com.

ferent stages of becoming addicted enhance the specificity of the different types of prevention. Targets of population-based prevention are those in Precontemplation and Contemplation stages of change, whereas at-risk prevention focuses on critical transitions from Contemplation to Preparation, Preparation to Action, and Action to Maintenance. Prevention aimed at those already afflicted with addictions should focus on those in the Action and Maintenance stages to provide early interventions, harm reduction, and, ultimately, addiction treatment options. However, once individuals develop well-maintained addictions, the focus should shift to stages of recovery.

Chapter 12

Designing Interventions for Recovery

To match the different tasks faced by clients moving through the stages of recovery, interventions must be dynamic and targeted to specific dimensions of change.

A COMMON PATHWAY TO QUITTING AN ADDICTION

Leaving an addictive behavior once it has become well maintained requires a journey through the stages of recovery described in the chapters in Part III. Although the journey could occur in a single attempt and a linear fashion, most often it is not rapid. Many individuals spend long periods of time in one or another of these stages, and most make a number of Action attempts before they successfully establish a lifestyle that is free of the addiction. For most addicted individuals who struggle to get free of their addiction, the journey follows what is more like a spiral path of movement through the stages of recovery. Forward successful movement toward change is often achieved only after cycling and recycling several times through the stages of Contemplation, Preparation, and Action before reaching stable recovery and finally exiting this spiral. Longitudinal research and the experiences of many formerly addicted individuals support this view of the journey to end an addiction. For some addicted individuals the journey is never successfully completed. Their lives are ended in one of the stages of change prior to Maintenance or termination. However, permanent change is not only possible but the norm for those who persist in learning how to move successfully through the stages of change (Carbonari et al., 1999; Moos et al., 1990).

Although this pathway to quitting an addiction has many common elements and is manifestly similar for all addictions, the actual passage through the stages and spiral of change is unique for each individual and for each behavioral addiction. This is probably the reason why it has been so difficult to predict the successful outcome for changing an addictive behavior (Donovan & Mattson, 1994). The difficulty predicting successful recovery lies partially in the reality that practically anyone can become addicted, which makes for a very heterogeneous group of addicts. It also lies partially in the multiplicity of behaviors to which one can become addicted. A third reason for failed prediction is that the course of change can be so variable and complicated. Precontemplators for change can utilize many different strategies for avoiding the prospect of change. Contemplators differ greatly in the number and strength of the costs and benefits they see in change and can spend variable amounts of time considering the question of change. In the Preparation stage, addicted individuals generate differing amounts of commitment and strategies or plans that are more or less effective. Action is taken in dissimilar environments, utilizing varied aids and treatments, and accompanied by diverse complicating problems in other areas of the addict's life. Relapse and the return to the addictive behavior occur with varying frequency and intensity and after unequal periods of successful change. Even after addicted individuals achieve some measure of maintained change, they differ in how well they are able to develop an alternative lifestyle and satisfying new activities that can protect the change and promote termination. The uniqueness of the journey through this common path of change for addictive behaviors poses challenges for addict, intervenor, and scientist.

The more we understand the process of addictive behavior change and identify both markers and strategies of successful transition through the stages, the better we can study and intervene in this process. The task of describing each of these stages of change is only a prelude to the work of discovering the mechanisms and the moderators of movement from one stage to the next in order to create a successful sequence of transitions. Although still incomplete, the picture of the process that is developing begins to identify the tasks and some of the mechanisms that are important in these transitions (Figure 12.1). This picture is beginning to take form from the static photos of our cross sectional research and the episodic views from our longitudinal research to create a dynamic view of the process. We still have a long way to go to understand how each addict moves through the stages of change in real time. However, our initial picture of the process of quitting an addictive behavior has many implications for designing programs and policies to assist addicted individuals in moving out of precontemplation and through the stages of recovery.

Stages of Change and Treatment Tasks

- Precontemplation
- Increase concern and hope for change

- Contemplation
- Tip the decisional balance

- Preparation
- Commitment and effective plan

- Action
- Problem solving; support self-efficacy

- Maintenance
- Prevent relapse; resolve context problems

FIGURE 12.1. A stage-based view of treatment tasks.

HELPING INDIVIDUALS MOVE THROUGH THE STAGES OF RECOVERY

One benefit to the stage view of changing behaviors is that individuals can label where they are in the process and indicate the current task that they face. In one of our first research projects on smoking cessation, a group of reviewers from the National Institutes of Health (NIH) visited the laboratory to evaluate the proposed project. One reviewer, a current smoker, took his nametag and wrote "Precontemplator" under his name. It let us know that, although he might ultimately give his approval for our study into the process of smoking cessation, he had no current consideration of changing his own smoking behavior. Simply understanding that change is a process with a series of stages with different tasks and goals creates a greater appreciation of the complexity of change and adjusts the focus of change attempts on more defined and doable parts of the process (Miller & Rollnick, 1991). Just being able to put a label on part of the process of change has been a welcome innovation to many lay and professional persons faced with the prospect of changing addictive and other health-related behaviors (Joseph et al., 1999; Kohler et al., 1999; Shaffer, 1992).

Labeling, however, is not the purpose of segmenting the process of change into the distinct stages. Rather, each of the stages presents intermediate tasks and goals for those who would change a particular behavior. Understanding how changers accomplish those tasks and reach other goals is to understand the process of moving from one stage to the next. Key factors that facilitate movement are decisional considerations (pros and cons, outcome expectancies), evaluations of temptation or vulnerability to engage in the behavior, self-efficacy to perform the particular behaviors needed to change, and, most importantly, the experiential and behavioral processes of change (Carbonari & DiClemente, 2000; DiClemente & Prochaska, 1998; DiClemente et al., 1985; Perz et al., 1996; Prochaska, Velicer, et al., 1994). Researchers using the TTM have examined these variables in detail across addictive behaviors from cigarettes to cocaine, alcohol, heroin, gambling, and obesity.

The finding that these dynamic factors vary systematically as individuals move through the stages of change has been the most important and helpful part of our entire research on quitting addictions. Identifying the stages and finding ways to influence the key factors have implications for interventions. To move through the early stages of change individuals must shift decisional considerations. Both negative consequences of the behavior and positive expectations about the change increase. These must also become more highly valued than the benefits of the behavior and the negative expectations for the change. In order to foster these shifts in decisional considerations, Precontemplators and Contemplators appear to increase use of experiential processes, particularly those that increase information and reevaluate the behavior and its consequences. Increasing commitment to change appears most critical during Preparation and Action stages. Increasing use of behavioral processes that modify the actual behavior and reinforce the change are most important in the Action and Maintenance stages, as is a growing sense of efficacy to perform the behaviors necessary to quit the addictive behavior. The lessening and ultimate fading of temptation to engage along with the solid sense of self-efficacy to abstain from the behavior seem to mark the termination of the process of change (DiClemente & Prochaska, 1998; Prochaska et al., 1992).

This information about the factors and the methods for achieving successful movement through the stages of change can be used to help individuals make successful changes (Prochaska, Norcross, & DiClemente, 1994) and to create innovative treatment materials and programs (Connors et al., 2001; DiClemente, Marinilli, Singh, & Bellino, 2001; Prochaska, DiClemente, Velicer, & Rossi, 1993; Velasquez et al., 2001; Velicer et al., 1993). Strong and replicated findings in the research and many anecdotal experiences of addicts and treatment providers support the contention that individuals who use appropriate processes and have a success profile on the dynamic change process indicators negotiate the journey through the stages and achieve successful change more often than those who use less appropriate processes and have lower scores on these markers (Carbonari & DiClemente, 2000). The secret of successful change of addictive behaviors is not just doing something or doing more of one thing. It seems to be doing "the right thing at the right time" (Perz et al., 1996). Addicted individuals, treatment programs, policymakers, and others who understand this should have a better chance of promoting successful transitioning through the stages of change.

Programs to Promote Individual Change

The process of change for addictive behaviors as described in the previous chapters and just recapped outlines the tasks and strategies needed to successfully negotiate the journey through the stages of recovery. This approach makes the case for an individualized approach to helping addicted individuals. However, the individualized journey does not negate the possibility of learning from others or using certain common techniques in groups (Velasquez et al., 2001). That is one of the benefits of having the common set of dynamic factors described earlier.

Miller and Rollnick (1991, 2002), in their book *Motivational Interviewing*, offer a good example of mixing a set of common techniques with a perspective on change that is individualized and based on the TTM. Motivational interviewing consists of strategies like reflective listening, rolling with resistance, supporting self-efficacy, and developing a change plan that allows for individual concerns and decisional considerations as well as for individual choice and responsibility (Bien, Miller, & Tonigan, 1993). Another example would be the multistage feedback program developed with funding from the National Cancer Institute for smokers in various stages of change (Prochaska et al., 1993). In this program, the feedback given to participants was based on the individual's responses to measures of the dimensions of change. The feedback was then personalized not only to the individual's stage of change, but also to each smoker's reported level of pros and cons, self-efficacy, and experiential and behavioral processes of change. The self-help book *Changing for Good* (Prochaska, Norcross, & DiClemente, 1994) is also based on the stages and offers advice and self-assessments designed to assist individuals to move forward a stage at a time to change addictive or health behaviors. In addition, there are new resources for addiction treatment that use the stages and processes of change to create group therapy modules (Velasquez et al., 2001), offer an overview of motivational strategies (Center for Substance Abuse Treatment Treatment Improvement Protocol No. 35), and give guidance to substance abuse professionals (Bishop, 2001; Connors et al., 2001). The TTM and the stage perspective definitely call for individualizing and personalizing interventions so they will facilitate movement through the stages of change.

A number of planners and programs are attempting to develop treatment programs and systems that are responsive to the process of change. Some programs are developing specific interventions for Precontemplators in response to large numbers of individuals being mandated to addiction treatment. Legal sanctions have greatly increased the numbers of Precontemplators who present themselves at various types of treatment programs predominantly in order to comply with sanctions and not necessarily to change. Some programs are developing pretreatment readiness courses that could be used to handle and prepare those not yet ready for change (Ingersol, Wagner, & Gharib, 2000). One cocaine treatment program runs a group for those who are not ready to change (Washton, personal communication, 1995). If a drug abuser comes to that program and wants to change, he or she is not allowed to enter this "not ready for change" group. One program for smokers consists only of a 2-hour motivational intervention that attempts to move clients into the Preparation stage and then lets them find their own way to change with or without the aid of self-help manuals. Other addiction-treatment programs select only those most prepared to change for their most intensive treatments. A number of programs, particularly in the area of smoking cessation and health promotion, are developing individualized feedback and monitoring systems in order to treat and track the progress of the person through the process of change (DiClemente, Marinilli, et al., 2001). Outcome evaluations and controlled trials of these approaches are only beginning. But the variety of individualized yet programmatic interventions is impressive and indicates that dynamic and programmatic matching can be accomplished.

Promoting Change: Group and Community Perspectives

Individualization of the process of change also offers interesting challenges and opportunities for those who take a larger group or community perspective on change. Different communities may or may not differ significantly in the number of addicts in various stages of recovery. For example, there are more smokers in the Precontemplation stage in Europe than there are in the United States (Dijkstra, DeVries, & Bakker, 1996; Etter, Perneger, & Ronchi, 1997). Within the United States there are slight regional differences in the number of smokers who report being in Precontemplation and Contemplation, while the percentage of smokers in various stages of change in Australia is similar to that in the United States (Owen, Wakefield, Roberts, & Esterman, 1992). An early attempt to compare stage status among different groups of smokers indicated that the population of current smokers often has approximately 30–40% in Precontemplation for smoking cessation, another 30–40% in Contemplation and about 20% in Preparation (Velicer et al., 1995). However, estimates of the distribution across stages of change vary greatly depending on attitudes, policies, and restrictions in the larger context of the society.

In response to diversity in stage status among addicts in various communities, program planning needs flexibility. When I chaired a committee entrusted with doing a needs-assessment for Harris County, Texas, we estimated the number of alcoholics and drug abusers in the county to be over 100,000. The number of treatment slots available in the county covered only about 10–15% of that number. At first, the group began to bemoan the lack of treatment facilities and argued that the county needed to create treatment slots to equal the number of addicts. However, this view reflected a static notion of both addiction and change. In actuality, the number of treatment slots needed were probably only slightly more than those already available. The real need for inpatient beds or intensive outpatient slots at any single point in time is probably best estimated to be about 10–20% of the addicted population, or those entering the Preparation and Action stages of recovery. If more intensive motivational interventions existed to prepare addicts for change and engage them in the process of change, we would expect the numbers of voluntary treatment seekers to increase dramatically. Likewise, if we criminalize the behavior and mandate treatment, greater treatment capacity would be needed.

There is an interesting interaction between the addicted individual and the larger environment that influences how many individuals are in each stage within a population. Societal context affects stage status for each addictive behavior. For example, the population of addicted cigarette smokers is segmented by stage according to a number of historical, epidemiological, and public policy factors. These include how long the practice of smoking has existed in the population, the number and intensity of public messages about smoking-related health problems, the amount and placement of cigarette advertising, visible consequences among peer cohorts of smokers, life expectancy of the population, and other more subtle factors like the status of women in the society. Although we are gaining in our knowledge of the process of change for each individual, we are not as far along in understanding the process of change in a total population of addicted individuals. Smoking cessation holds great promise for understanding this process if we can get the needed data not only here in the United States but also in some countries of Europe, Asia, South America, and Africa where there are differing levels of smoking prevalence and stage distribution.

Understanding the population of addicted individuals in terms of the stages of change also can assist in evaluating cultural and societal pressures to change and give direction to planning treatment and intervention efforts. I have been involved in several large-scale research projects that had as a goal changing the smoking, eating, and drinking behaviors of large numbers of individuals. Several interesting ones involved intervening with large numbers of workers in unions and at worksites scattered across extended areas of the country. There was minimal ability to individualize the interventions. However, we used the template of the stages to orchestrate intervention materials and strategies that first attempted to evoke motivation, then promote action, and finally create support for maintaining success or for recycling through the stages for those unable to achieve successful cessation. Evidence for the effectiveness of these approaches was mixed, and the approaches did not always do better than the control condition (DiClemente, 1993b; Sorenson et al., 1996). Although sequencing according to the stages appears to be a logical intervention strategy, it may be too difficult to achieve individualization in such large-scale interventions. Identifying subgroups and specific strategies for these subgroups is one thing; reaching these subgroups and implementing the tailored strategies can be a real challenge.

Prochaska and colleagues at the University of Rhode Island Cancer Prevention Research Center appear to be having greater success by being proactive (Prochaska, DiClemente, Velicer, & Rossi, 1993; Prochaska & Velicer, 1997b). They reach out to individuals in various stages of change in order to deliver stage specific messages and interventions. They have used a random-digit dialing procedure to reach smokers and individuals with various other health-risk behaviors in all the various stages of change in order to promote movement through the stages. Current reports are that they have been successful in reaching large numbers of individuals in early stages of change who would not come to a treatment program and that they have been able to move a certain proportion of these individuals forward with minimal interventions (DiClemente & Prochaska, 1998; Goldberg et al., 1994). Proactive approaches that reach out to individuals in early stages of change appear to be more feasible than was first thought (Rollnick et al., 1992; Yahne & Miller, 1999). Many Precontemplators are not necessarily unreachable, particularly if the approach is respectful and specifically directed to that individual. These initial reports need to be confirmed and results repeated. Not all clinical trials of these types of interventions have supported their effectiveness (Joseph et al., 1999). There may be specific limitations and cultural differences in the individualization process. However, proactive approaches that can be individualized offer a promising strategy. They are an example of the kind of dynamic strategies called for by the TTM to assist in quitting addictive behaviors.

A different type of proactive approach currently being used in the war on drugs in the United States is the increasing use of court-mandated referral for treatment. These proactive interventions may be effective in getting individuals to consider and move toward change (Anglin & Hser, 1992; Wild et al., 1998). However, most of the interventions being used are action-oriented, not stage-based. Because all that really can be mandated is the offender's presence at a mandatory number of sessions or events, mandating treatment often produces attendance at treatment sessions but not always effective, intentional change (Joe, Simpson, & Broome, 1998; Schottenfeld, 1989; Speiglman, 1997).

Mandating interventions better adapted to the offender's stage of change might increase their effectiveness. Participants can be helped to work through the tasks of the early stages of change in order to benefit from the more action-oriented strategies. Ensuring that there are individualized follow-ups and active support for change once the mandate is lifted could also assure the continuation of any gains and progress. Once released from these external controls, the individual must have the internal mechanisms to sustain the gains and to continue the change (Anglin & Hser, 1992; El-Bassel et al., 1998).

Another example of proactive strategies involves recent efforts to provide addiction treatment while individuals are incarcerated. Incarceration creates an artificial and structured environment in which to offer a treatment program. That is not necessarily bad, but does pose serious problems for the intentional process of change. Prison can eliminate addictive behaviors by restricting access to the addictive substance (drug) or opportunities to engage in the addictive behavior (gambling). However, change is experienced as imposed, not chosen. As discussed previously, imposed change differs from intentional change in the nature of the process of change. Imposed change and extrinsic motivation can be effective in producing short-term change. However, it often does so without engaging the intentional process of change and intrinsic motivation needed to create successful, free-standing, sustained change, as demonstrated with pregnant women who stop smoking for the pregnancy and abstain from smoking for many months, only to return to it soon after the birth of the baby (DiClemente, Dolan-Mullen, & Windsor, 2000; Solomon, Secker-Walker, Skelly, & Flynn, 1996; Stotts, DiClemente, Carbonari, & Mullen, 2000; Stotts et al., 1996). This pattern is similar to that of prisoners who demonstrate cessation during imprisonment and return to the addictive behaviors soon after release. The challenge for prison-based addictive behavior treatment programs is to engage the intentional process of change in a restricted environment so prisoners accomplish tasks of Contemplation and Preparation (Ryan & Deci, 2000). Release into a less restricted or unrestricted environment needs to find them prepared for Action.

ENLISTING SOCIETAL RESOURCES
TO PROMOTE THE RECOVERY PROCESS

The larger community creates community norms and can create an environment conducive to producing movement through the stages of recovery. Although ultimately it is the responsibility of the individual to make stage transitions and successfully quit an addictive behavior, the larger community can have an important influence on the individual at various points in the process of change. It is helpful to frame the question of how a community can promote change of addictive behaviors in a stage-based manner. What programs and practices in a community will foster movement from Precontemplation to Contemplation, from Contemplation to Preparation, from Preparation to Action, and from Action to Maintenance and Termination? What is needed from the community varies for these different transitions.

There are ways to influence drug addicted individuals in the Precontemplation and Contemplation stages of recovery. Although often not ready to enter treatment, these individuals can be reached and possibly moved by various social strategies as they go about their lives in the communities in which they live. For example, consequences can be important motivators to get the Precontemplator and particularly the Contemplator to consider change if they are administered in a manner that is informed by what we know about rewards and punishments (Klingemann, 1991; Krampen, 1989). Punishments work best when they are immediate and linked to the target behavior, but they tend to suppress rather than eliminate behaviors. Although punishment is not usually an effective intrinsic motivator for intentional change, it is very clear that consequences that are given too late, inconsistently administered, and not perceived as connected to the addictive behavior will have little or no impact on the process of recovery.

Reaching out with concern can be used along with or instead of consequences. For example, there is clear evidence that a significant number of trauma center and emergency room patients have alcohol and drug involvement (Soderstrom et al., 1997). However, routine screening for these problems is not in place, and often no one even discusses the role that the addiction played in the current emergency. However, there are significant new studies and efforts to reach out to take advantage of this window of opportunity to influence the process of recovery (DiClemente & Soderstrom, 2001; Gentilello et al., 1999).

Despite the evidence that consequences and early interventions are effective, most communities provide punishments that fail to take advantage of the opportunity to increase addicts' motivation to change. There are hundreds and thousands of DWI arrests every year in each of the 50 states across the United States. Under pressure from Mothers Against Drunk Driving (MADD) and other lobbying groups, most judges will mandate some type of education and evaluation. However, there is often no uniform enforcement of these procedures and no long-term follow-up or check-in procedure that could proactively reach out to any of these individuals who have ongoing problems (Wagenaar, O'Malley, & LaFond, 2001). Most Precontemplators are able to respond to pressure and clean up their act for a short period of time. The real test of change comes in the longer term. Reminders and check-ups could continue to reach out and potentially raise the awareness of such individuals and move them forward in the process of change.

The goals of policies and programs for the Precontemplator should be to shorten the time spent in Precontemplation and to hasten serious consideration of change and decision making. Zero tolerance should mean never ignoring an addictive behavior problem in an individual whenever and wherever the problem becomes obvious to the society. Zero tolerance should *not* mean that we criminalize every appearance of use or create a growing class of criminals who use drugs and have not the means to get the kind of lawyers who could successfully elude the criminal charge.

Similar strategies can be used for those in the Contemplation stage of change. What gets individuals to seriously consider changing any particular behavior are personal considerations and consequences. Policies cannot mandate Contemplation but can provide the kinds of consequences and practices that would increase the probability that the individual would engage in Contemplation. Private reflection time and personal feedback about the extent of the problem and the nature of the consequences is often more helpful than jail time for many Contemplators. Involvement of family and significant others in the process would give the individual additional opportunities for feedback if it could be done in a nonconfrontational, facilitative manner (Stanton, 1997).

For individuals more prepared to change who have made a firm decision to change, offering an array of options that could assist the individual to take effective action should be the goal of the policymaker. For this ready-for-action group, delays and obstacles in offering treatment caused by insufficient beds, waiting lists, or attitudes of treatment personnel can significantly interfere with the process of change. Adequate funding from legislatures for the array of treatment options needed by substance abusers would most seriously impact individuals in the Preparation and Action stages of change (Sobell & Sobell, 1999).

The challenge for the Action and Maintenance stages of recovery is providing support for the active attempt to change and creating appropriate reinforcements for cessation and treatment. Society should reinforce cessation as much as it tries to punish abuse. Policies should reflect the reality of relapse and recycling. Programs cannot be judged solely on the single outcome of continuous abstinence while also realistically interacting with the process of changing addictive behaviors. For example, programs that seek out the least motivated substance abusers and make some significant contact that can increase Contemplation and Preparation should be evaluated and rewarded based on these outcomes. Punishment should be integrated with treatments that acknowledge recycling through the stages of change. Persistence and patience should be the watchwords of policies related to promoting change.

Patience does not mean pampering or coddling the abuser. Policymakers and punishment providers need to understand how difficult it is to change an addictive behavior and allow for multiple attempts and different types of problem solving. They need clear delineation of the role of punishment and how it can be used to benefit the process of change. In venues other than criminal justice, drug abusers and addicted individuals should be treated similarly to any individuals with chronic conditions. Individuals suffering from diabetes, high cholesterol, asthma, and obesity have as much trouble maintaining change in their behaviors as those who are addicted (McLellan et al., 1995; Zimmerman, Olsen, & Bosworth, 2000). Persistent efforts to motivate, educate, and create technologies and support systems that produce lasting change should be the hallmarks of social policy, proscriptions, and procedures aimed at recovery from addictive behaviors.

ORCHESTRATING INTERVENTIONS TO MIRROR THE PROCESS OF CHANGE

Addicted individuals can spend extended periods in one particular stage of change. They often get stuck in Precontemplation and Contemplation stages and take months or years to successfully complete these tasks in the process. The opposite is also true. Some individuals move rapidly through the stages, often precipitated by some dramatic or tragic event. The more time-intensive, deliberate path seems to be the one that most addicted individuals follow, yet the literature is filled with the swifter, more dramatic, conversion types of changes as well. One middle-aged male smoker was comfortably smoking with no real thought of quitting when he learned of his best friend and colleague dying of a massive heart attack while playing golf. Within a week he had quit smoking and began watching his diet carefully. The effectiveness of both rapid and time-intensive transitioning is ultimately gauged by successful maintenance of change over time. However, there is no theoretical reason to consider rapid movement that accomplishes the tasks of each stage any less effective than more deliberate movement. Although we are just beginning to get better data on conversion types of changers (Miller & C'deBaca, 2001), I do not believe this type of change represents a separate process of change. Many of the reports of these quantum changers demonstrated thoughts and actions that represent transitioning through the stages.

Whether treatment programs focus on promoting rapid, conversion-type changes or more deliberate transitioning through the stages, they need to orchestrate interventions so that they coincide with the stage status and tasks of the clients making the change. This requires an approach different from many current treatment programs that are designed to offer one or two types of services and not to modify or shift interventions as individuals move through the various stages of change. One of the most important implications of taking a stage-and-process approach to changing addictive behaviors is that intervenors should change approaches as clients move through the stages (DiClemente et al., 1992).

Eclectic Treatments and the Client Process of Change

Luckily, most treatment programs are eclectic in their orientation. The techniques that most therapists or counselors employ often represent multiple processes of change. Therefore, clients who receive multicomponent interventions can use or discard the parts that are not consistent with their stage status. In many ways clients may shape the behavior of the therapist as much or more than the therapists shape the behavior of the clients. One option for offering interventions that mirror the process of change is to continue to offer multicomponent treatments and let clients take what they need. It would be helpful if counselors openly describe the process of change in terms of stages and then tell the clients that they should pick and choose techniques offered that match best with what they need. However, this seems an inefficient intervention delivery system, and there is a better one.

Dynamic Treatment Matching

The best way to mirror the process of change is to have a dynamic treatment protocol that can respond to being stuck at various stages as well as to movement through the stages of change. Techniques and strategies that engage specific processes of change should be matched to the current stage of change and the dynamic processes and markers of that stage (Velasquez et al., 2001). Strategies should shift if they are ineffective in engaging the appropriate processes of change or when the client moves forward or recycles backward through the stages of change. The therapist can assess the effectiveness of strategies from reported and observed behavior of the client both during and between treatment sessions (Connors et al., 2001). The process of change is coextensive with the life space of the individual and not confined to the time spent in the treatment setting. In fact, what the client is doing between sessions is much more important than what occurs during the treatment session (Prochaska & DiClemente, 1984).

Shifts in stage status can occur during the actual treatment session, outside the session, or after the treatment has ended. I am reminded of a client who came back to see me 1 year after our first consultation. Life events had finally convinced her that our discussion the previous year had merit and that the problem was a real one that needed changing. The responsibility of the therapist or counselor is to promote stage-appropriate tasks and movement to the next stage. The client must do the work to make the transition possible.

Orchestration is the best term that I can think of to characterize how to create programs and treatments that mirror the process of change. Orchestras are composed of many different instruments that can be organized and create moving unified sound or can be disorganized and create cacophony like the "noise" they create while tuning up. The same is true of our efforts to help addicted individuals successfully negotiate the stages of behavior change to an addiction-free life. Often our current addiction treatment efforts sound more like the cacophony of the orchestra warming up than a coordinated symphony. We have judges ordering individuals to treatment, therapists wanting to treat only motivated clients, hostile confrontation of those not ready for change, programs that want clients to conform to their needs rather than the other way around, discharging of the difficult client, offering substitute drugs to everyone, and discarding of treatment failures. Paying more attention to the entire process of change represented by all the stages of change, identifying the strategies that best suit the tasks of each stage, and creating an interactive and dynamic intervention system could help to create a more harmonious intervention delivery system for addictive behaviors.

ADDRESSING THE CONTEXT OF CHANGE

Addicted individuals often have serious problems in multiple areas of their lives. Treatment programs and personnel who focus only on the addiction have a myopic view that ignores the addictive behavior's integration into the entire life of the individual. Sometimes, however, a single-minded approach is very helpful. AA suggests that alcoholics focus solely on changing the drinking and ignore other problems until they have achieved at least a year of sobriety (Alcoholics Anonymous, 1952). However, this is not always feasible. Sooner or later the treatment provider must step back and examine how all systems—physical, psychological, and social—are involved in movement toward successful recovery. Failure to address the context in which change happens is often counterproductive because the context plays an important role in sustaining addiction or recovery.

The problem-by-stage matrix introduced in Chapter 11 (see Figure 11.2) can enrich the perspective of the treatment provider. This matrix offers a holistic picture of the client in the context of his or her current life situation. Thus, the alcohol-dependent client whose current excessive drinking is partially a response to the death of a problematic parent and who may have been divorced for several years and estranged from his or her children would differ from the alcohol-dependent client drinking the same amount who is experiencing serious marital and family problems and who has a serious mental illness. Addicted individuals differ not only in the severity and extent of their engagement in the addictive behavior, but also in the number and intensity of additional problem areas in their lives, how integrated these problems are with the addictive behavior, and how ready the addicted individuals are to face and change these additional problems. Moving through the stages of change for the addictive behavior often has to be coordinated with movement through the stages for other problem areas. Thus, a dynamic treatment approach would not only address the addictive behavior but also life's contextual problems that would interfere with making successful, sustained change of the addictive behavior (McLellan et al., 1993, 1997; Schmidt & Weisner, 1999; Tucker, Vuchinich, & Pukish, 1995).

The preceding description of a dynamic and comprehensive intervention system would be complicated and demanding. However, treatment systems currently being used for addiction that are more focused on severity of the addiction and less focused on the process of change are no less complicated. In fact, the current system of treatment is often more complicated and demanding than the proposed new system. Lack of coordinated services that track the client and lack of resources to deal with contextual problems create barriers to change for the addicted individual and demoralizing problems for treatment personnel.

Shifting from the current to a new system would require significant changes. To be worth it, the costs of that change must be outweighed by the benefits and the costs of not changing. Would an orchestrated system of treatment be more problematic than the current system? I invite the reader to examine the dropout rates, long-term success rates, and the problems of the current system before rejecting the suggestions contained in this chapter and book.

SUMMARY

Effective policy and programs to assist the addicted individual to move successfully toward full and lasting recovery from an addiction should begin with an insider's view of recovery. We should be guided by the process of how very dedicated, seemingly hopelessly addicted addicts become healthy and contributing members of society. The perspective offered by the dimensions of change, stages, processes, markers, and context of change provides one way to capture this recovery process. Societal restrictions, punishments, programs, and services should be designed to interact with these dimensions of change in ways that promote successful recovery. Patience and persistence are critical not only for the individual addict but also for a society that hopes to promote recovery. Whether we use the TTM's view or another, the path through the process of recovery should guide policymakers and program developers.

Chapter 13

Research on Addiction
and Change

Research and evaluation studies will not advance knowledge or improve interventions unless they are designed to be sensitive to the process of human behavior change for becoming addicted and recovering from an addiction.

ADVANCING THE RESEARCH AGENDA

The process of human intentional behavior change offers a unique, dynamic view of how one becomes addicted and how one negotiates recovery. What is new and exciting about the change perspective is that it can provide a continuous, integrated view of the entire process of entering and exiting from addictions. It allows the field to move from a static, linear, and dichotomous view of addiction to one that incorporates the nuances of developmental, longitudinal, multidimensional change perspectives. Viewing addiction and recovery in this way offers addiction researchers and program evaluators an overview that organizes multiple dimensions and influences and provides an integrative perspective for the multidisciplinary viewpoints needed to adequately address addiction.

Addiction research has become more sophisticated and extensive over the past 20 years (Donovan & Marlatt, 1988; Glantz & Pickens, 1992; Leshner, 1997; McCrady & Epstein, 1999). However, as noted in Chapter 1, the field lacked a way to integrate the complex relationships among different end points, risk and protective factors, and unique dimensions of the different addictive behaviors. Now, the various tasks identified in the stage of change transitions provide a dynamic framework for examining the interactions of the important biological, psychological and social factors involved in addiction and recovery. The cognitive/experiential and behavioral processes of change constitute measurable mechanisms that build a bridge between multidimensional influential factors and the specific transitions through the stages. The markers of change identify important mediators of the process of change that can be used as indicators of specific transitions and end points in their own right. The context of change outlines areas of functioning that constitute risk and protective factors. These areas should be evaluated to see how they interact with specific stage transitions in order to estimate their impact on the process of addiction and recovery.

These dimensions of change challenge scientists and evaluators to examine addiction and recovery in light of the process of intentional behavior change. By incorporating the process and its dimensions, research can address three main deficits in many of the current studies.

1. First of all, many studies fail to make critical distinctions among change dimensions in the questions addressed and types of populations studied. Is the sample of individuals recruited into the study representative of the entire population in all stages of change or do they primarily come from one or two stages? How relevant is the examination of the phenomenon of interest among participants who represent different stages? Do two studies differ because they have recruited samples from different stages of addiction or recovery?

2. A second deficit is that studies often examine inappropriate or unlikely end points that may have little variance in some populations, seriously limiting their ability to find predictors or differences among treatment and control groups. Although it may be rather easy to get at expectations of fourth graders about alcohol consumption, measuring actual consumption is problematic. Almost all these students will be in the earliest stages for acquisition of drinking behavior, so consumption as an outcome is not informative. Is long-term behavior change a realistic short-term goal for addicted individuals in Precontemplation for recovery? Using total abstinence that is sustained over 6 months as the only relevant outcome for a program that recruits mostly Precontemplators seems particularly unfair, as does comparing programs that have dramatically different mixes of clients in terms of their stages of change using a single behavioral outcome.

3. A third deficit involves the lack of process research and measures that focus on how, not whether, this or that result was found. Etiological research most often measures only prevalence of use and not stage status or movement of the population through the stages of addiction or recovery. Treatment research often fails to measure important critical markers and processes of change that could explain how a treatment did or did not operate as expected (Longabaugh & Wirtz, 2001).

This chapter examines several broad areas of intervention and evaluation research and reviews how the process of change perspective and
the dimensions of change can enrich these endeavors. It concludes with
an exploration of how the TTM can contribute to some current special
topics of interest including cultural competence, pharmacological treatments, harm reduction, and dual diagnosis.

OUTCOME RESEARCH

The task of specifying and validating outcomes for addiction prevention
and treatment programs is a challenging one. The coveted goal for prevention programs has been stopping people from ever engaging in or experimenting with any addictive behaviors. On the treatment side, the
gold standard for recovery has been total abstinence. However, total
avoidance or total abstinence from all addictive behaviors is difficult to
achieve and problematic to validate, even with sophisticated biochemical
or other objective markers (Babor, Steinberg, Anton, & Del Boca, 2000;
Del Boca, Babor, & McKee, 1994; Miller & Del Boca, 1994). For many
individuals, abstaining from any experimentation does not allow for experiences that could lead to a firm determination to not become involved
with this or that addictive behavior. Achieving total abstinence after one
has become addicted is often a long-term goal that is achieved only after
many attempts to change. Even for those who are considered successfully recovered, the abstinence they achieve is not always total (Cisler &
Zweben, 1999; Project MATCH Research Group, 1997a; Vaillant,
1995). Moreover, neither total avoidance nor total abstinence takes into
account the fact that individuals can engage in self-regulated use.

Defining realistic behavioral goals for addiction and recovery becomes more challenging but conceptually clearer if we can frame the
behavioral goals in the context of the process of change (Velicer,
Prochaska, Rossi, & Snow, 1992). In order to stage a behavior it is critically important to clearly define what constitutes Action and distinguish
it from Maintenance for that behavior. For example, self-regulated use
of alcohol can be defined as never having a drinking occasion where the
individual drinks more than four or five drinks. That definition, then,
becomes the Action criterion, and maintained self-regulated use would
consist of more than 6 months of drinking responsibly without an excessive drinking occasion. If cutting down on cigarettes so that only smoking on weekends is defined as success, then this pattern of smoking
behavior becomes the Action criterion. If not driving after drinking is the
goal, successfully achieving this pattern of behavior becomes the Action
criterion. If total abstinence from heroin is the goal, then total absti-

nence from heroin but not necessarily from marijuana or nicotine is the Action criterion. Staging intentional behavior change requires specificity in the behavioral target. If researchers are very clear about the specifics of the intended behavioral outcome, they could examine in greater detail the process of addictive behavior change. Although staging behaviors and classifying individuals into distinct stages is difficult (Carey, Purnine, Maisto, Carey, & Barnes, 1999; Littell & Girvin, 2002; Miller & Tonigan, 1996; Sutton, 2001), it is worth the effort to divide the population according to the various tasks of the stages when possible. At minimum, identifying individuals at various points in this process of readiness and motivation to change is more helpful than simply measuring the actual behavior (Carney & Kivlahan, 1995; Connors et al., 2001; DiClemente & Prochaska, 1998; Edens & Willoughby, 2000; Joe et al., 1998; Rothfleisch, 1997).

Specifying the Action criterion, however, is only the first step in being able to examine the multiple outcomes related to the process of change involved in addiction. The specificity of tasks, goals, processes, and markers related to the different stages of change offer a rich array of alternative starting points and outcomes for researchers. In fact, when examining addictive behaviors, researchers should be required to report the starting points as well as the outcome or end points on these dimensions for participants in their research. For example, specifying as an outcome the drinking of any alcohol during a 1-month follow-up is not as useful if the group studied consists of children all in Precontemplation than if it consisted of adults in Preparation or Action for use. For the former, expectations, decisional considerations, beliefs, intentions, and efficacy to avoid would be more appropriate outcomes to evaluate before and after an intervention. Outcomes for any type of prevention or intervention program must be consistent conceptually and practically with participants' status in the process of becoming addicted or achieving recovery.

Often researchers attempt to manage initial discrepancy in exposure or stage status by statistically covarying baseline values of these important characteristics. However, this type of procedure often can remove important information, as it attempts to make the groups equivalent on certain characteristics when it should be precisely those differences that we examine. Most often the key question of the research is precisely how the prevention programs, for example, work for different groups of individuals: those who come into the study already exposed, those considering use, or those who have no intention to use. Removing variance associated with these differences can be counterproductive. Luckily, statistical methods able to handle multiple constructs and multiple markers of single constructs as well as how these change over time are continually being refined in order to examine complex interactions across time (Collins & Horn, 1991). Tracking the journey to successful change of addictive behaviors necessitates complex, longitudinal, interactive analyses (Bryk & Raudenbush, 1987; Collins & Sayer, 2001; Francis, Fletcher, Stuebing, Davidson, & Thompson, 1991)

Examples from some recent research can illustrate the importance of stage status and process of change measures. Project MATCH, a large multisite clinical trial to evaluate the effectiveness of matching client characteristics with specific treatments, examined a variety of process and outcome measures (DiClemente, Carroll, Connors, & Kadden, 1994). One study evaluated the effect of the working alliance (client and therapist perceptions of the mutuality in bond, task, and goals) on drinking outcomes of clients. These researchers found a significant small effect of higher working alliance scores, measured at the second session of treatment, on the frequency and intensity of drinking in the year following treatment (Carroll et al., 1998). However, a subsequent study examined the impact of the client's initial stage or readiness to change on both the working alliance and treatment outcomes. This study found that readiness to change not only predicted both client and therapist ratings of the alliance but significantly moderated the effect of working alliance on drinking outcomes (Connors et al., 2000). Thus, individuals who were more ready to change when they came into treatment rated their working alliance with the therapist more highly and had better outcomes. Other analyses demonstrated that client readiness to change prior to treatment and not treatment type predicted drinking outcomes up to 3 years posttreatment and predicted engagement in the cognitive/experiential and behavioral processes of change during and at the end of treatment and successful movement through the process of change to achieve abstinence (Carbonari & DiClemente, 2000; DiClemente, Carbonari, Zweben, et al., 2001; Project MATCH Research Group, 1997a, 1998a). Initial stage status influenced treatment and change mechanisms as well as drinking outcomes.

Prevention programs and research also need to be aware of the impact of the initial stage status of participants. Several studies that targeted children in early stages of engagement in an addictive behavior found little change in actual behavior over time (Gritz et al., 1998; Werch, Carlson, Owen, DiClemente, & Carbonari, 2001). However, the research has been able to detect subtle attitudinal differences in these types of populations (Hudmon et al., 1997; Werch et al., 2001). Werch (2001) has argued that the initial staging is critical in organizing and targeting prevention programming precisely because of the potential impact of stage status on prevention outcomes. It also seems to be true that not only are outcomes influenced by initial stage status, but outcomes should be differentiated based on stage status of the individuals who enter the program. Studying only behavioral outcomes for individuals in early stages of change often fails to yield enough variance to examine statistical significance. More subtle measures of the dimensions of change could provide greater sensitivity with which to examine engagement or prevention outcomes.

In addition to the behavioral outcome of engaging in the addictive behavior, addiction and recovery involve biochemical and brain dimensions, socioenvironmental influences, and psychological processes (Leshner, 1997). It is becoming clearer that these biological, psychological, and social factors play important but somewhat different roles depending on whether the change process is one of engagement in or cessation of an addiction (Donovan & Marlatt, 1988; Glantz & Pickens, 1992; McCrady & Epstein, 1999). More importantly, however, the research is also beginning to indicate that the impact and importance of each of these multidimensional aspects can vary with the individual's stage of change and can interact with the other dimensions of change (V. B. Brown, Melchior, Panter, Slaughter, & Huba, 2000; Clements-Thompson, Klesges, Haddock, Landon, & Talcott, 1998; DiClemente, 1999b; Pollak, Carbonari, DiClemente, Niemann, & Mullen, 1998; Willoughby & Edens, 1996). Thus primary and secondary outcomes should be viewed in the context of the dimensions of change described in the TTM.

PROGRAM EVALUATION

The sensitivity and specificity provided by the dimensions of change also can enrich program evaluations. There are broad ranges of activities that are classified as either prevention or treatment programs in the field of addictive behaviors. All of these programs exist in a broader context of cultural and social factors that influence the process of change. This context of change interacts with the process of change and certainly affects movement through the stages of change for the individuals who are touched by these programs. Thus, program evaluations should consider both the context of change and the other dimensions of change in order to assess program impact.

There are several specific recommendations that can be made to those involved in program evaluation in prevention and treatment of addictive behaviors. First, programs to be evaluated should be asked to provide an accurate description based on the dimensions of change of the population served and the types of outcomes desired. Evaluations should be specifically designed to evaluate relevant dimensions rather than using a "one size fits all" evaluation protocol. Programs whose modal clients are predominantly in Precontemplation for quitting co-caine, perceive themselves as hopelessly addicted, are homeless, and have multiple complicating problems and few resources in the context of change should not be evaluated solely on cocaine abstinence. Moreover, they should not be compared with the Betty Ford Clinic or other pro-grams that attract more motivated, competent clients with access to sig-nificantly more resources in various areas of the context of change. Pro-grams can always look better in terms of outcomes if they are allowed to eliminate those clients who are in earlier stages of change, those who have poorer prognosis, and those who have multiple problems (Ryan, Plant, & O'Malley, 1995). However, if programs cannot be selective and provide no barriers to screen out the less motivated, outcome expecta-tions for their clients should focus on realistic goals related to the stages, processes, markers, and context of change.

Evaluators should examine the entire process of change in order to identify types of outcomes that are relevant to the program. A detoxifi-cation program should be evaluated on how successful it is in stabilizing a client and motivating the client to engage in treatment or move toward recovery. A long-term residential treatment program can be evaluated on movement through the stages of change that have occurred not only for the target behavior but also for contextual areas of functioning in the life of an addicted individual (McLellan et al., 1993, 1997; Schmidt & Weisner, 1999). Brief treatment programs should be evaluated on how effectively they promote movement through the stages of change and modify the target behavior and not simply whether they have achieved abstinence (Myers, Brown, Tate, Abrantes, & Tomlinson, 1999). Smok-ing cessation programs aimed at pregnant women should be evaluated on how they have succeeded in protecting the baby during the pregnancy and not necessarily whether they produced postpartum cessation (DiClemente, Dolan-Mullen, & Windsor, 2000; Stotts et al., 1996; Windsor et al., 2000). Dual-diagnosis programs should be evaluated on types of outcomes as well as on process of change dimensions related to each of the two problems (Bellack & DiClemente, 1999; Blume & Schmaling, 1997; Carey, Purnine, Maisto, Carey, & Barnes, 1999). Inappropriate program goals and failure to evaluate critical, program-specific outcomes do a disservice to the programs evaluated, making it difficult to compare outcomes across programs, to identify best prac-tices, and to offer specific recommendations for improving services.

Finally, program evaluation should examine short-term as well as long-term outcomes. The process of change is one marked by movement back and forth through the stages as well as cycling and recycling through the stages. Programs that plant seeds should not be evaluated in the same time frame as those that harvest the grain. Every treatment program, for example, wants to be the last treatment program that was associated with the successful recovery for this addicted individual. However, at any given point in time, many of the clients in any single treatment program have been through many other treatments. Almost 50% of the 952 clients who participated in the Project MATCH outpatient treatment research had prior inpatient treatment. To pretend that all the other treatments did nothing and that the final treatment program should receive all the credit for recovery is foolhardy. It is as difficult to apportion out the credit for an addict's recovery as it is to assess the blame for an adolescent moving forward to become addicted. Multiple influences and experiences play a role in movement through the process of change. Program evaluators who ignore this reality are destined to examine only a small part of the picture.

PROCESS RESEARCH

One of the most important implications of the TTM of intentional behavior change both for outcome researchers and for program evaluators is the need to integrate process research into every study. Often there has been a distinction made between outcome research that concentrates on intervention effectiveness and process research that focuses on mechanisms of action. That distinction is blurred when one views addiction and recovery as a process of change. Sometimes process variables can be viewed as outcomes and some behavioral outcomes are clearly part of the process of addiction or recovery. Decisional balance, for example, can be viewed as an important marker of movement as well as an outcome of change. The same is true of the processes of change, self-efficacy, temptation, and contextual areas of change. Research can examine which techniques successfully engender a specific experiential or behavioral process of change or use that process as an outcome variable (Daniels, 1998). Another research project could look at which processes are related to producing behavioral outcomes like smoking abstinence (Perz et al., 1996). Similarly, an episode of experimentation with a substance can be evaluated as an outcome in its own right but can also be seen as part of Contemplation stage activity. A failed quit attempt can be seen as a relapse outcome or as a contribution to preparing a more effective Action plan. The distinction between process and outcome, however, continues to be useful. Researchers should examine mediators and moderators of specific outcomes in order to understand how the process of change operates (Baron & Kenny, 1986; Bryk & Raudenbush, 1987; Francis et al., 1991; Longabaugh & Wirtz, 2001). Nevertheless, the distinction between process and outcome research should be reexamined in light of the process of change perspective proposed in this volume. Instead of a more traditional view of process research as examining the process of treatment, I would urge a focus on the process of change. In order to obtain a truly comprehensive picture of the process of addiction and recovery we must examine the process of intentional behavior change instead of focusing exclusively on mechanisms of treatment or therapy relationship variables (Cooney, Babor, DiClemente, & Del Boca, 2002; DiClemente, Carroll, Miller, Connors, & Donovan, 2002).

The Project MATCH Research Group made a commitment to understand process of treatment and process of change as well as drinking outcomes in its evaluation of the matching hypotheses (DiClemente, Carroll, Connors, & Kadden, 1994; DiClemente, Carroll, et al., 1994; Longabaugh & Wirtz, 2001). The three treatments in the study were chosen because they were different in how they conceptualized change and in the techniques used to produce change (Donovan et al., 1994). These differences were confirmed when objective observers rated session tapes and found significant differences in the activities of therapists consistent with the specific treatment philosophies (Carroll et al., 1998). However, when delivered responsibly and competently in outpatient and aftercare settings, these three different treatments produced similar outcomes (Project MATCH Research Group, 1997a, 1997b, 1998a, 1998b). More relevant for our discussion of the process of change is that all three of these treatments interacted with process variables of self-efficacy, behavioral processes of change, and stage of change in exactly the same manner (DiClemente, Carbonari, Zweben, et al., 2001; DiClemente, Carbonari, Daniels, et al., 2001; DiClemente, Carroll, Miller, Connors, & Donovan, 2002). Moreover, as individuals made changes in their drinking, there were accompanying changes in reported stage-related attitudes and behaviors. Those who were successful in moving into recovery endorsed at the end of treatment greater commitment to stop drinking, less struggling with relapse, higher levels of self-efficacy and more use of behavioral processes of change (Carbonari & DiClemente, 2000). Process dimensions rather than treatment type were related to the specific outcomes of frequency and intensity of drinking and ultimately to recovery as far out as 3 years after treatment (Project MATCH Research Group, 1998a).

In creating the over 20 matching hypotheses that were tested in this trial, the researchers made a commitment to a process analysis to examine change dimensions and treatment mechanisms. Hypothesis teams were required to specify the mechanisms of action as well as types of matches that would produce optimal outcomes (Longabaugh & Wirtz, 2001). In most cases not only were the hypothesized matching outcomes not supported, but also there was little evidence to support the mechanisms and mediators assumed by investigators and the literature to be the causal mechanisms that would create the matching of client characteristic and treatment. In reviewing the evaluations of the causal chains hypothesized by the various teams, Longabaugh & Wirtz (2001) concluded that our understanding of the mechanisms of action for various treatments is still rather primitive and that we do not understand how treatments and their interactions with clients succeed or fail. Many of the more stable characteristics of clients were not very predictive of drinking outcomes and did not interact with the treatments as hypothesized. However, they noted in the final chapter of the causal chain monograph that the dimensions of change related to the process of change were consistently and logically related to outcomes and served as interim markers of long-term recovery (Carbonari & DiClemente, 2000; Project MATCH Research Group, 1998a; Longabaugh & Wirtz, 2001).

One clear implication of these findings from Project MATCH is that, in order to be able to understand program effectiveness and addiction outcomes, researchers must focus on the dimensions of the change process as well as the outcomes, intervention programs, or strategies that are of interest. Such a focus could enable the field to patch together views of the process of change from different studies and examine how interventions and programs interact with the process of addiction and recovery. In order to advance the understanding of addiction and recovery every study should include enough information to be able to compare samples of participants on some basic dimensions of change and not simply on demographic or addiction severity variables. Every study should try to include some interim measures of the dimensions of change and attempt to obtain important process assessments for at least three time points in order to be able to evaluate changes over time. Finally, every study of prevention and intervention activities should be required to offer a causal chain that explains the reasoning of the researchers and include measures to accomplish an analysis of the hypothesized causal chain.

POLICY RESEARCH

Societies and governments are rightfully concerned about addictive behaviors. For the most part, however, they have used moral, legal, and medical models with which to view and attack the problem (Donovan & Marlatt, 1988). A process of change perspective and the TTM of intentional behavior change in particular offer real advantages over these other models as a framework for developing and evaluating policy strategies to reduce initiation and to promote sustained cessation.

A suggestion that emanates from this addiction and change analysis is to examine current and proposed policies and social engineering strategies for each addictive behavior to see exactly where in the process of change they would have beneficial or detrimental effect. Ideally, this exercise could be accomplished while suspending judgments about the morality and legality of each of the individual addictive behaviors, at least for the duration of the exercise. Legality and morality concerns often cloud our ability to look across addictive behaviors to get an overall view of strategies and policies. Of course, legality and illegality are critical dimensions and ultimately must be considered. However, part of the problem with our strategies and policies to manage addictive behaviors has been the inconsistencies and anomalies created because of distinctions based on legality. Moreover, these distinctions have influenced policy research and restricted the types of questions that are examined. In order to adequately evaluate the value of their laws and strategies, policymakers need to examine their efforts to regulate and control all addictive behaviors, including alcohol, nicotine, marijuana, heroin, cocaine, prescription drugs, and gambling without blinders imposed by the restriction that this one is legal, this one illegal.

Conflicts of interest and mixed messages are abundant in our societal policies and laws with regard to many different addictive behaviors. A recent editorial piece on the tobacco settlement published in the Baltimore Sun by Dave Barry, cartoonist and satirist, illustrates the problem. He pointed out that as a result of the currently proposed settlement between the tobacco companies and the United States, tobacco companies would now have to admit that they produce a product that kills people and that from now on they could do this only under the watchful eye of the Federal Drug Administration. Moreover, the tobacco companies would have to pay large sums of monies to the lawyers and the government that would come from the profits they made from continuing to sell these products to people in our country and throughout the world. On the other hand, the government would continue to subsidize farmers who grow tobacco and receive large sums of revenues from the taxes on the sale of tobacco products.

Policy confusion and conflicts also abound with regard to alcohol consumption and gambling behavior. Governments are in the business of regulating and promoting, restricting and providing access to these behaviors all at the same time. Liquor licenses and alcohol taxes provide important sources of revenue and an ability to control the sale and distribution of alcohol. Gambling provides the most recent example of the multiple roles of government with regard to an addictive behavior. Recently, lottery officials in Maryland were criticized for going to shopping malls where senior citizens were walking and demonstrating to them how easy it was to play the lottery. State lotteries often advertise and entice individuals to play the lottery in order to gain revenue for worthwhile projects in education, child care, and the like. In fact, most lotteries were marketed to the citizens of the states that adopted them as means of gaining revenue for important social agendas. This is done with the knowledge that such access would increase the numbers of addicted gamblers and create addiction. In some states, enlightened legislators recognizing both sides of the coin have dedicated a percentage of the revenue for a hot line and treatment referral service for problem gamblers. These policies with their inherent contradictions play an important role in the attempts by societies to manage addictive behaviors and pose great difficulties for policy researchers seeking to examine the impact of any single policy.

Conflicted societal and government relationships with each of the various addictive behaviors can influence the initiation and maintenance of the problematic behaviors and impact the process of recovery. Acknowledging the conflicted and multiple relationships would mark the beginning of society emerging from a Precontemplation stage with regard to changing practices to reflect a more thoughtful and coordinated set of strategies and policies. Leaders must consider the pros and cons of each of the strategies they propose. For every proposed policy related to addictive behaviors legislative staffers should be required to develop a list of potentially positive and negative influences on the process of addiction and recovery. This decision-making list should be presented to the lawmakers and discussed in the development of any policy. Action plans should be tested out in various settings and evaluated for their impact on engagement or recovery. This evaluation and implementation process will take time and energy. However, such a process is critical to developing sane and successful addiction control strategies. Policymakers will have to work through the tasks of Contemplation and Preparation before taking Action. They will have to curb desires to provide a quick fix or to respond reflexively to a particular event. The notion that whatever is done in good faith cannot be harmful is misguided. Every strategy and policy has the potential to increase and to decrease the frequency of engagement in addictive behaviors as well as the pain and suffering that result from them. Only information generated through research and program evaluation that address key questions can effectively guide policymakers.

What follows is one example of a policy analysis on the medical use of marijuana that evaluates the impact of such a policy from a process of change perspective. Such an analysis generates clearly researchable questions that could guide the formation and implementation of policy on medical marijuana.

The issue facing policymakers is whether to legalize the smoking of marijuana for the relief of nausea and other symptoms of pain and discomfort related to chronic administration of cancer medications or treatment of other chronic conditions. Proponents believe that this is a humane act with little or no impact on the drug abuse problem. Critics argue that this is simply a foot-in-the-door strategy to promote the argument for legalization of marijuana use in this country. The analysis focuses on how making or failing to make policy could impact engagement in or recovery from an addictive behavior.

An Impact Analysis on Engagement

Allowing or not allowing medical use of marijuana raises many questions about how each of these options would influence the process of becoming addicted. Will viewing marijuana as a medicine increase its attractiveness to the young adolescent or adult in the Precontemplation or Contemplation stage with regard to marijuana use? Does medical use legitimize its use in other situations? On the other hand, will banning medical use create a criminalization of a use that will be viewed as overreaching by a significant segment of the population? Will this perception foster a lack of credibility in policy or policymakers that can set the stage for some rebellious backlash in attitudes about marijuana use? Is medical marijuana destined to produce dependent use that extends across the individual's lifestyle and creates an addiction? What are the consequences of this dependence, if medical marijuana is legal or if it is illegal? Will dependence on marijuana that is created by medical use influence positively or negatively personal or social consequences? Can individuals who will use marijuana medicinally keep its use under self-regulatory, situational control? What impact would use of marijuana by the patient have on other peers, family members, or acquaintances in terms of their potential for moving through the stages of initiation of marijuana use? If we make medicinal use illegal, will we be able to enforce this ban? Will we create a black market in marijuana for medicinal purposes that would create an industry dedicated to increasing use? Can we regulate the distribution of the substance and create a legal but limited access that would be limited to medicinal use? Answers to these questions could enlighten policymakers to the risks and benefits of such a policy on the stages of Addiction.

An Impact Analysis on Recovery

A similar set of questions could evaluate the impact of such a policy on individuals in various recovery stages. Would individuals using medicinal marijuana become physically and psychologically dependent on the drug and considered addicted? How easily can they stop after medicinal use is no longer appropriate? Do we have many cases of individuals who have used medical marijuana for a time then quit and remained drug-free for long periods of time? Will it make a difference if they have a history of prior use of marijuana or other drugs? What are comparable policies related to other addictive behaviors? In the United States many individuals are legally prescribed mood- and mind-altering drugs with dependence potential for long periods of time. Would medical marijuana be most like methadone maintenance treatment that involves chronic administration of a psychoactive substance to avoid the physical and social consequences of heroin addiction? Or would it be more similar to prescription narcotics that are prescribed for pain on a short- or long-term basis regardless of the addiction potential and that seem to cause little long-term addiction when used specifically for pain (Stine & Kosten, 1999)? Or would medical marijuana be more like nicotine products, like Nicorette gum and the nicotine patch, that are now available over the counter? How would medical marijuana affect those who are already addicted to one or another addictive behavior? Would prescription of this medicinal marijuana be contraindicated for individuals who have a history of drug abuse or dependence or who have a history of abusing marijuana?

Objective, research-based answers to these questions can provide an estimate of the impact of any specific policy change on the initiation of marijuana dependence as well as on the process of recovery from addiction to marijuana. The answers to these questions also offer ideas on how to make a policy that would decrease the potential for any unwanted increase in the initiation of marijuana use among others in the immediate and larger environment. For example, calling it medical marijuana may clarify its difference with the illegal street version of the substance. Offering indications and counterindications for prescribing this medicinal regimen could possibly regulate some use without making all use by all individuals illegal. On the other hand, continuing to criminalize a use for which there are potentially documented medical benefits could undermine the credibility and impact of prevention efforts.

A comprehensive impact assessment of this type from the perspective of addiction and change could offer useful guidance to policymakers and replace heated exchanges of opinions with enlightened debates about the impact of the policy. What is needed is a research agenda that can inform the decisions. Understanding the policy impact on the naive nonuser or novice marijuana user and the process of initiation as well as on the addicted marijuana user and the process of recovery could also indicate how to implement it in a way that would maximize utility and minimize harm. Similar impact analyses and research strategies could be done for policies related to other addictive behaviors such as legalizing casino gambling, taxing cigarettes, creating lotteries, changing the drinking age, lowering legal blood alcohol concentrations, or introducing slot machines at racetracks.

SPECIAL TOPICS

Cultural Competence

How do ethnic and cultural differences affect the process of change in addiction and recovery? This is an interesting question that requires a complex answer informed by sensitive and sensible research. The first question that must be answered is whether there are unique factors or aspects of specific cultures or subgroups that would invalidate the application of the stages, processes, or markers of change of the TTM. For example, it is clear that there are biological and sociological risk and protective factors that are unique to certain ethnic subgroups. Asians have a genetic flushing response to exposure to alcohol that could have a protective effect (Segal, 1992). Alaskan and Native Americans have both biological/genetic and sociological factors that are also specific to their engagement in drinking (Castro et al., 1999; Reback, 1992; Walker et al., 1996). These risk and protective factors constitute unique cultural elements that can retard or promote movement forward through the stages of Precontemplation, Contemplation, and Preparation for alcohol consumption. Although important, these factors do not appear to necessitate a separate model of change for African Americans, Asians, or Native Americans because the TTM is being used with these populations (Center for Substance Abuse Treatment, 1999; Griffin, Gilliand, Perez, Helitzer, & Carter, 1999; Schorling, 1995).

Another set of questions that could invalidate the cross-cultural application of this intentional behavior change model concern the assumptions of the model and whether these assumptions would be applicable across ethnic or cultural subgroups. For example, a colleague who was discussing implementing a motivational interviewing and stages-of-change smoking cessation project in China suggested that the Chinese doctors that she encountered seemed to have little difficulty understanding and using the concept of stages of smoking cessation but balked at the emphasis on patient responsibility and choice contained in the motivational interviewing perspective. It seems that the doctors believed that patients should simply comply with their advice. The doctors were reluctant to spend time to discuss decision making and barriers to change with the client. The strong emphasis on authority and familial decision making in contrast to personal decision making in some societies and subcultures certainly challenges an intentional process of change. However, even in these cultures personal choice seems to play a significant role in the change process. Certainly, cultural differences in viewing the role of authority figures and ancestral influences would require a sophisticated understanding of how intentional behavior change operates in that society. However, there does not appear to be a society or subgroup where intentional change and personal decision making are completely inoperative. For individuals becoming addicted or recovering in more traditional cultures the societal and family systems in their context of change would be particularly salient. Research on these cultural dimensions and what they mean for the process of change is just beginning. However, at this point it seems that although the importance of social and familial influences on the decision-making process would have to be evaluated to address cultural influences, most cultures and subcultures would not necessitate a separate model of change. The possible exception might be repressive societies where there is little or no choice and behavior change is imposed by force and punishment. Even in this case the problem would be the lack of opportunity for intentional in contrast to imposed change rather that the inappropriateness of an intentional change model.

Cultural competence would require adaptation in the dimensions of change rather than a complete rethinking of the process of change. There is growing support for using this model of addictive behavior change in many different countries around the world. The stages of change, in particular, have been successfully adapted to be used in Australia, Canada, China, Germany, Great Britain, Greece, Ireland, Italy, Japan, the Netherlands, New Zealand, South America, Spain,Switzerland, and other countries (Etter et al., 1997; Keller et al., 1999; Kohler et al., 1999; Miller & Heather, 1998; Schmid & Gmel, 1999; Weinstein et al., 1998). Although much of the research on the model to date has been conducted in English-speaking populations, there are numerous addiction programs and research projects based on the model in non-English-speaking countries of Brazil, China, Germany, Greece, Italy, the Netherlands, Norway, Spain, and others.

My experiences and reading in the area of cultural influences lead me to the conclusion that the basic dimensions of change and the view of the process of change offered by the TTM are compatible with different cultural perspectives. Intentional behavior change is an important element that contributes to becoming addicted or to moving into recovery no matter what the culture or ethnic group. However, there are important differences that should be taken into account as one attempts to apply the model to specific subgroups of individuals. These subgroups could be classified according to religion, country of origin, gender, ethnic background, or cultural identity. There may be important differences that affect the process of change even among individuals within the similar ethnic or language subgroups (e.g., Hispanics who come from Mexico and those who come from Puerto Rico). However, examining cross-cultural decision making, the processes of change, self-efficacy, and the stages of change to determine empirically whether and how much adaptation is needed could provide information about differences among subgroups and subcultures. Cultural adaptations of the TTM of intentional behavior change in addictions, in fact, can provide a rich source of conceptual and clinical questions to advance our understanding of the process of change and of what it means to be culturally competent.

There are some obvious areas of adaptation that should be examined in every culture or subgroup where the model is applied. The marker of decisional balance should be evaluated to make sure that it contains the considerations and situations that reflect subgroup differences. Finding the value system and culturally relevant influences that promote movement from Precontemplation to Contemplation involves examining the cultural background and learning history of the individual and his or her social group. First-generation immigrants would differ from fifth-generation landowners, African Americans from Hispanics. The value system that the individual brings to the Contemplation stage is critical in decision making. How the behavior fits in or is discrepant with the cultural origins and upbringing of the individual can make a big difference in whether the individual adopts or stops the behavior.

Understanding cultural and subgroup influences and values can also be helpful in creating experiences and developing techniques that can successfully engage the cognitive/experiential and behavioral processes of change needed to move through the stages. Engaging self-reevaluation and environmental reevaluation requires approaches and conversations that are personally relevant and culturally sophisticated. Engaging emotional arousal/dramatic relief and social liberation involves understanding the value of emotions and the relevant social norms in the culture. Longshore, Grills, and Annon (1999) developed an innovative treatment engagement research project for Los Angeles drug-addicted African American youth that incorporated a solid understanding of African American cultural roots. Their treatment entry strategy used two counselors, because a one-to-one counseling setting was not as culturally appropriate, and a location where they could cook food and discuss the client's addiction problem in the context of a meal. This program was more successful in engaging clients in terms of stage movement and treatment entry when compared with a traditional triage system of engagement and referral (Longshore et al., 1999). There are also interesting anecdotes of how counselors use cultural considerations to engage addicted individuals in the process of change. Other reported cultural adaptations are Native American counselors using sweat lodges in their treatments in order to engage and move their clients through the stages and Hispanic counselors focusing on family of origin issues in promoting reasons for recovery (Center for Substance Abuse Treatment Treatment Improvement Protocol No. 35, p. 85, 1999).

Cultural competence also includes avoiding some problematic techniques that do not fit with a client's culture. For example, a highly affect-laden approach where counselors or clients hug or touch each other would be problematic for many Asian clients, whose sense of personal space and appropriate distance could be violated in such a setting. Finding and using messages and techniques that can sensitively engage cognitive/experiential processes of change while respecting the values and cultural practices of clients is a critical component for cultural competence.

In a similar manner it is important to understand the environment, social network, and social systems that exist in subcultures and groups in order to effectively engage behavioral processes of change and to comprehend the context of change. There are practices and rituals among subcultures that could influence the processes of reinforcement management, helping relationship, and self-liberation as well as the conditioning processes of stimulus control and counterconditioning. Assertiveness training, group treatment, and self-help groups may not be appropriate or effective in cultures that value self-effacement and privacy. There may be culturally sensitive ways to teach relaxation using either Eastern or Western techniques. There may be specific important individuals from whom praise and reinforcement would be particularly potent. Understanding the social environment could also assist in creating efficacy probes that would include situations and scenarios that would be unique to the particular client from a subculture. Similarly, knowledge of the culture of any particular majority or minority group would assist intervenors in understanding unique problems or issues that could arise in the various areas of functioning in the context of change.

Cultural competence in promoting the process of change requires an understanding of the values, practices, social influences, and social structure of a subgroup in order to be able to engage the appropriate processes of change, to understand the client's perspective in his or her decisional considerations, and to assist in restructuring the environment. Understanding cultural and ethnic customs and practices can assist researchers, counselors, and program developers to avoid labeling as pathological cultural practices which are acceptable in that subculture and which help them problem solve issues that arise in the context of change. Ultimately, the individual who is moving through the stages of addiction or recovery must comprehend and integrate the relevant cultural considerations and influences into his or her process of change. The challenge for the counselor and the researcher is to find out for whom and how particular cultural influences and factors play a role in the process of change (O'Connor, Carbonari, & DiClemente, 1996). Then they can adjust their efforts to more effectively incorporate cultural considerations in their research and interventions to prevent or promote movement through the stages of change for addiction or recovery.

Medications and Pharmacological Interventions

A significant amount of effort and energy is being dedicated to developing medications that can assist individuals to stop using substances or quit addictive behaviors (Barber & O'Brien, 1999). There are several types of pharmacological aids. Some medications try to block the effect of the substance or addictive behavior so there is no high (naltrexone, ondonsetrim, acamprosate). Other pharmacological agents try to substitute a less problematic substance or delivery system for the addictive behavior or substance (nicotine replacement, methadone maintenance). Some substances are used to create negative reactions when combined with the drug in order to promote abstinence and discourage relapse (disulfiram or Antabuse). Finally, there are medications to treat associated conditions or to relieve the distress of withdrawal effects.

One of the interesting, underresearched issues in the field of addiction treatment is how these medications interact with the process of change. Discussions of medication effects often concentrate on the biological mechanisms that are affected by the particular medication or pharmacological agent and how these are related to the biological actions of cocaine, heroin, or alcohol (Allen & Litten, 1999). Most medications are tested in efficacy trials using a backdrop of some type of psychosocial intervention as well as the medication. The efficacy of nicotine substitutes, for example, has been tested with a behavioral change package given to the participants. Medications to manage alcohol and drug cravings have been examined, usually in combination with a cognitive-behavioral group treatment (Johnson et al., 2000) or a brief motivational intervention (Volpicelli, Pettinati, McClellan, & O'Brien, 2001). Participants given placebos are also given the psychosocial intervention so that in order for the medication to be approved the active medication effect must exceed that of placebo and psychosocial treatment. However, little is done to separate out the effects due to either the placebo or the medication from the effects of the psychosocial treatments. Thus, there is little understanding of how psychosocial treatments interact with pharmacological agents in terms of compliance with dosage and the research protocol or in terms of movement through the process of change (Beitman et al., 1994; DiClemente & Scott, 1997). This seems to be particularly important because recent evidence indicates that placebos may produce effects through sometimes similar, sometimes dissimilar neurological mechanisms in the brain (Holden, 2002; Mayberg et al., 2002).

Using medications and other agents to counter substance abuse offers a unique opportunity to examine many interesting questions about the process of change and how these agents interact with the intentional process of behavior change. One central question that can be addressed is that of intrinsic and extrinsic motivation and how they interact (DiClemente, Bellino, & Neavins, 1999). Many individuals who seek pharmacotherapy for their addiction are looking for an external aid that can make them stop smoking, drinking, or drugging. Some are really expecting a miracle despite warnings against such expectations from the prescribing professionals. Thus, medication can interfere with the process of intentional behavior change if it is viewed as an extrinsic agent that will make the change for the individual instead of as an aid and part of a more comprehensive change plan.

Medications can have a variable impact on the process of change. They can undermine or inflate self-efficacy, enable individuals to begin to make a change without a decisional balance sufficient to support change, or discourage use of essential behavioral processes of change. On the other hand, medications can play a significant role in helping clients achieve successful recovery by decreasing temptation to use, supporting stimulus control by helping them avoid cues or by decreasing cues to drink or drug, providing enhanced counterconditioning effects by reducing negative emotions, and offering an individual short-term support that enable clients to increase confidence to abstain and to establish alternate reinforcers that can support long-term change. How medications interact with movement through the stages for each individual poses intriguing questions that demand more sophisticated research designs that can examine these potential interactions.

Existing research studies on the effectiveness of medication do provide some clues to figuring out the interactions between medications and intentional behavior change. Compliance with medication is a critical indicator of success in pharmacological trials and is related to motivation and making a commitment to a plan of change (Monti, Rohsenhow, et al., 2001). Many medication trials are of brief duration (3–4 months) and measure outcomes primarily during the time of active dosing of the medication. Thus they examine mostly Action and not always the effects of the medication on Maintenance of change. This is particularly true for those medications not designed to be substitutes for the addictive behavior, like methadone. Finally, many medication trials require a "wash out" period where the individual must stop using the substance for a period of time (a couple of days to a week or two) before they are allowed to go on the medication in order to prevent drug interactions and side effects of such interactions (Johnson et al., 2000). However, this requires clients to demonstrate some self-control of the addictive behavior even before the medication is administered. How this "wash out" period interacts with decision making and how it may necessitate the use of behavioral processes of change prior to the initiation of medication would make a fascinating area of study. It may be that individuals who are able to do this are more motivated and have more intact self-control systems than many of the individuals who fail to get into these medication trials. In any case, there are significant interactions between pharmacological interventions and how they are studied and many different elements of the process of intentional behavior change.

There are numerous research questions that remain to be answered in this area. How does the entry stage of the individual seeking pharmacotherapy interact with future success? Is the placebo effect in drug trials simply a reflection of self-change? How does the belief that a client has a pharmacological aid to help make a change affect the change process for those who have no active medication? The most tempted individuals would seem to need a pharmacological aid the most. However, they may be the least likely to be able to enter a medication trial because they may fail the wash out period. Is this true? What stage of change would be most appropriate for entry into a medication trial? Can we change decisional considerations with a quit attempt that is supported by medication? How does the individual who has been able to stay away from the addictive behavior with the aid of some pharmacological intervention transition into using psychosocial behavioral processes of change once the chemical aid is removed? What effects do the different types of pharmacological aids (substitutes, blockers, and negative reaction inducers) have on the process of intentional behavior change? Long-term administration of methadone substitutes dependence on one type of substance for another. What is the impact of substitution on the process of change for the targeted addictive behavior (heroin) and for other nontargeted addictive behaviors? Finally, what are the best ways to integrate medication into the process of recovery and how can we create a synergy between the intentional change process and the biological effects created by the pharmacological agent? This is an exciting series of questions that could launch significant new areas of research.

Harm Reduction

Harm reduction approaches to addiction include a wide range of intervention strategies that have as a common theme minimizing risk or harm associated with the addictive behavior and offering healthier choices to those who are engaged in an addictive behavior (MacCoun, 1998). Harm reduction efforts began initially in reaction to the AIDS epidemic and the need to reduce risky behaviors that contribute to HIV infection, like needle sharing by drug abusers (E. T. Miller, Turner, & Marlatt, 2001). Advocates suggested that distributing clean needles and offering bleach and other ways to cleanse needles would prevent the spread of infections and thereby reduce harm. Harm reduction strategies, however, are widespread across addictive behaviors (see Chapter 11). Designated driver initiatives, free taxi rides home after drinking, warning addicts about tainted cocaine supplies, methadone maintenance programs, attempts to create safer cigarettes, training bartenders not to serve already intoxicated patrons, and Breathalyzer-controlled ignition systems are all harm reduction programs for individuals who are actively engaged in an addictive behavior. Often harm reduction prevention programs are directed at individuals who are in the earlier stages of acquisition for an addictive behavior (Baer, 1993; Marlatt et al., 1998). Initiatives such as reducing risky binge drinking among college students, providing condoms in the restrooms of places where alcohol is sold, testing substances prior to use to make sure of purity, and guaranteed rides after proms and parties for students who are drinking illegally are directed at those who may be experimenting or learning how to self-manage drinking or drug use so that they will not experience irrevocable harm in the process (E. T. Miller et al., 2001).

Critics of harm reduction strategies argue that these strategies promote use and fail to preach abstinence as the best or only harm reduction strategy (MacCoun, 1998). However, as in the earlier discussion on policymaking, the real test of harm reduction strategies is how much harm they prevent and how much impact they have on the process of addiction and recovery. Once again legality complicates the questions and the answers. One of the biggest issues in harm reduction is that it often operates alongside of laws that prohibit the addictive behavior. Although it is illegal to be served and drink alcohol if you are under age 21 in most states, offering free rides to intoxicated students who are under 21 years of age is a viable harm reduction strategy. Methadone and needle exchanges required separate laws that allow their distribution to heroin-addicted individuals. Teaching 19- and 20-year-old college students how to drink responsibly often is complicated by the legal drinking age (Baer, 1993; Baer, Marlatt, & McMahon, 1993). Nevertheless, the key questions to be addressed in the research on harm reduction strategies should focus on how these interventions interact with the process of change involved in becoming addicted and in getting into recovery.

Although there is growing evidence of the effectiveness of needle exchange programs in reducing the incidence of STD and HIV infections (Marlatt & Tapert, 1993), there continue to be concerns about this type of harm reduction program. Both critics and advocates could make better arguments based on research analyzing the impact of these programs on the process of change for addiction and recovery (Bowen & Trotter, 1995).

An Impact Analysis of Needle Exchange on Addiction

What is the impact of needle exchange programs on individuals who are not those already addicted to heroin or cocaine? Do needle exchanges increase the number of individuals using injection drugs? Will this program increase experimentation or use of drugs because it heightens the awareness of injection drug use to the uninitiated Contemplators or makes it seem safer to individuals in the Preparation or Action stages of initiation? How do the drug addicts who use the needle exchange view the program and talk about the program to other, nonusing individuals? Will this encourage those in action for using some drugs to become injection heroin addicts? Will the impact of this program be different if the intervention is generated out of concern for the drug abuser rather than a concern about stopping the spread of HIV to nonabusing populations?

An Impact Analysis of Needle Exchange on Recovery

Many argue that offering clean needles to injection drug users condones drug use and sends the wrong message to drug abusers. However, this opinion appears driven more by sentiment and values than by data. How does this program interact with the process of recovery from addiction? Does providing a safer way to continue to use a drug prolong Precontemplation for change? Would getting a drug user to be concerned about the dangers to health that are related to injecting drugs increase the cons of drug use and move him or her to Contemplation of recovery? Does the added safety of the needles prolong the time spent in Contemplation and reduce the salience of the dangers of using, thus tilting the decisional balance against change? Can the needle exchange programs be used to bring messages and to increase motivation that would promote cessation of heroin and other injected drug use? Are the individuals who take part in the needle exchange always in early stages of recovery? Is it better to have access to drug abusers who are not in treatment than to ignore them until they come to the treatment providers? Will proactive contact increase the speed of movement through the stages of recovery? Do we have effective interventions for Precontemplating and Contemplating drug abusers that could be brought to bear while distributing the needles?

Once research can answer some of these questions or similar ones about needle exchange programs, then we can evaluate the true impact as well as the benefits and risks of harm reduction strategies. Even if a program of harm reduction does not move an individual forward in the process of recovery, it can be useful in light of the harm avoided coupled with the lack of any seriously negative effects either in stopping addicts from going through the stages of recovery or in getting uninitiated individuals into problems with the addictive behavior. Moreover, it is important to note that harm reduction is not the opposite of abstinence and that abstinence is a harm reduction strategy. In fact, getting individuals to consider the harm or consequences related to their engaging in the addictive behavior can actually increase Contemplation stage activities and contribute to the reevaluation that would be needed to move forward in the stages of recovery (DiClemente, 1999a).

Comorbidity and Dual Diagnosis

Current state and federal funding procedures usually separate addiction treatment from treatment of mental disorders. The ensuing dilemma created by this dualistic provider system has been that individuals who have both diagnosable mental illness and addiction disorders have difficulty finding comprehensive services and pose problems for providers. However, comorbidity, that is, the existence of two or more diagnosable problems, is not a new phenomenon. Individuals with addictions often have multiple serious problems in addition to the addiction. Some of these are diagnosable as medical problems and others as mental health problems that range from anxiety and depression to schizophrenia and manic–depression to posttraumatic stress and psychopathic or other personality disorders (American Psychiatric Association, 1994; Rosenthal & Westreich, 1999). The problem of comorbidity has been institutionalized in the current term, dual diagnosis. However, dual diagnosis is only a label created in order to alert treatment systems that at least two problems need attention and that there is a need to coordinate their efforts. The reality is that many individuals have multiple problems at clinical or preclinical levels that span the areas of addictive behaviors and mental health. The plight of the multiply diagnosed individual poses interesting and researchable questions about the process of change involved in addiction and recovery.

Mental health problems are a recognizable risk factor involved in the process of becoming addicted (Rosenthal & Westreich, 1999). The psychotropic effects of drugs and alcohol provide significant reinforcing effects, particularly for people troubled by anxiety, depression, fears, mania, and psychotic symptoms. Distressed individuals suffering from these conditions learn to abuse substances more quickly and have fewer protective factors and resources to support self-regulation. These emotional and psychological conditions can impact the process of change by influencing decisional considerations, interfering with cognitive/experiential and behavioral processes of change, undermining self-efficacy, and increasing temptations to engage in the addictive behavior. How this vulnerability operates to move individuals forward through the stages of addiction is the key to understanding the high comorbidity prevalence of addiction in the mentally ill (Regier et al., 1990).

On the other hand, addictive behaviors can trigger or contribute to the development of psychiatric disorders. Psychotropic substances create altered brain and mood states that most often are ephemeral and last only as long as the drug's biologically active life. However, at times drug effects can trigger severe reactions that last well beyond the drug-taking incident. Many initial psychotic breaks in individuals who later become diagnosed with schizophrenia or manic–depression co-occur with drug or alcohol use, although it is not always clear whether drug use simply provided an occasion or was a contributory cause to the psychotic symptoms and emerging mental illness (Muesser et al., 1992). The interplay between mental illness and addiction is complicated and reciprocal. The interaction is best understood in light of the process of becoming addicted in order to tease apart effects of decision making, impaired judgment, behavioral engagement, and progression to addiction.

Once an individual has become addicted and has a serious mental illness, the challenge becomes one of trying to see how to engage the process of recovery for the two chronic conditions of addiction and mental illness. The TTM views the process of recovery from both types of problems as similar. The mental illness may require continual medication management and compliance with medication as well as other behavior changes as the target of the change process (Prochaska & DiClemente, 1984). However, the dually diagnosed individual would have to access the intentional process of behavior change in order to manage the mental illness as well as to recover from addiction (Ziedonis & Trudeau, 1997). Some concerns have been raised as to whether individuals with serious mental illness can access the intentional process of change in order to move into recovery from the addiction (Bellack & DiClemente, 1999). Research is needed to determine the extent to which the process of change is similar across the different domains of problems presented by dually diagnosed individuals.

Some of the initial research in this area supports the existence of an intentional process of change among dually diagnosed individuals with alcohol and drug problems. Velasquez and colleagues (1999) found that psychiatric symptoms interacted with the change dimensions of the TTM. Specifically, psychiatric severity increased temptation to drink and reduced behavioral coping among a sample of dually diagnosable individuals. Moreover, the dimensions of change focused on their drinking problems demonstrated interrelationships that paralleled those found with other, non-dually diagnosed alcohol-abusing and -dependent populations. Hagedorn's recent study (2000) examined decisional considerations related to alcohol abuse in a dually diagnosed sample of individuals with chronic schizophrenia and alcohol problems. She replicated the structure of the alcohol decisional balance scale and found that, although there are some unique pro and con considerations for dually diagnosed populations, the basic elements of decision making were similar in structure and relationship with other change dimensions to that found in other samples of alcohol abusers. Alan Bellack and I are currently examining this process of change for individuals who are dually diagnosed with schizophrenia and cocaine abuse and comparing them with individuals who have a chronic, nonschizophrenia, serious mental illness and cocaine abuse. Initial results support the use of this intentional process of addictive behavior change even among these dually diagnosed individuals (Bellack, Gearon, & DiClemente, 2001). Clearly, the intentional behavior change process is significantly disrupted when there is an active psychotic episode. However, when psychotic symptoms are managed and under some control, the change process for recovery from addiction appears to be operative and the change dimensions of the TTM to be relevant.

Additional research is needed to understand the interplay between the dual problems of dually diagnosed individuals as well as to tease apart the interactions between addictive behaviors and mental illness involved in the addiction and recovery process. A recent vignette that appeared in the *Consumer's Corner* (2001, pp. 26–27) described the experience of an individual who achieved abstinence from alcohol and drugs for over 13 years. However, during that time he continued to be a Precontemplator for change with regard to his mental illness. Only after several divorces and other problems that occurred while he remained abstinent from alcohol and drugs did he acknowledge that the addiction was not the only problem and that his manic–depression was a problem that needed to be addressed. Individuals can be in different stages for each disorder. Successfully maintained change in one does not necessarily guarantee readiness to change another.

Dually diagnosed individuals bring clearly into focus how multiple problems and the context of change can influence the process of recovery from addiction. Most often, dually diagnosed individuals have multiple problems that have different behavior change targets and need different types of interventions. Aggressive case management that continues over long periods of time seems to be the only effective strategy to manage multiple problems that require effective action in order to move the individuals forward to successful behavior change on multiple fronts (Higgins, 1999; Minkoff, 1989; Osher & Kofoed, 1989).

A FINAL NOTE

The universal nature of the intentional behavior change process helps the clinician and researcher to avoid a myopic focus on a single addictive behavior and a quixotic search for a separate change process for every problem. The important dimensions of change outlined in the TTM of change provide the tools with which to examine the process of intentional behavior change. This process can help us to understand the pathways into and out of addictions and offers a framework for the development and design of research that can sensitively explore the phenomena of addiction and change. In addition, the specificity and generalizability of the change dimensions provide a way to focus in on specific behavioral changes without losing a more holistic perspective. Research on addictions should respect both the specificity of the behavior change and the universality of the change process. The TTM and the intentional behavior change process offer a unique perspective that can enrich outcome and process research, program evaluation, and policy research. Moreover, current critical issues in the field of addictions, like cultural competence, dual diagnosis, harm reduction, and pharmacotherapy could benefit from research that is sensitive to this process of change and incorporates change dimensions of the TTM. Although this model has been in existence for 20 years, its application to the process of addiction and recovery continues to offer new insights and yield important new information about addiction and change.

References

Abrams, D. B., Herzog, T. A., Emmons, K. M., & Linnan, L. (2000). Stages of change versus addiction: a replication and extension. *Nicotine and Tobacco Research, 2*(3), 223–229.

Abrams, D. B., Orleans, C. T., Niaura, R. S., Goldstein, M. G., Prochaska, J. O., & Velicer, W. (1996). Integrating individual and public health perspectives for treatment of tobacco dependence under managed health care: A combined stepped-care and matching model. *Annals of Behavioral Medicine, 18,* 290–304.

Adesso, V. J. (1985) Cognitive factors in alcohol and drug abuse. In M. Galizio & S. Maisto (Eds.), *Determinants of substance abuse: Biological, psychological and environmental factors* (pp. 179–208). New York: Plenum Press.

Alcoholics Anonymous. (1952). *Twelve steps and twelve traditions.* New York: Alcoholics Anonymous World Services.

Alcoholics Anonymous. (1976). *Alcoholics Anonymous (The Blue Book).* New York: Alcoholics Anonymous World Services.

Allen, J. P., & Litten, R. Z. (1999). Treatment of drug and alcohol abuse: An overview of major strategies and effectiveness. In B. S. McCrady & E. E. Epstein (Eds.), *Addictions: A comprehensive guidebook* (pp. 385–398). New York: Oxford University Press.

American Psychiatric Association. (1980). *Diagnostic and statistical manual of mental disorders* (3rd ed.). Washington, DC: Author.

American Psychiatric Association. (1994). *Diagnostic and statistical manual of mental disorders* (4th ed.). Washington, DC: Author.

Anglin, M. D., & Hser, Y. (1992). Drug abuse treatment. In R. R. Watson (Ed.), *Drug abuse treatment* (pp. 1–36). Totowa, NJ: Humana Press.

Babor, T., & Del Boca, F. (Eds.). (2002). *Treatment matching in alcoholism.* New York: Cambridge University Press.

Babor, T. F., Steinberg, K., Anton, R., & Del Boca, F. (2000). Talk is cheap: Measuring drinking outcomes in clinical trials. *Journal of Studies on Alcohol, 61,* 55–63.

Baer, J. S. (1993). Etiology and secondary prevention of alcohol problems with young adults. In J. S. Baer, G. A. Marlatt, & R. J. McMahon (Eds.), *Addictive behaviors across the lifespan: Prevention, treatment and policy issues* (pp. 111–137). Newbury Park, CA: Sage.

Baer, J. S., Kivlahan, D. R., Blume, A. W., McKinght, P., & Marlatt, G. A. (2001). Brief intervention for heavy drinking college students: 4-year follow-up and natural history. *American Journal of Public Health, 91*, 1310–1316.

Baer, J. S., Marlatt, G. A., & McMahon R. J. (Eds.). (1993). *Addictive behaviors across the lifespan: Prevention, treatment and policy issues.* Newbury Park, CA: Sage.

Bailey, S. L., & Rachal, J. V. (1993). Dimensions of adolescent problem drinking. *Journal of Studies on Alcohol, 54*(5), 555–565.

Bandura, A. (1977). The anatomy of stages of change [Editorial]. *American Journal of Health Promotion, 12*, 8–10.

Bandura, A. (1986). *Social foundations of thought and action: A social cognitive theory.* Englewood Cliffs, NJ: Prentice-Hall.

Bandura, A. (1997). *Self-efficacy: The exercise of control.* New York: Freeman.

Barber, W. S., & O'Brien, C. P. (1999). Pharmacotherapies. In B. S. McCrady & E. E. Epstein (Eds.), *Addictions: A comprehensive guidebook* (pp. 3747–369). New York: Oxford University Press.

Baron, R. M., & Kenny, D. A. (1986). The moderator–mediator variable distinction in social psychological research: Conceptual, strategic, and statistical considerations. *Journal of Personality and Social Psychology, 51*, 1173–1182.

Barrett, R. J. (1985). Behavioral approaches to individual differences in substance abuse: Drug-taking behavior. In M. Galizio & S. A. Maisto (Eds.), *Determinants of substance abuse: Biological, psychological and environmental factors* (pp. 125–178). New York: Plenum Press.

Beattie, M., & Longabaugh, R. (1999). General and alcohol-specific social support following treatment. *Addictive Behaviors, 24*(5), 593–606.

Beck, A. T., Wright, F. D., Newman, C. F., & Liese, B. S. (1993). *Cognitive therapy of substance abuse.* New York: Guilford Press.

Becker, M. H., & Maiman, L. A. (1975). Socio-behavioral determinants of compliance with health and medical care recommendations. *Medical Care, 13*, 10–24.

Begleiter, H., & Porjesz, B. (1999). What is inherited in the predisposition toward alcoholism? A proposed model. *Alcoholism: Clinical and Experimental Research, 23*, 1125–1135.

Beitman, B. D., Beck, N. C., Deuser, W., Carter, C., Davidson, J., & Maddock, R. (1994). Patient stages of change predicts outcome in a panic disorder medication trial. *Anxiety, 1*, 64–69.

Belding, M., Iguchi, M., & Lamb, R. J. (1996). Stages of change in methadone maintenance: Assessing the convergent validity of two measures. *Psychology of Addictive Behaviors, 10*, 157–166.

Bellack, A. S., & DiClemente, C. C. (1999) Treating substance abuse among patients with schizophrenia. *Psychiatric Services, 50*(1), 75–80.

Bellack, A. S., Gearon, J., & DiClemente, C. C. (2001, May). *The process of change in substance abuse in schizophrenia.* Poster presented at the International Congress on Schizophrenia, Whistler, British Columbia, Canada.

Bergin, A. E., & Garfield, S. L. (1994). *Handbook of psychotherapy and behavior change* (4th ed.). New York: Wiley.

Bien, T. H., Miller, W. R., & Tonigan, J. S. (1993). Brief interventions for alcohol problems: A review. *Addiction, 88*(3), 315–336.

Biener, L., Aseltine, R. H., Cohen, B., & Anderka, M. (1998). Reactions of adult and teenaged smokers to the Massachusetts Tobacco Tax. *American Journal of Public Health, 88*, 1398–1391.

Bishop, F. M. (2001). *Managing addictions: Cognitive, emotive and behavioral techniques.* Northvale, NJ: Jason Aronson.

Blume, A. W., & Schmaling, K. B. (1997). Specific classes of symptoms predict readiness to change scores among dually diagnosed patients. *Addictive Behaviors, 22*(5), 625–630.

Bobo, J. K., & Husten, C. S. (2000). Sociocultural influences on smoking and drinking. *Alcohol Research and Health World, 24*, 225–232.

Botvin, G. J., Baker, E., Dusenbury, L., Botvin, E. M., & Diaz, T. (1995). Long-term follow-up results of a randomized drug abuse prevention trial in a white middle class population. *Journal of the American Medical Association, 273*(14), 1106–1112.

Bowen, A., & Trotter, R. (1995). HIV risk in intravenous drug users and crack cocaine smokers: Predicting stage of change for condom use. *Journal of Consulting and Clinical Psychology, 63*, 238–248.

Brown, S. (1985). *Treating the alcoholic: A developmental model of recovery.* New York: Wiley.

Brown, S., & Yalom, I. D. (Eds.). (1995). *Treating alcoholism.* San Francisco, CA: Jossey-Bass.

Brown, S. A. (1993). Recovery patterns in adolescent substance abuse. In J. S. Baer, G. A. Marlatt, & R. J. McMahon (Eds.), *Addictive behaviors across the lifespan: Prevention, treatment and policy issues* (pp. 161–183). Newbury Park, CA: Sage.

Brown, S. A., Carello, P. D., Vik, P. W., & Porter, R. J. (1998). Change in alcohol effect and self-efficacy expectancies during addiction treatment. *Substance Abuse, 19*(4), 155–168.

Brown, S. A., Creamer, V. A., & Stetson, B. A. (1987). Adolescent alcohol expectancies in relation to personal and parental drinking patterns. *Journal of Abnormal Psychology, 96*, 117–121.

Brown, S. A., Goldman, M. S., & Christiansen, B. A. (1985). Do alcohol expectancies mediate drinking patterns of adults. *Journal of Consulting and Clinical Psychology, 53*, 512–519.

Brown, S. A., Goldman, M. S., Inn, A., & Anderson, L. R. (1980). Expectations of reinforcement from alcohol: Their domain and relation to drinking patterns. *Journal of Consulting and Clinical Psychology, 48*, 419–426.

Brown, V. B., Melchior, L. A., Panter, A. T., Slaughter, R., & Huba, G. J. (2000) Women's steps of change and entry into drug abuse treatment: A multidimensional stages of change model. *Journal of Substance Abuse Treatment, 18*(3), 231–240.

Brown, V. B., Ridgely, S. M., Pepper, R. M. S., Levine, L. S., & Ryglewicz, H. (1989). The dual crisis: Mental illness and substance abuse. *American Psychologist, 44*(3), 565–569.

Brownell, K., Marlatt, G. A., Lichtenstein, E., & Wilson, C. T. (1986). Understanding and preventing relapse. *American Psychologist, 41*, 765–782.

Bryk, A. S., & Raudenbush, S. W. (1987). Application of hierarchical linear models to assessing change. *Psychological Bulletin, 101*, 147–158.

Cadoret, R. J. (1992). Genetic and environmental factors in the initiation of drug use and the transition to abuse. In M. Glantz & R. Pickens (Eds.), *Vulnerability to drug abuse* (pp. 99–113). Washington, DC: American Psychological Association.

Cappell, H., & Greeley, J. (1987). Alcohol and tension reduction: An update on research and theory. In H. T. Blane & K. E. Leonard (Eds.), *Psychological theories of drinking and alcoholism* (pp. 15–89). New York: Guilford Press.

Carbonari, J. P., & DiClemente, C. C. (2000). Using Transtheoretical Model profiles to differentiate levels of alcohol abstinence success. *Journal of Consulting and Clinical Psychology, 68*(5), 810–817.

Carbonari, J. P., DiClemente, C. C., & Sewell, K. B. (1999). Stage transitions and the Transtheoretical "stages of change" model of smoking cessation. *Swiss Journal of Psychology, 58*(2), 134–144.

Carey, K. B., Purnine, M. M., Maisto, S. A., & Carey, M. P. (1999). Assessing readiness to change substance abuse: A critical review of instruments. *Clinical Psychology: Science and Practice, 6*, 245–266.

Carey, K. B., Purnine, M. M., Maisto, S. A., & Carey, M. P., Barnes, K. L. (1999). Decisional balance regarding substance use among persons with schizophrenia. *Community Mental Health Journal, 35*(4), 289–299.

Carney, M. M., & Kivlahan, D. R. (1995). Motivational subtypes among veterans seeking substance abuse treatment: Profiles based on stages of change. *Psychology of Addictive Behaviors, 9*, 1135–1142.

Carroll, K. M., Connors, G. J., Cooney, N. L., DiClemente, C. C., Donovan, D. M., Kadden, R. R., Longabaugh, R. L., Rounsaville, B. J., Wirtz, P. W., & Zweben, A. (1998). Internal validity of Project MATCH treatments: Discriminability and integrity. *Journal of Consulting and Clinical Psychology, 66*, 290–303.

Castaneda, C. (1984). *The fire within*. New York: Simon & Schuster.

Castro, F. G., Proescholdbell, R. J., Abeita, L., & Rodriquez, D. (1999). Ethnic and cultural minority groups. In B. S. McCrady & E. E. Epstein (Eds.), *Addictions: A comprehensive guidebook* (pp. 499–526). New York: Oxford University Press.

Center for Substance Abuse Treatment Treatment Improvement Protocol Number 35. (1999). *Enhancing motivation for change in substance abuse treatment* (DHHS Publication No. SMA 99-3354). Washington, DC: U.S. Government Printing Office.

Cermak, T. L. (1986). *Diagnosing and treating co-dependence: A guide for professionals who work with chemical dependents, their spouses and children*. Minneapolis, MN: Johnson Institute Books.

Chassin, L., Curran, P. J., Hussong, A. M., & Colder, C. R. (1996). The relations of parent alcoholism to adolescent substance use: A longitudinal follow-up study. *Journal of Abnormal Psychology, 105*, 70–80.

Chassin, L., Presson, C. C., Pitts, S. C., & Sherman, S. J. (2000). The natural history of cigarette smoking from adolescence to adulthood: Multiple trajectories and their psychosocial correlates. *Health Psychology, 19*(3), 223–231.

Chassin, L., Presson, C. C., Sherman, S. J., & Edwards, D. A. (1990). The natural history of cigarette smoking: Predicting young adult outcomes from adolescent smoking. *Health Psychology, 9*(6), 701–716.

Chassin, L., Presson, C. C., Sherman, S. J., & Edwards, D. A. (1991). Four pathways to young-adult smoking status: Adolescent social-psychological antecedents in a midwestern community sample. *Health Psychology, 10,* 409–418.

Chassin, L., Rogosch, F., & Barrera, M. (1991). Substance use and symptomatology among adolescent children of alcoholics. *Journal of Abnormal Psychology, 100*(4), 449–463.

Choi, W. S., Ahluwalia, J. S., & Nazir, N. (2002). Adolescent smoking cessation: Implications for relapse sensitive interventions. *Archives of Pediatric Adolescent Medicine, 156*(6), 625–626.

Cialdini, R. B. (1988). *Influence: Science and practice* (2nd ed.). Boston: Scott Foresman.

Cisler, R. A., & Zweben, A. (1999). Development of a composite measure for assessing alcohol treatment outcome: Operationalization and validation. *Alcoholism: Clinical and Experimental Research, 23*(2), 263–271.

Clark, L. F., Aaron, L., Littleton, M., Pappas-Deluca, K., Avery, J. B., & McKleroy, V. S. (1999). Stress, coping, social support and illness. In J. M. Raczynski & R. J. DiClemente (Eds.), *Handbook of health promotion and disease prevention* (pp. 123–148). New York: Kluwer Academic/Plenum Press.

Clayton, R. R. (1992) Transitions in drug use: Risk and protective factors. In M. Glantz & R. Pickens (Eds.), *Vulnerability to drug abuse* (pp. 15–51). Washington, DC: American Psychological Association.

Clayton, R., Cattarelo, A., & Johnstone, B. (1996). The effectiveness of Drug Abuse Resistance Education (Project DARE): 5-year follow-up results. *Preventive Medicine, 25,* 307–318.

Clements-Thompson, M., Klesges, R. C., Haddock, K., Lando, H., & Talcott, W. (1998). Relationships between stages of change in cigarette smokers and healthy lifestyle behavior in a population of young military personnel during forced smoking abstinence. *Journal of Consulting and Clinical Psychology, 66*(6) 1005–1011.

Cohen, S., & Lichtenstein, E. (1990). Partner behaviors that support quitting smoking. *Journal of Consulting and Clinical Psychology, 58,* 304–309.

Collins, L. M., & Horn, J. L. (1991). *Best methods for the analysis of change.* Washington, DC: American Psychological Association.

Collins, L. M., & Sayer, A. G. (2001). *New methods for the analysis of change.* Washington, DC: American Psychological Association.

Collins, R. L., Lapp, W. M., Emmons, K. M., & Isaac, L. M. (1990). Endorsement and strength of alcohol expectancies. *Journal of Studies on Alcoholism, 51,* 336–342.

Collins, R. L., Parks, G. A., & Marlatt, G. A. (1985). Social determinants of alcohol consumption: The effects of social interaction and model status on the self-administration of alcohol. *Journal of Consulting and Clinical Psychology, 53,* 189–200.

Connors, G. J., DiClemente, C. C., Dermen, K. H., Kadden, R., Carroll, K. M., &

Frone, M. R. (2000). Predicting the therapeutic alliance in alcoholism treatment. *Journal of Studies on Alcohol, 61*(1), 139–149.

Connors, G. J., Donovan, D. M., & DiClemente, C. C. (2001). *Substance abuse treatment and the stages of change: Selecting and planning interventions.* New York: Guilford Press.

Connors, G. J., Longabaugh, R., & Miller, W. R. (1996). Looking forward and back to relapse: Implications for research and practice. *Addiction, 91,* S191–S196.

Connors, G. J., Maisto, G. A., & Dermen, K. H. (1992). Alcohol-related expectancies and their applications to treatment. In R. R. Watson (Ed.), *Alcohol abuse treatment: Drug and alcohol abuse reviews 3* (pp. 203–231). Totowa, NJ: Humana Press.

Connors, G. J., & Tarbox, A. R. (1985). Macroenvironmental factors as determinants of substance use and abuse. In M. Galizio & S. A. Maisto (Eds.), *Determinants of substance abuse: Biological, psychological, and environmental factors* (pp. 283–314). New York: Plenum Press.

Consumer's Corner. (2001). Please don't label me crazy. *Dual Networker: Quarterly Publication of the Dual Diagnosis Recovery Network, 2*(1), 26–27.

Coombs, R. H., & Zeidonis, D. (Eds). (1995). *Handbook on drug abuse prevention.* New York: Allyn & Bacon.

Cooney, N. L., Babor, T. F., DiClemente, C. C., & Del Boca, F. K. (2002). Clinical and scientific implications of Project MATCH. In T. F. Babor & F. K. Del Boca (Eds.), *Treatment matching in alcoholism* (pp. 222–237). London: Cambridge University Press.

Cooper, P. J. (1995). Eating disorders and their relationship to mood and anxiety disorders. In K. D. Brownell & C. G. Fairburn (Eds.), *Eating disorders and obesity: A comprehensive handbook* (pp. 159–164). New York: Guilford Press.

Costa, P. T., & McCrae, R. R. (1992). Normal personality inventories in clinical assessment: General requirements and potential for using the NEO Personality Inventory. *Psychological Assessment, 4,* 5–13.

Cox, W. M. (1985). Personality correlates of substance abuse. In M. Galizio & S. A. Maisto (Eds.), *Determinants of substance abuse: Biological, psychological and environmental factors* (pp. 209–246). New York: Plenum Press.

Cox, W. M. (1987). Personality theory and research. In H. T. Blane & K. E. Leonard (Eds.), *Psychological theories of drinking and alcoholism* (pp. 55–89). New York: Guilford Press.

Crabbe, J. C., McSwigan, J. D., & Belnap, J. K. (1985). The role of genetics in substance abuse. In M. Galizio & S. A. Maisto (Eds.), *Determinants of substance abuse: Biological, psychological and environmental factors* (pp. 13–64). New York: Plenum Press.

Craighead, W. E., Craighead, L. W., & Ilardi, S. S. (1995). Behavior therapies in historical perspective. In B. Bongar & L. E. Beutler (Eds.), *Comprehensive textbook of psychotherapy* (pp. 64–83). New York: Oxford University Press.

Curry, S., Wagner, E. H., & Grothaus, L. C. (1990). Intrinsic and extrinsic motivation for smoking cessation. *Journal of Consulting and Clinical Psychology, 58,* 310–316.

Curry, S. J., Kristal, A. R., & Bowen, D. J. (1992). An application of the stage model of behavior change to dietary fat reduction. *Health Education Research*, 7(1), 97–105.

Daniels, J. W. (1998). *Coping with the health threat of smoking: An analysis of the Precontemplation stage of smoking cessation.* Unpublished doctoral dissertation, Psychology Department, University of Maryland, Baltimore County.

Deas, D., Riggs, P., Langenbucher, J., Goldman, M., & Brown, S. (2000). Adolescents are not adults: Developmental considerations in alcohol users. *Alcoholism: Clinical and Experimental Research*, 24(2), 232–237.

Del Boca, F. K., Babor, T. F., & McRee, B. (1994). Reliability enhancement and estimation in multisite clinical trials. *Journal of Studies on Alcohol*, Suppl. 12, 130–136.

DeLeon, G. (1999). Therapeutic communities. In B. S. McCrady & E. E. Epstein (Eds.), *Addictions: A comprehensive guidebook* (pp. 306–327). New York: Oxford University Press.

DeLeon, J. (1996) Smoking and vulnerability for schizophrenia. *Schizophrenia Bulletin*, 22(3), 405–409.

DiClemente, C. C. (1978). *Perceived processes, change on the cessation of smoking and the maintenance of that change.* Unpublished doctoral dissertation, University of Rhode Island.

DiClemente, C. C. (1981). Self efficacy and smoking cessation maintenance: A preliminary report. *Cognitive Therapy and Research*, 5(2), 175–187.

DiClemente, C. C. (1991). Motivational interviewing and the stages of change. In W. R. Miller & S. Rollnick, *Motivational interviewing: Preparing people to change addictive behavior* (pp. 191–202). New York: Guilford Press.

DiClemente, C. C. (1993a). Alcoholics Anonymous and the structure of change. In W. R. Miller & B. McCrady (Eds.), *Alcoholics Anonymous and research* (pp. 79–97). New Brunswick, NJ: Rutgers Center of Alcohol Studies.

DiClemente, C. C. (1993b). Changing addictive behaviors: A process perspective. *Current Directions in Psychological Science*, 2(4), 101–106.

DiClemente, C. C. (1994). If behaviors change, can personality be far behind? In T. Heatherton & J. Weinberger (Eds.), *Can personality change?* (pp. 175–198). Washington, DC: American Psychological Association.

DiClemente, C. C. (1999a). Motivation for change: Implications for substance abuse. *Psychological Science*, 10(3), 209–213.

DiClemente, C. C. (1999b). Prevention and harm reduction for chemical dependency: A process perspective. *Clinical Psychology Review* (Special issue: Prevention of children's behavioral and mental health problems: New horizons for psychology), 19(4), 473–486.

DiClemente, C. C., Bellino, L. E., & Neavins, T. M. (1999). Motivation for change and alcoholism treatment. *Alcohol Health and Research World*, 23(2), 86–92.

DiClemente, C. C., Carbonari, J. P., Daniels, J. W., Donovan, D. M., Bellino, L. E., & Neavins, T. M. (2001). Self-efficacy as a matching hypothesis: Causal chain analysis. In R. Longabaugh & P. W. Wirtz (Eds.), *Project MATCH: A priori matching hypotheses, results, and mediating mechanisms* (National Institute on Alcohol Abuse and Alcoholism Project MATCH Monograph Series, Vol. 8, pp. 239–259). Rockville, MD: National Institute on Alcohol Abuse and Alcoholism.

DiClemente, C. C., Carbonari, J. P., Montgomery, R., & Hughes, S. (1994). The Alcohol Abstinence Self-Efficacy Scale. *Journal of Studies on Alcohol, 55*, 141–148.

DiClemente, C. C., Carbonari, J. P., & Velasquez, M. M. (1992). Alcoholism treatment mismatching from a process of change perspective. In R. R. Watson (Ed.), *Treatment of drug and alcohol abuse* (pp. 115–142). Totowa, NJ: Humana Press.

DiClemente, C. C., Carbonari, J., Zweben, A., Morrel, T., & Lee, R. E. (2001). Motivation hypothesis causal chain analysis. In R. Longabaugh & P. W. Wirtz (Eds.), *Project MATCH: A priori matching hypotheses, results, and mediating mechanisms* (National Institute on Alcohol Abuse and Alcoholism Project MATCH Monograph Series, Vol. 8, pp. 206–222). Rockville, MD: National Institute on Alcohol Abuse and Alcoholism.

DiClemente, C. C., Carroll, K. M., Connors, G. J., & Kadden, R. M. (1994). Process assessment in treatment matching research. *Journal of Studies on Alcohol*, Suppl. 12, 156–162.

DiClemente, C. C., Carroll, K. M., Miller, W. R., Connors, G. J., & Donovan, D. M. (2002). A look inside treatment: Therapist effects, the therapeutic alliance, and the process of intentional behavior change. In T. F. Babor & F. K. Del Boca (Eds.), *Treatment matching in alcoholism* (pp. 166–183). London: Cambridge University Press.

DiClemente, C. C., Dolan-Mullen, P., & Windsor, R. (2000). The process of pregnancy smoking cessation: Implications for interventions. *Tobacco Control, 9*(Suppl. 3), 16–21.

DiClemente, C. C., Fairhurst, S. K., & Piotrowski, N. A. (1995). The role of self-efficacy in the addictive behaviors. In J. Maddux (Ed.), *Self-efficacy, adaptation and adjustment: Theory, research and application* (pp. 109–142). New York: Plenum Press.

DiClemente, C. C., & Hughes, S. O. (1990). Stages of change profiles in alcoholism treatment. *Journal of Substance Abuse, 2*, 217–235.

DiClemente, C. C., Marinilli, A. S., Singh, M., & Bellino, L. E. (2001). The role of feedback in the process of health behavior change. *American Journal of Health Behavior, 25*, 217–227.

DiClemente, C. C., & Prochaska, J. O. (1982). Self-change and therapy change of smoking behavior: A comparison of processes of change in cessation and maintenance. *Addictive Behaviors, 7*, 133–142.

DiClemente, C. C., & Prochaska, J. O. (1985). Processes and stages of change: Coping and competence in smoking behavior change. In S. Shiffman & T. A. Wills (Eds.), *Coping and substance abuse* (pp. 319–342). New York: Academic Press.

DiClemente, C. C., & Prochaska, J. O. (1998). Toward a comprehensive, trans-theoretical model of change: Stages of change and addictive behaviors. In W. R. Miller & N. Heather (Eds.), *Treating addictive behaviors* (2nd ed., pp. 3–24). New York: Plenum Press.

DiClemente, C. C., Prochaska, J. O., Fairhurst, S., Velicer, W. F., Velasquez, M., & Rossi, J. (1991). The process of smoking cessation: An analysis of Precontemplation, Contemplation and Preparation. *Journal of Consulting and Clinical Psychology, 59*(2), 295–304.

DiClemente, C. C., Prochaska, J. O., & Gibertini, M. (1985). Self-efficacy and the stages of self-change smoking. *Cognitive Therapy and Research, 9*(2), 181–200.

DiClemente, C. C., & Scott, C. W. (1997). Stages of change: Interaction with treatment compliance and involvement. In L. S. Onken, J. D. Blaine, & J. J. Boren (Eds.), *Beyond the therapeutic alliance: Keeping the drug-dependent individual in treatment* (NIDA Monograph No. 165, pp. 131–156). Rockville, MD: National Institute on Drug Abuse.

DiClemente, C. C., & Soderstram, C. (2001, March). *Intervening with alcohol problems in emergency medicine settings.* Paper presented at the CDC-sponsored meeting "Alcohol Problems among Emergency Department Patients: Research on Identification and Intervention." Washington, DC.

DiClemente, C. D., Story, M., & Murray, K. (2000). On a roll: The process of initiation and cessation of problem gambling among adolescents. *Journal of Gambling Studies, 16*(2/3), 289–313.

DiClemente, C. C., & Velasquez, M. (2002). Motivational interviewing and the stages of change. In W. R. Miller & S. Rollnick (Eds.), *Motivational interviewing: Preparing people for change* (2nd ed., pp. 201–216). New York: Guilford Press.

Dijkstra, A., DeVries, H., & Bakker, M. (1996). Pros and cons of quitting, self-efficacy, and the stages of change in smoking cessation. *Journal of Consulting and Clinical Psychology, 64,* 758–763.

Dodes, L. M., & Khantzian, E. J. (1991). Individual psychodynamic psychotherapy. In R. J. Frances & S. I. Miller (Eds.), *Clinical textbook of addictive disorders* (pp. 391–405). New York: Guilford Press.

Dolan-Mullen, P., DiClemente, C., Velasquez, M., Timpson, S., Groff, J., Carbonari, J., & Nicol, L. (2000). Enhanced prenatal case management for low income smokers. *Tobacco Control, 9*(Suppl. 3), 75–77.

Donovan, D. M. (1996). Assessment issues and domains in the prediction of relapse. *Addiction, 91*(Suppl.), S29–S36.

Donovan, D. M., & Chaney, E. F. (1985). Alcoholic relapse: Models and methods. In G. A. Marlatt & J. R. Gordon (Eds.), *Relapse prevention: Maintenance strategies in the treatment of addictive behaviors* (pp. 351–416). New York: Guilford Press.

Donovan, D. M., Kadden, R. M., DiClemente, C. C., Carroll, K. M., Longabaugh, R., Zweben, A., & Rychtarik, R. (1994). Issues in the selection and development of therapies in alcoholism treatment matching research. *Journal of Studies on Alcohol,* Suppl. 12, 138–148.

Donovan, D. M., & Marlatt, G. A. (Eds.). (1988). *Assessment of addictive behaviors.* New York: Guilford Press.

Donovan, D. M., & Mattson, M. E. (1994). Alcoholism treatment matching research: Methodological and clinical approaches. *Journal of Studies on Alcohol,* Suppl. 12, 5–14.

Donovan, D. M., & Rosengren, D. B. (1999). Motivation for behavior change and treatment among substance abusers. In J. A. Tucker, D. M. Donovan, & G. A. Marlatt (Eds.), *Changing addictive behavior: Bridging clinical and public health strategies* (pp. 127–159) New York: Guilford Press.

Dunn, M. E., & Goldman, M. S. (1996). Empirical modeling of an alcohol expectancy memory network in elementary school children as a function of grade. *Experimental and Clinical Pharmacology, 4*(2), 209–217.

Dunn, N. J., Seilhamer, R. A., Jacob, T., & Whalen, M. (1992). Comparisons of retrospective and current reports of alcoholics and their spouses on drinking behavior. *Addictive Behaviors, 17*(6), 543–555.

Ebaugh, H. R. F. (1988). *Becoming an EX: The Process of Role Exit.* Chicago: University of Chicago Press.

Edens, J. F., & Willoughby, F. W. (2000). Motivational patterns of alcohol dependent patients: A replication. *Psychology of Addictive Behaviors, 14*(4), 397–400.

El-Bassel, N., Schilling, R. F., Ivanoff, A., Chen, D. R., Hanson, M., & Bidassie, B. (1998). Stages of change profiles among incarcerated drug-abusing women. *Addictive Behaviors, 23*(3), 389–394.

Ellis, A., & Dryden, W. (1987). *The practice of rational-emotive therapy.* New York: Springer.

Ennett, S. T., Tabler, N. S., Ringwolt, C. L., & Fliwelling, R. L. (1994). How effective is drug abuse resistance education? A meta-analysis of Project DARE outcome evaluations. *American Journal of Public Health, 84,* 1394–1401.

Erikson, E. H. (1963). *Childhood and society* (2nd ed.). New York: Norton.

Etter, J. F., Perneger, T. V., & Ronchi, A. (1997). Distributions of smokers by stage: International comparisons and associations with smoking prevalence. *Preventive Medicine, 26,* 580–585.

Fairburn, C. G., & Brownell, K. (Eds.). (2002). *Eating disorders and obesity* (2nd ed.). New York: Guilford Press.

Fals-Stewart, W., O'Farrell, T. J., & Hooley, J. M. (2001). Relapse among married or cohabiting substance-abusing patients: The role of perceived criticism. *Behavior Therapy, 32,* 787–801.

Farkas, A. J., Pierce, J. P., Zhu, S. H., Rosbrook, B., Gilpin, E. A., Berry, C., & Kaplan, R. M. (1996). Addiction versus stages of change models in predicting smoking cessation. *Addiction, 91*(9), 1271–1280.

Feldman, H. L., Damron, D., Anliker, J., Ballesteros, M., Langenberg, P., DiClemente, C. C., & Havas, S. (2000). The effect of Maryland WIC 5-a-day promotion program on participant's stage of change for fruit and vegetable consumption. *Health Education and Behavior, 27*(5), 649–663.

Festinger, L. (1957). *A theory of cognitive dissonance.* Stanford, CA: Stanford University Press.

Fiore, M. C., Jorenby, D. E., & Baker, T. B. (1997). Smoking cessation: Principles and practice based upon the AHCPR Guideline, 1996. *Annals of Behavioral Medicine, 19*(3), 213–219.

Fitzgerald, T. E., & Prochaska, J. O. (1989). Nonprogressing profiles in smoking cessation: What keeps people refractory to self-change? *Journal of Substance Abuse, 2,* 93–111.

Fletcher, A. M. (2001). *Sober for good: New solutions for drinking problems—Advice from those who have succeeded.* New York: Houghton Mifflin.

Francis, D. J., Fletcher, J. M., Stuebing, K. K., Davidson, K. C., & Thompson, N.

M. (1991). Analysis of change: Modeling individual growth. *Journal of Consulting and Clinical Psychology, 59*, 27–37.

Freud, S. (1949). *An outline of psychoanalysis* (J. Strachey, Trans.). New York: Norton.

Fromme, K., & Dunn, M. E. (1992). Alcohol expectancies, social and environmental cues as determinants of drinking and perceived reinforcement. *Addictive Behaviors, 17*, 167–177.

Fromme, K., Stroot, E., & Kaplan, D. (1993). Comprehensive effects of alcohol: Development and psychometric assessment of a new expectancy questionnaire. *Psychological Assessment, 5*(1), 19–26.

Galanter, M. (1999). *Network therapy for alcohol and drug abuse.* New York: Guilford Press.

Galizio, M., & Maisto, S. A. (Eds.). (1985). *Determinants of substance abuse: Biological, psychological and environmental factors.* New York: Plenum Press.

Gentilello, L. M., Rivara, F. P., Donovan, D. M., Jurkovich, G. J., Daranciang, E., Dunn, C. W., Villaveces, A., Copass, M., & Ries, R. R. (1999). Alcohol interventions in a trauma center as a means of reducing the risk of injury recurrence. *Annals of Surgery, 230*, 473–483.

Giancola, P. R., & Tarter, R. E. (1999). Executive cognitive functioning and risk for substance abuse. *Psychological Science, 10*(3) 203–205.

Glantz, M., & Pickens, R. (Eds.). (1992). *Vulnerability to drug abuse.* Washington, DC: American Psychological Association.

Glanz, K., Patterson, R. E., Kristal, A. R., DiClemente, C. C., Heimendinger, J., Linnan, L., & Ockene, J. (1994). Stages of change in adopting healthy diets: Fat, fiber and correlates of nutrient intake. *Health Education Quarterly, 21*(4), 499–519.

Goldberg, D. N., Hoffman, A. M., Farinha, M. F., Marder, D. C., Tinson-Mitchem, L., Burton, D., & Smith, E. G. (1994). Physician delivery of smoking cessation advice based on the stages of change model. *American Journal of Preventive Medicine, 10*(5), 267–274.

Goldfried, M. R. (1980). Toward a delineation of therapeutic change principles. *American Psychologist, 35*, 991–999.

Goldman, M. S. (1999). Risk for substance abuse: Memory as a common etiological pathway. *Psychological Science, 10*(3), 196–198.

Goldman, M. S., Del Boca, F. K., & Darkes, J. (1999). Alcohol expectancy theory: The application of cognitive neuroscience. In K. E. Leonard & H. T. Blane (Eds.), *Psychological theories of drinking and alcoholism* (2nd ed., pp 203–246). New York: Guilford Press.

Gordis, E. (2000, July). From genes to geography: The cutting edge of alcohol research. *Alcohol Alert* (No. 48). Rockville MD: National Institute on Alcohol Abuse and Alcoholism.

Grant, B. F., & Dawson, D. A. (1999). Alcohol, drug use, abuse, and dependence: Classification, prevalence and comorbidity. In B. S. McCrady & E. E. Epstein (Eds.), *Addictions: A comprehensive guidebook* (pp. 9–29). New York: Oxford University Press.

Greaves, G. B. (1980). An existential theory of drug dependence. In D. J. Lettieri, M. Sayers, & H. W. Pearson (Eds.), *Theories on drug abuse: Selected contem-*

porary perspectives (NIDA Research Monograph No. 30, pp. 24–28; DHHS Publication No. ADM 80-967). Rockville, MD: National Institute on Drug Abuse.

Griffin, J. A., Gilliland, S. S., Perez, G., Helitzer, D., & Carter, J. S. (1999). Participant satisfaction with a culturally appropriate diabetes education program: The Native American Diabetes Project. *Diabetes Education, 25*(3), 351–363.

Grimley, D. M., Riley, G. E., Bellis, J. M., & Prochaska, J. O. (1993, December). Assessing the stages of change and decisionmaking for contraceptive use for the prevention of pregnancy, sexually transmitted diseases, and Acquired Immunodeficiency Syndrome. *Health Education Quarterly, 20*(4), 455–470.

Gritz, E. R., Prokhorov, A. V., Hudmon, K. S., Chamberlain, R. M., Taylor, W. C., DiClemente, C. C., Johnston, D. A., Hu, S., Jones, L. A., Jones, M. M., Rosenblum, C. K., Ayars, C. L., & Amos, C. I. (1998). Cigarette smoking in a multiethnic population of youth: Methods and baseline findings. *Preventive Medicine, 27*(3), 365–384.

Hagedorn, H. (2000). *Application of the Transtheoretical Model of behavior change to cessation of alcohol use in patients with schizophrenia.* Unpublished doctoral dissertation, Department of Psychology, University of Maryland, Baltimore County.

Haug, N. (2002). *Motivational enhancement for smoking cessation among pregnant drug abusing women.* Unpublished doctoral dissertation, University of Maryland, Baltimore County.

Heather, N., Rollnick, S., & Bell, A. (1993). Predictive validity of the Readiness to Change to Change Questionnaire, *Addiction, 88,* 1667–1677.

Hesselbrock, M. N., Hesselbrock, V. M., & Epstein, E. E. (1999). Theories of etiology of alcohol and other drug use disorders. In B. S. McCrady & E. E. Epstein (Eds.), *Addictions: A comprehensive guidebook* (pp. 50–74). New York: Oxford University Press.

Higgins, S. T. (1997). The influence of alternative reinforcers on cocaine use and abuse: A brief review. *Pharmacology, Biochemistry and Behavior, 57,* 419–427.

Higgins, S. T. (1999). Potential contributions of the community reinforcement approach and contingency management to broadening the base of substance abuse treatment. In J. A. Tucker, D. M. Donovan, & G. A. Marlatt (Eds.), *Changing addictive behavior: Bridging clinical and public health strategies* (pp. 283–306). New York: Guilford Press.

Hinson, R. E. (1985). Individual differences in tolerance and relapse: A Pavlovian conditioning perspective. In M. Galizio & S. A. Maisto (Eds.), *Determinants of substance abuse: Biological, psychological and environmental factors* (pp. 101–124). New York: Plenum Press.

Holden, C. (2002, February 8). Neuroscience: Drugs and placebos look alike in the brain. *Science, 295*(5557), 947.

Holder, H. (1999). Prevention aimed at the environment. In B. S. McCrady & E. E. Epstein (Eds.), *Addictions: A comprehensive guidebook* (pp. 573–594). New York: Oxford University Press.

Horn, D. (1976). A model for the study of personal choice behavior. *International Journal of Health Education, 19,* 89–98.

Hudmon, K. S., Prokhorov, A. V., Koehly, L. M., DiClemente, C. C., & Gritz, E. R. (1997). Psychometric properties of the decisional balance scale and temptations to try smoking inventory in adolescents. *Journal of Child and Adolescent Substance Abuse, 6*(3), 1–18.

Hunt, W. A., Barnett, L. W., & Branch, L. G. (1971) Relapse rates in addiction programs. *Journal of Clinical Psychology, 90,* 586–600.

Hurt, R. D., Dale, L. C., McClain, F. L., Eberman, K. M., Offord, K. P., Bruce, B. K., & Lauger, G. G. (1992). A comprehensive model for treatment of nicotine dependence in a medical setting. *Medical Clinics of North America, 76,* 495–514.

Ingersol, K. S., Wagner, C. C., & Gharib, S. (2000). *Motivational groups for community substance abuse programs.* Richmond, VA: Mid-Atlantic Addiction Technology Transfer Center.

Isenhart, C. (1994). Motivational subtypes in an inpatient sample of substance abusers. *Addictive Behaviors, 19,* 463–475.

Institute of Medicine. (1990). *Broadening the base of treatment for alcohol problems.* Washington, DC: National Academy Press.

Janis, I. L., & Mann, L. (1977). *Decision making.* New York: Free Press.

Jessor, R., & Jessor, S. L. (1977). *Problem behavior and psychosocial development.* New York: Academic Press.

Jessor, R., & Jessor, S. (1980). A social-psychological framework for studying drug use. In U. S. Department of Health and Human Services, *Theories on drug abuse: Contemporary perspectives* (NIDA Research Monograph No. 30, pp. 102–109; DHHS Publication No. ADM 80-967). Washington, DC: U.S. Government Printing Office.

Jessor, R., Van Den Bos, J., Vanderryn, J., Costa, F. M., & Turbin, M. S. (1995). Protective factors in adolescent problem behavior: moderator effects and developmental change. *Developmental Psychology, 31,* 923–933.

Joe, G. W., Simpson, D. D., & Broome, K. M. (1998). Effects of readiness for drug abuse treatment on client retention and assessment of process. *Addiction, 93*(8), 1177–1190.

Johnson, B. A., Roache, J. D., Javors, M. A., DiClemente, C. C., Cloninger, C. R., Prihoda, T. J., Bordnick, P. S., Ait-Daoud, N., & Hensler, J. (2000). Ondansetron for reduction of drinking among biologically predisposed alcoholic patients. *Journal of the American Medical Association, 284*(8), 963–971.

Johnson, B. D. (1980). Toward a theory of drug subcultures. In D. J. Letteri, M. Sayers, & H. W. Pearson (Eds.), *Theories on drug abuse: Selected contemporary perspectives* (NIDA Research Monograph No. 30, pp. 110–119; DHHS Publication No. ADM 80-967). Washington, DC: National Institute on Drug Abuse.

Johnson, E. O., van den Bree, M. B. M., Uhl, G. R., & Pickens, R. W. (1996). Indicators of genetic and environmental influences in drug abusing individuals. *Drug and Alcohol Dependence, 41,* 17–23.

Joseph, J., Breslin, C., & Skinner, H. (1999). Critical perspectives on the Transtheoretical Model and stages of change. In J. A. Tucker, D. M. Donovan, & G. A. Marlatt (Eds.), *Changing addictive behavior: Bridging clinical and public health strategies* (pp. 160–190). New York: Guilford Press.

Kandel, D. B. (1975). Stages in adolescent involvement in drug use. *Science, 190,* 912–914.

Kandel, D. B., & Davies, M. (1992). Progression to regular marijuana involvement: Phenomenology and risk factors for near daily use. In M. Glantz & R. Pickens (Eds.), *Vulnerability to drug abuse* (pp. 211–254) Washington, DC: American Psychological Association.

Kaplan, H. B., & Johnson, R. J. (1992). Relationships between circumstances surrounding initial illicit drug use and escalation of use: Moderating effects of gender and early adolescent experiences. In M. Glantz & R. Pickens (Eds.), *Vulnerability to drug abuse* (pp. 299–358). Washington, DC: American Psychological Association.

Keller, S., Nigg, C. R., Jakle, C., Baum, E., & Basler, H. (1999). Self-efficacy, decisional balance and the stages for smoking cessation in a German sample. *Swiss Journal of Psychology, 5*(2), 101–110.

Khantzian E. J. (1980). An ego/self theory of substance dependence: A contemporary psychoanalytic perspective. In U. S. Department of Health and Human Services, *Theories on drug abuse: Contemporary perspectives* (NIDA Research Monograph No. 30, pp. 29–33; DHHS Publication No. ADM 80-967). Washington, DC: U.S. Government Printing Office.

King T., & DiClemente, C. C. (1993, November). *A decisional balance measure for assessing and predicting drinking behavior.* Poster presented at the 26th annual convention of the Association for Advancement of Behavior Therapy, Atlanta GA.

Klingemann, H. (1991). The motivation for change from problem alcohol and heroin use. *British Journal of Addiction, 86,* 727–744.

Kohler, C. C., Grimley, D., & Reynolds, K. (1999). Theoretical approaches guiding the development and implementation of health promotion. In J. M. Raczynski & R. J. DiClemente (Eds.), *Handbook of health promotion and disease prevention* (pp. 23–50). New York: Kluwer Academic/Plenum.

Krampen, G. (1989). Motivation in the treatment of alcoholism. *Addictive Behaviors, 14*(2), 197–200.

Kreuter, M. W., Strecher, V. J., & Glassman, B. (1999). One size does not fit all: The case for tailoring print materials. *Annals of Behavioral Medicine, 21*(4), 276–283.

Lazarus, R., & Folkman, S. (1985). *Stress, appraisal and coping.* New York: Springer.

Lee, R. (1998). *Understanding motivation for two kinds of physical activity among older adolescent college students.* Unpublished doctoral dissertation, University of Maryland, Baltimore County.

Lee, R., & DiClemente, C. C. (2000). Ecological influences on exercise behavior and motivational readiness. *Annals of Behavioral Medicine, 22,* S213.

Leeds, J., & Morgenstern, L. (1995). Psychoanalytic theories of substance abuse. In F. Rotgers, D. S. Keller, & J. Morgenstern (Eds.), *Treating substance abuse: Theory and technique* (pp. 68–83). New York: Guilford Press.

Leigh, B. C., & Stacy, A. W. (1993). Alcohol expectancies: Scale construction and predictive utility in higher order confirmatory models. *Psychological Assessment, 5,* 216–229.

Leonard, K. E., & Blane, H. T. (Eds.). (1999). *Psychological theories of drinking and alcoholism* (2nd ed.). New York: Guilford Press.

Leonard, K. E., & Mudar, P. J. (2000). Alcohol use in the year before marriage: Alcohol expectancies and peer drinking as proximal influences on husband and wife alcohol involvement. *Alcoholism: Clinical and Experimental Research, 24*(11), 1666–1679.

Leshner, A. I. (1997). Addiction is a brain disease, and it matters. *Science, 278,* 45–47.

Lettieri, D. J., Sayers, M., & Pearson, H. W. (Eds.). (1980). *Theories on drug abuse: Selected contemporary perspectives* (NIDA Research Monograph No. 30; DHHS Publication No. ADM 80-967). Rockville, MD: National Institute on Drug Abuse.

Liepman, M. R. (1993). Using family influence to motivate alcoholics to enter treatment: The Johnson Institute intervention approach. In T. J. O'Farrell (Ed.), *Treating alcohol problems: Marital and family interventions* (pp. 54–77). New York: Guilford Press.

Liskow, B. I., & Goodwin, D. W. (1987). Pharmacological treatment of alcohol intoxication, withdrawal, and dependence: A critical review. *Journal of Studies on Alcohol, 48*(4), 356–370.

Littell, J. H., & Girvin, H. (2002). Stages of change: A critique. *Behavior Modification, 26,* 223–273.

Litten, R. Z., Allen, J., & Fertig, J. (1996). Pharmacotherapies for alcohol problems: A review with focus on developments since 1991. *Alcoholism: Clinical and Experimental Research, 20*(5), 859–876.

Lohr, J. B., & Flynn, K. (1992). Smoking and schizophrenia. *Schizophrenia Research, 8,* 93–102.

Longabaugh, R., & Wirtz, P. W. (Eds). (2001). *Project MATCH: A priori matching hypotheses, results, and mediating mechanisms* (National Institute on Alcohol Abuse and Alcoholism Project MATCH Monograph Series, Vol. 8). Rockville, MD: National Institute on Alcohol Abuse and Alcoholism.

Longabaugh, R., Wirtz, P. W., Beattie, M. C., Noel, N., & Stout, R. (1995). Matching treatment focus to patient social investment and support: 18-month follow-up results. *Journal of Consulting and Clinical Psychology, 63,* 296–307.

Longabaugh, R., Wirtz, P. W., Zweben, A., & Stout, R. (1998). Network support for drinking: Alcoholics Anonymous and long-term matching effects. *Addiction, 93,* 1313–1333.

Longabaugh, R., Wirtz, P. W., Zweben, A., & Stout, R. (2001). Network support for drinking. In R. Longabaugh & P. W. Wirtz (Eds.), *Project MATCH: A priori matching hypotheses, results, and mediating mechanisms* (National Institute on Alcohol Abuse and Alcoholism Project MATCH Monograph Series, Vol. 8, pp. 260–275). Rockville, MD: National Institute on Alcohol Abuse and Alcoholism.

Longshore, D., Grills, C., & Annon, K. (1999). Effects of a culturally congruent intervention on cognitive factors related to drug-use recovery. *Substance Use and Misuse, 34*(9), 1223–1241.

Lukoff, I. F. (1980). Toward a sociology of drug use. In U. S. Department of Health and Human Services, *Theories on drug abuse: Contemporary perspectives* (NIDA Research Monograph No. 30, pp. 201–211; DHHS Publication No. ADM 80-967). Washington, DC: U.S. Government Printing Office.

Lynam, D. R., Milich, R., Zimmerman, R., Novak, S. P., Logan, T. K., Martin, C., Leukfield, C., & Clayton, R. R. (1999). Project DARE: No effects at 10 year follow-up. *Journal of Consulting and Clinical Psychology, 67,* 467–471.

MacCoun, R. J. (1998). Toward a psychology of harm reduction. *American Psychologist, 53,* 1199–1208.

Maisto, S. A., Carey, K. B., & Bradizza, C. M. (1999). Social learning theory. In K. E. Leonard & H. T. Blane (Eds.), *Psychological theories of drinking and alcoholism* (2nd ed., pp. 106–163). New York: Guilford Press.

Mann, L. M., Chassin, L., & Sher, K. J. (1987). Alcohol expectancies and the risk for alcoholism. *Journal of Consulting and Clinical Psychology, 55*(3), 411–417.

Marcus, B. H., Rossi, J. S., Selby, V. C., Niaura, R. S., & Abrams, D. B. (1992). The stages and processes of exercise adoption and maintenance in a worksite sample. *Health Psychology, 11*(6), 386–395.

Marlatt, G. A., Baer, J. S., Kivlahan, D. R., Dimeff, L. A., Larimer, M. E., Quigley, L. A., Somers, J. M., & Williams, E. (1998). Screeing and brief interventions for high-risk college student drinkers: Results from a 2-year follow-up assessment. *Journal of Consulting and Clinical Psychology, 66,* 604–615.

Marlatt, G. A., & Gordon, J. R. (Eds.). (1985). *Relapse prevention.* New York: Guilford Press.

Marlatt, G. A., & Tapert, S. F. (1993). Harm reduction: Reducing the risks of addictive behaviors. In J. S. Baer, G. A. Marlatt, & R. J. McMahon (Eds.), *Addictive behaviors across the lifespan: Prevention, treatment and policy issues* (pp. 111–137). Newbury Park, CA: Sage.

Mattson, M. E., Del Boca, F. K., Carroll, K. M., Cooney, N. L., DiClemente, C. C., Donovan, D., Kadden, R. M., McRee, B., Rice, C., Rycharik, R. G., & Zweben, A. (1998). Compliance with treatment and follow-up protocols in Project MATCH: Predictors and relationship to outcome. *Alcoholism: Clinical and Experimental Research, 22*(6), 1328–1339.

Mayberg, H. S., Silva, J. A., Brannan, S. K., Tekell, J. L., Mahurin, R. K., McGinnis, S., & Jerabek, P. A. (2002). The functional neuroanatomy of the placebo effect. *American Journal of Psychiatry, 159*(5), 728–737.

McBride, C. M., Curry, S. J., Lando, H. A., Pirie, P. L., Grothaus, L. C., Nelson, J. C. (1999). Prevention of relapse in women who quit smoking during pregnancy. *American Journal of Public Health, 89*(5), 706–711.

McCarty, D. (1985). Environmental factors in substance abuse: The microsetting. In M. Galizio & S. A. Maisto (Eds.), *Determinants of substance abuse: Biological, psychological and environmental factors* (pp. 247–291). New York: Plenum Press.

McCrady, B. S., & Epstein, E. E. (Eds.). (1999). *Addictions: A comprehensive guidebook.* New York: Oxford University Press.

McCrady, B. S., & Miller, W. R. (Eds.). (1993). *Research on Alcoholics Anony-*

mous: Opportunities and alternatives. New Brunswick, NJ: Rutgers Center of Alcohol Studies.

McGue, M., Pickens, R. W., & Svikis, D. S. (1992). Sex and age effects on the inheritance of alcohol problems: A twin study. *Journal of Abnormal Psychology, 101*(1), 3–17.

McGurrin, M. C. (1992). *Pathological gambling: Conceptual, diagnostic and treatment issues.* Sarasota, FL: Professional Resource Press.

McLellan, A., Arndt, I., Metzger, D., Woody, G., & O'Brien, C. (1993). The effects of psychosocial services in substance abuse treatment. *Journal of the American Medical Association, 269*(15), 1953–1959.

McLellan, A. T., Grissom, G., Zanis, D., & Brill, P. (1997). Problem–service "matching" in addiction treatment: A prospective study in four programs. *Archives of General Psychiatry, 54*, 730–735.

McLellan, A. T., Luborsky, L., & O'Brien, C. P. (1986). Alcohol and drug abuse treatment in three different populations: Is there improvement and is it predictable? *American Journal of Drug and Alcohol Abuse, 12*, 101–120.

McLellan, A. T., Woody, G. E., Metzger, D. J., McKay, J., Alterman, A. I., & O'Brien, C. P. (1995). Evaluating the effectiveness of treatments for substance use disorders: Reasonable expectations, appropriate comparisons. In D. Fox (Ed.), *The Milbank Foundation volume on health policy issues.* New York: Milbank Foundation Press.

Mellers, B. A., Schwartz, A., & Cooke, A. D. J. (1998). Judgment and decision-making. *Annual Review of Psychology, 49*, 447–477.

Merikangas, K. R., Rounsaville, B. J., & Prusoff, B. A. (1992). Familial factors in vulnerability to drug abuse. In M. Glantz & R. Pickens (Eds.), *Vulnerability to drug abuse* (pp. 75–98). Washington, DC: American Psychological Association.

Meyers, R. J., & Smith, J. E. (1995). *Clinical guide to alcohol treatment: The community reinforcement approach.* New York: The Guilford Press.

Miller, E. T., Turner, A. P., & Marlatt, G. A. (2001). The harm reduction approach to the secondary prevention of alcohol problems in adolescents and young adults. In P. M. Monti, S. M. Colby, & T. A. O'Leary (Eds.), *Adolescents, alcohol and substance abuse: Reaching teens through brief interventions* (pp. 58–79). New York: Guilford Press.

Miller, W. R. (1985). Motivation for treatment: A review with special emphasis on alcoholism. *Psychological Bulletin, 98*(1), 84–107.

Miller, W. R., Benefield, R. G., & Tonigan, J. S. (1993). Enhancing motivation for change in problem drinking: A controlled comparison of two therapist styles. *Journal of Consulting and Clinical Psychology, 61*(3), 455–461.

Miller, W. R., & Brown, J. M. (1991). Self-regulation as a conceptual basis for the prevention and treatment of addictive behaviors. In N. Heather, W. R. Miller, & J. Greeley (Eds.), *Self-control and the addictive behaviours.* New York: Maxwell Macmillan Publishing Australia.

Miller, W. R., & C'deBaca, J. (2001). *Quantum change.* New York: Guilford Press.

Miller, W. R., & Del Boca, F. K. (1994). Measurement of drinking behavior using the Form 90 family of instruments. *Journal of Studies on Alcohol,* Suppl. 12, 112–118.

Miller, W. R., & Heather, N. (Eds.). (1998). *Treating addictive behaviors* (2nd ed.). New York: Plenum Press.

Miller, W. R., & Hester, R. K. (1986). The effectiveness of alcoholism treatment: What research reveals. In W. R Miller & N. Heather (Eds.), *Treating addictive behaviors: Processes of change* (pp. 121–174). New York: Plenum Press.

Miller, W. R., & Kurtz, E. (1994). Models of alcoholism used in treatment: Contrasting AA and other perspectives with which it is often confused. *Journal of Studies on Alcohol, 55,* 159–166.

Miller, W. R., & Rollnick, S. (1991). *Motivational interviewing: Preparing people to change addictive behavior.* New York: Guilford Press.

Miller, W. R., & Rollnick, S. (2002). *Motivational interviewing* (2nd ed.). New York: Guilford Press.

Miller, W. R., Sovereign, R. G., & Krege, B. (1988). Motivational interviewing with problem drinkers: II. The Drinker's Check-up as a preventive intervention. *Behavioural Psychotherapy, 16,* 251–258.

Miller, W. R., & Tonigan, J. S. (1996). Assessing drinkers' motivation for change: The stages of change readiness and treatment eagerness scale (SOCRATES). *Psychology of Addictive Behaviors, 10,* 81–89.

Miller, W. R., Zweben, A., DiClemente, C. C., & Rychtarik, R. G. (1992). *Motivational Enhancement Therapy manual: A clinical research guide for therapists and individuals with alcohol abuse and dependence.* Rockville, MD: National Institute on Alcohol Abuse and Alcoholism.

Minkoff, K. (1989). An integrated treatment model for dial diagnosis of psychosis and addiction. *Hospital and Community Psychiatry, 40*(10), 1031–1036.

Minuchin, S. (1974). *Families and family therapy.* Cambridge, MA: Harvard University Press.

Minuchin, S., Rosman, S. L., & Baker, L. (1978). *Psychosomatic families.* Cambridge, MA: Harvard University Press.

Montgomery, R. P. G. (1991). *The relationship between physiological and psychological dependence in the maintenance and modification of nicotine addiction.* Unpublished master's thesis, Department of Psychology, University of Houston.

Monti, P. M., Colby, S. M., & O'Leary, T. A. (Eds.). (2001). *Adolescents, alcohol and substance abuse: Reaching teens through brief interventions.* New York: Guilford Press.

Monti, P. M., Rohsenhow, D. J., Colby, S. M., & Abrams, D. B. (1995). Smoking among alcoholics during and after treatment: Implications for models, treatment strategies, and policy. In J. B. Fertig & J. P. Allen (Eds.), *Alcohol and tobacco: From basic science to clinical practice* (NIDA Monograph No. 30, pp. 187–206; NIH Publication No. 95-3931. Rockville, MD: National Institute on Drug Abuse.

Monti, P. M., Rohsenhow, D. J., Swift, R. M., Gulliver, S. B., Colby, S. M., Mueller, T. I., Brown, R. A., Gordon, A., & Abrams, D. B. (2001). Naltrexone and cue exposure with coping and communication skills training for alcoholics: Treatment process and 1–year outcomes. *Alcoholism, Clinical and Experimental Research, 25,* 1634–1647.

Moos, R. H., Finney, J. W., & Cronkite, R. C. (1990). *Alcoholism treatment: Context, process, and outcome.* New York: Oxford University Press.

Morgenstern, J., Labouvie, E., McCrady, B. S., Kahler, C. W., Frey, R. M. (1997). Affiliation with Alcoholics Anonymous after treatment: A study of its therapeutic effects and mechanisms of action. *Journal of Consulting and Clinical Psychology, 65*(5), 768–777.

Mueser, K. T., Bellack, A. S., & Blanchard, J. J. (1992). Comorbidity of schizophrenia and substance abuse: Implications for treatment. *Journal of Consulting and Clinical Psychology, 60*, 845–856.

Mullen, P. D., Richardson, M. A., Quinn, V. P., & Ershoff, D. H. (1997). Postpartum return to smoking: Who is at risk and when. *American Journal of Health Promotion, 11*(5), 323–330.

Myers, M. G., Brown, S. A., Tate, S., Abrantes, A., & Tomlinson, K. (1999). Toward brief interventions for adolescents with substance abuse and comorbid psychiatric problems. In P. M. Monti, S. M. Colby, & T. A. O'Leary (Eds.), *Adolescents, alcohol and substance abuse: Reaching teens through brief interventions* (pp. 275–296). New York: Guilford Press.

Nathan, P. E. (1988). The addictive personality is the behavior of the addict. *Journal of Consulting and Clinical Psychology, 56*(2), 183–188.

National Academy of Sciences, Committee on the Social and Economic Impact of Pathological Gambling. (1999). *Pathological gambling: A critical review.* Washington, DC: National Academy Press.

Newcomb, M. D. (1992). Understanding the multidimensional nature of drug use and abuse: The role of consumption, risk factors and protective factors. In M. Glantz & R. Pickens (Eds.), *Vulnerability to drug abuse* (pp. 255–298). Washington, DC: American Psychological Association.

Newcomb, M. D., & Bentler, P. M. (1988). *Consequences of adolescent drug use: Impact on the lives of young adults.* Newbury Park, CA: Sage.

Newcomb, M. D., Scheier, L. M., & Bentler, P. M. (1993). Effects of adolescent drug use on adult mental health: A prospective study of a community sample. *Experimental and Clinical Psychopharmacology, 1*, 215–241.

Newlin, D. B., Miles, D. R., van den Bree, M. B., Gupman, A. E., & Pickens, R. W. (2000). Environmental transmission of DSM-IV substance use disorders in adoptive and step families. *Alcoholism: Clinical and Experimental Research, 24*(12), 1785–1794.

Nowinski, J. (1999). Self-help groups for addictions. In B. S. McCrady & E. E. Epstein (Eds.), *Addictions: A comprehensive guidebook* (pp. 287–305). New York: Oxford University Press.

Nowinski, J., Baker, S., & Carroll, K. (1992). *Twelve step facilitation therapy manual: A clinical research guide for therapists treating individuals with alcohol abuse and dependence* (NIAAA Project MATCH Monograph Series, Vol. 1). Rockville, MD: National Institute on Alcohol Abuse and Alcoholism.

O'Connor, E., Carbonari, J. P., & DiClemente, C. C. (1996). Gender and smoking cessation: A factor structure comparison of processes of change. *Journal of Consulting and Clinical Psychology, 64*, 130–138.

O'Farrell, T. J., & Fals-Stewart, W. (1999). Treatment models and methods: Family models. In B. S. McCrady & E. E. Epstein (Eds.), *Addictions: A comprehensive guidebook* (pp. 287–305). New York: Oxford University Press.

Orford, J. (1985) *Excessive appetites: A psychological view of addictions.* New York: Wiley.

Orleans, C. T., & Slade, J. (Eds.). (1993). *Nicotine addiction: Principles and management.* New York: Oxford University Press.

Osher, F. C., & Kofoed, L. (1989). Treatment of patients with psychiatric and substance use disorders. *Hospital and Community Psychiatry, 40* (10), 1025–1030.

Owen, N., Wakefield, M., Roberts, L., & Esterman, A. (1992). Stages of readiness to quit smoking: Population prevalence and correlates. *Health Psychology, 11,* 413–417.

Page, J. B., Fletcher, J., & True, W. R. (1988). Psychosociocultural perspectives on chronic cannabis use: The Costa Rican follow-up. *Journal of Psychoactive Drugs, 20*(1), 57–65.

Pallonen, U. E., Prochaska, J. O., Velicer, W. F., Prokhorov, A. V., & Smith, N. F. (1998). Stages of acquisition and cessation for adolescent smoking: An empirical integration. *Addictive Behaviors, 23*(3), 303–324.

Pandina, R. J., Johnson, V., & Labouvie, E. W. (1992). Affectivity: A central mechanism in the development of drug dependence. In M. Glantz & R. Pickens (Eds.), *Vulnerability to drug abuse* (pp. 179–210) Washington, DC: American Psychological Association.

Peele, S. (1985). *Meaning of addiction: Compulsive experience and its interpretation.* Lexington, MA: Lexington Books.

Pentz, M. A. (1985). Social cognitions and self-efficacy as determinants of substance use in adolescence. In S. Shiffman & T. A. Wills (Eds.), *Coping and substance abuse* (pp. 117–142). New York: Academic Press.

Perz, C. A., DiClemente, C. C., & Carbonari, J. P. (1996). Doing the right thing at the right time? Interaction of stages and processes of change in successful smoking cessation. *Health Psychology, 15,* 462–468.

Pickens, R. W., Elmer, G. I., LaBuda, M. C., & Uhl, G. R. (1996). Genetic vulnerability to substance abuse. In C. R. Schuster & M. J. Kuhar (Eds.), *Handbook of experimental pharmacology: Vol. 118. Pharmacological aspects of drug dependence: Toward an integrated neurobehavioral approach* (pp. 3–52). Heidelberg, Germany: Springer-Verlag.

Pollak, K. I., Carbonari, J. P., DiClemente, C. C., Niemann, Y. F., & Mullen, P. D. (1998). Causal relationships of processes of change and decisional balance: Stage specific models for smoking. *Addictive Behaviors, 23*(4), 437–448.

Prochaska, J. O. (1979). *Systems of psychotherapy: A transtheoretical analysis.* Homewood, IL: Dorsey Press.

Prochaska, J. O., & DiClemente, C. C. (1982). Transtheoretical therapy: Toward a more integrative model of change. *Psychotherapy: Theory, Research and Practice, 19*(3), 276–288.

Prochaska, J. O., & DiClemente, C. C. (1983). Stages and processes of self-change of smoking: Toward an integrative model of change. *Journal of Consulting and Clinical Psychology, 51,* 390–395.

Prochaska, J. O., & DiClemente, C. C. (1984). *The Transtheoretical approach: Crossing the traditional boundaries of therapy.* Malabar, FL: Krieger.

Prochaska, J. O., & DiClemente, C. C. (1985). Common processes of change in smoking, weight control and psychological distress. In S. Shiffman & T. A. Wills (Eds.), *Coping and substance abuse* (pp. 345–362). New York: Academic Press.

Prochaska, J. O., & DiClemente, C. C. (1986). Toward a comprehensive model of change. In W. R. Miller & N. Heather (Eds.), *Treating addictive behaviors: Processes of change* (pp. 3–27). New York: Plenum Press.

Prochaska, J. O., & DiClemente, C. C. (1992). Stages of change in the modification of problem behavior. In M. Hersen, R. Eisler, & P. M. Miller (Eds.), *Progress in behavior modification* (Vol. 28, pp. 184–214). Sycamore, IL: Sycamore.

Prochaska, J. O., & DiClemente, C. C. (1998). Comments, criteria and creating better models. In W. R. Miller & N. Heather (Eds.), *Treating addictive behaviors* (2nd ed., pp. 39–45). New York: Plenum Press.

Prochaska, J. O., DiClemente, C. C., & Norcross, J. C. (1992). In search of how people change: Applications to the addictive behaviors. *American Psychologist, 47,* 1102–1114.

Prochaska, J. O., DiClemente, C. C., Velicer, W. F., Ginpil, S., & Norcross, J. C. (1985). Predicting change in smoking status for self-changers. *Addictive Behaviors, 10,* 395–406.

Prochaska, J. O., DiClemente, C. C., Velicer, W. F., & Rossi, J. S. (1993). Standardized, individualized, interactive and personalized self-help programs for smoking cessation. *Health Psychology, 12,* 399–405.

Prochaska, J. O., & Norcross, J. C. (1999). *Systems of psychotherapy: A transtheoretical analysis.* Pacific Grove, CA: Brooks/Cole.

Prochaska, J. O., Norcross, J. C., & DiClemente, C. C. (1994). *Changing for good.* New York: Morrow.

Prochaska, J. O., & Velicer, W. F. (1997a). Response: Misinterpretations and misapplications of the Transtheoretical Model. *American Journal of Health Promotion, 12,* 11–12.

Prochaska, J. O., & Velicer, W. F. (1997b). The transtheoretical model of health behavior change. *American Journal of Health Promotion, 12*(1), 38–48.

Prochaska, J. O., Velicer, W. F., DiClemente, C. C., & Fava, J. (1988). Measuring processes of change: Applications to the cessation of smoking. *Journal of Consulting and Clinical Psychology, 56*(4), 520–528.

Prochaska, J. O., Velicer, W. F., DiClemente, C. C., Guadagnoli, J. O., & Rossi, J. S. (1991). Patterns of change: Dynamic typology applied to smoking cessation. *Multivariate Behavioral Research, 26,* 83–107.

Prochaska, J. O., Velicer, W. F., Rossi, J. S., Goldstein, M. G., Marcus, B. H., Rakowski, W., Fiore, C., Harlow, L. L., Redding, C. A., Rosenbloom, D., & Rossi, S. R. (1994). Stages of change and decisional balance for twelve problem behaviors. *Health Psychology, 13*(1), 39–46.

Project MATCH Research Group. (1997a). Matching alcoholism treatments to client heterogeneity: Project MATCH post-treatment drinking outcomes. *Journal of Studies on Alcohol, 58*(1), 7–29.

Project MATCH Research Group. (1997b). Project MATCH secondary a priori hypotheses. *Addiction, 92*(12), 1671–1698.

Project MATCH Research Group. (1998a). Matching alcoholism treatments to client heterogeneity: Project MATCH three-year drinking outcomes. *Alcoholism Clinical and Experimental Research, 22,* 1300–1311.

Project MATCH Research Group. (1998b). Therapist effects in three treatments for alcohol problems. *Psychotherapy Research, 8*(4), 455–474.

Quigley, L. A., & Marlatt, G. A. (1996). Drinking among young adults: Prevalence, patterns, and consequences. *Alcohol Health and Research World, 20,* 185–191.

Quigley, L. A., & Marlatt, G. A. (1999). Relapse prevention: Maintenance of change after initial treatment. In B. S. McCrady & E. E. Epstein (Eds.), *Addictions: A comprehensive guidebook* (pp. 370–384). New York: Oxford University Press.

Raczynski, J. M., & DiClemente, R. J. (1999). *Handbook of health promotion and disease prevention.* New York: Kluwer Academic/Plenum.

Rakowski, W., Ehrich, B., Dube, C. E., & Pearlman, D. N. (1997). Screening mammography and constructs from the Transtheoretical Model: Associations using two definitions of the stages of adoption. *Annals of Behavioral Medicine, 18*(2), 91–100.

Reback, H. (1992). Alcohol and drug use among American minorities. In J. E. Trimble, C. S. Bolek, & S. J. Niemcryk (Eds.), *Ethnic and multicultural drug abuse: Perspectives on current research.* (pp. 23–58). New York: Haworth Press.

Regier, D. A., Farmer, M. E., Rae, D. S., Locke, B. Z., Keith, S. J., Judd, L. L., & Goodwin, F. K. (1990). Comorbidity of mental disorders with alcohol and other drugs. *Journal of the American Medical Association, 264,* 2511–2518.

Roberts, A. J., & Koob, G. J. (1997). The neurobiology of addiction: An overview. *Alcohol Health and Research World, 21*(2), 101–143.

Robins, L. (1974). A follow-up study of Vietnam veterans' drug use. *Journal of Drug Issues, 4,* 61–63.

Robins, L. N. (1979). Addict careers. In R. L. DuPont, A. Goldstein, & J., O'Donnell (Eds.), *Handbook on drug abuse* (pp. 325–336). Rockville, MD: National Institute on Drug Abuse.

Robins, L. N. (1980). The natural history of drug abuse. In U.S. Department of Health and Human Services, *Theories on drug abuse: Contemporary perspectives* (NIDA Research Monograph No. 30, pp. 215–225; DHHS Publication No. ADM 80-967). Washington, DC: U.S. Government Printing Office.

Robins, L. N., Helzer, J. E., & Davis, D. H. (1975). Narcotic use in Southeast Asia and afterward. *Archives of General Psychiatry, 2,* 955–961

Rogers, C. R. (1954). *Psychotherapy and personality change.* Chicago: University of Chicago Press.

Rogers, E. M. (1995). *Diffusion of innovations* (4th ed.). New York: Free Press.

Rollnick, S., Heather, N., & Bell, A. (1992). Negotiating behaviour change in medical settings: The development of brief motivational interviewing. *Journal of Mental Health, 1,* 25–39.

Rollnick, S., Mason, P., & Butler, C. (1999). *Health behavior change*. London: Churchill Livingstone.

Rosenthal, R. N., & Westreich, L. (1999). Treatment of persons with dual diagnoses of substance abuse disorders and other psychological problems. In B. S. McCrady & E. E. Epstein (Eds.), *Addictions: A comprehensive guidebook* (pp. 439–476) New York: Oxford University Press.

Rotgers, F., Keller, D. S., & Morgenstern, J. (Eds.). (1996). *Treating substance abuse: Theory and technique*. New York: Guilford Press.

Rothfleisch, J. (1997). *Comparison of two measures of stages of change among drug abusers*. Unpublished doctoral dissertation, University of Houston.

Ryan, R. M., & Deci, E. L. (2000). Self-determination theory and the facilitation of intrinsic motivation, social development, and well-being. *American Psychologist, 55,* 68–78.

Ryan, R. M., Plant, R. W., & O'Malley, S. (1995). Initial motivations for alcohol treatment: Relations with patient characteristics, treatment involvement, and dropout. *Addictive Behaviors, 20*(3), 279–297.

Rychtarik, R. G., Connors, G. J., Whitney, R. B., McGillicuddy, N. B., Fitterling, J. M., & Wirtz, P. W. (2000). Treatment settings for persons with alcoholism: Evidence for matching clients to inpatient versus outpatient care. *Journal of Consulting and Clinical Psychology, 68*(2), 277–289.

Sanjuan, P. M., & Langenbucher, J. W. (1999). Age-limited populations: Youth, adolescents, and older adults. In B. S. McCrady & E. E. Epstein (Eds.), *Addictions: A comprehensive guidebook*. (pp. 477–498). New York: Oxford University Press.

Sarason, B. R., Sarason, I. G., & Pierce, G. R. (1990). *Social support: An interactive view*. New York: Wiley.

Scheier, L. M., Botvin, G. J., & Griffin, K. W. (2001). Preventive intervention effects on developmental progression in drug use: Structural equation modeling analyses using longitudinal data. *Prevention Science, 2*(2), 91–112.

Schinke, S. P., Botvin G. J., & Orlandi, M. A. (1991). *Substance abuse in children and adolescents: Evaluation and intervention*. Newbury Park, CA: Sage.

Schmid, H., & Gmel, G. (1999). Identification and characteristics of clusters of smokers within the early stages of change. *Swiss Journal of Psychology, 58*(2) 111–122.

Schmidt, L. A., & Weisner, C. M. (1999). Public health perspectives on access and need for substance abuse treatment. In J. A. Tucker, D. M. Donovan, & G. A. Marlatt (Eds.), *Changing addictive behavior: Bridging clinical and public health strategies* (pp. 67–96). New York: Guilford Press.

Schorling, J. B. (1995). The stages of chnge of rural African-American smokers. *American Journal of Preventive Medicine, 11*(3), 170–177.

Schottenfeld, R. S. (1989). Involuntary treatment of substance abuse disorders—impediments to success. *Psychiatry, 52*(2), 164–176.

Schuckit, M. A. (1980). A theory of alcohol and drug abuse: A genetic approach. In D. J. Lettieri, M. Sayers, & H. W. Pearson (Eds.), *Theories on drug abuse: Selected contemporary perspectives* (NIDA Research Monograph No. 30, pp. 297–302; DHHS Publication No. ADM 80-967). Rockville, MD: National Institute on Drug Abuse.

Schuckit, M. A. (1995). A long-term study of sons of alcoholics. *Alcohol Health and Research World, 19*, 172–175.

Schuckit, M. A., Goodwin, D. W., & Winokur, G. A. (1972). A half-sibling study of alcoholism. *American Journal of Psychiatry, 128*, 1132–1136.

Schulenberg, J., Maggs, J. L., Steinman, K. J., & Zucker, R. A. (2001). Development matters: Taking the long view on substance abuse etiology and intervention during adolescence. In P. M. Monti, S. M. Colby, & T. A. O'Leary (Eds.), *Adolescents, alcohol, and substance abuse: Reaching teens through brief interventions* (pp. 19–57). New York: Guilford Press.

Schulenberg, J., Wadsworth, K. N., O'Malley, P. M., Bachman, J. G., & Johnston, L. D. (1996). Adolescent risk factors for binge drinking during the transition to young adulthood: Variable and pattern-centered approaches to change. *Developmental Psychology, 32*, 659–674.

Segal, B. (1992). Ethnicity and drug-taking behavior. In J. E. Trimble, C. S. Bolek, & S. J. Niemcryk (Eds.), *Ethnic and multicultural drug abuse: Perspectives on current research* (pp. 269–312). New York: Haworth Press.

Selvini-Palazzoli, M. (1974). *Self-starvation: From the intrapsychic to the transpersonal approach.* London: Chaucer.

Shaffer, H. J. (1992). The psychology of stage change: The transition form addiction to recovery. In J. H. Lowison, P. Ruiz, R. B. Millman, & J. G. Langrod (Eds.), *Substance abuse: A comprehensive textbook* (2nd ed., pp. 100–105). Baltimore, MD: Williams & Wilkins.

Shedler, J., & Block, J. (1990). Adolescent drug use and psychological health: A longitudinal inquiry. *American Psychologist, 45*, 612–630.

Sheehan, T., & Owen, P. (1999). The disease model. In B. S. McCrady & E. E. Epstein (Eds.), *Addictions: A comprehensive guidebook* (pp. 268–286). New York: Oxford University Press.

Sher, K. J. (1987). Stress response dampening. In K. E. Leonard & H. T. Blane (Eds.), *Psychological theories of drinking and alcoholism* (2nd ed., pp. 227–271). New York: Guilford Press.

Sher, K. J. (1993). Children of alcoholics and the intergenerational transmission of alcoholism: A biopsychosocial perspective. In J. S. Baer, G. A. Marlatt, & R. J. McMahon (Eds.), *Addictive behaviors across the lifespan: Prevention, treatment and policy issues* (pp. 3–33). Newbury Park, CA: Sage.

Sher, K. J., Walitzer, K. S., Wood, P. K., & Brent, E. E. (1991). Characteristics of children of alcoholics: Putative risk factors, substance use and abuse, and psychopathology. *Journal of Abnormal Psychology, 111*, 427–448.

Shiffman, S. (1982). Relapse following smoking cessation: A situational analysis. *Journal of Consulting and Clinical Psychology, 50*, 71–86.

Shiffman, S., Hickcox, M., Paty, J. A., Gnys, M., Kassel, J. D., & Richards, T. J. (1997). The abstinence violation effect following smoking lapses and temptations. *Cognitive Therapy and Research, 21*(5), 497–523.

Shiffman, S., & Wills, T. A. (Eds.). (1985). *Coping and substance abuse.* New York: Academic Press.

Simpson, D. D., & Joe, G. W. (1993). Motivation as a predictor of early dropout from drug abuse treatment. *Psychotherapy, 30*, 357–368.

Simpson, D. D., Joe, G. W., & Lehman, W. E. K. (1986). *Addiction careers: Sum-*

mary of studies based on the DARP 12–year follow-up (DHHS Publication No. ADM 86-1420). Rockville, MD: National Institute on Drug Abuse.

Simpson, D. D., & Sells, S. B. (1982). *Evaluation of drug abuse treatment effectiveness: Summary of the DARP follow-up research* (DHHS Publication No. ADM 82-12109). Rockville, MD: National Institute on Drug Abuse.

Skinner, B. F. (1938). *The behavior of organisms: An experimental analysis.* New York: Appleton-Century-Crofts.

Skinner, B. F. (1953). *Science and human behavior.* New York: Macmillan.

Slade, J. (1999) Nicotine. In B. S. McCrady & E. E. Epstein (Eds.), *Addictions: A comprehensive guidebook* (pp. 162–170). New York: Oxford University Press.

Sloane, R. B., Staples, F. R., Cristol, A. H., Yorkston, N. J., & Whipple, K. (1975). *Psychotherapy versus behavior therapy.* Cambridge, MA: Harvard University Press.

Smart, R. G. (1980). An availability-proneness theory of illicit drug abuse. In D. J. Lettieri, M. Sayers, & H. W. Pearson (Eds.), *Theories on drug abuse: Selected contemporary perspectives* (NIDA Research Monograph No. 30, pp. 46–49; DHHS Publication No. ADM 80-967). Rockville, MD: National Institute on Drug Abuse.

Smith, G. T., & Anderson, K. G. (2001). Personality and learning factors combine to create risk for adolescent problem drinking: A model and suggestions for intervention. In P. M. Monti, S. M. Colby, & T. A. O'Leary (Eds.), *Adolescents, alcohol, and substance abuse: Reaching teens through brief interventions* (pp. 109–144). New York: Guilford Press.

Smith, K. J., Subich, L. M., & Kolodner, C. (1995). The Transtheoretical Model's stages and processes of change and their relation to premature termination. *Journal of Counseling Psychology, 42,* 34–39.

Snow, M., Prochaska, J., & Rossi, J. (1994). Processes of change in Alcoholics Anonymous: Maintenance factors in long-term sobriety. *Journal of Studies on Alcohol, 55,* 362–371.

Sobell, L. C., Cunningham, J. A., Sobell, M. B., & Toneatto, T. (1993). A life-span perspective on natural recovery (self-change) from alcohol problems. In J. S. Baer, G. A. Marlatt, & R. J. McMahon (Eds.), *Addictive behaviors across the life span.* Newbury Park, CA: Sage.

Sobell, M. B., & Sobel, L. C. (1999). Stepped care for alcohol problems: An efficient method for planning and delivering clinical services. In J. A. Tucker, D. M. Donovan, & G. A. Marlatt (Eds.), *Changing addictive behavior* (pp. 331–343). New York: Guilford Press.

Soderstrom, C. A., Smith, G. S., Dischinger, P. C., McDuff, D. R., Hebel, J. R., Gorelick, D. A., Kerns, T. J., Shiu, H., & Read, K. M. (1997). Psychoactive substance use disorders among seriously injured trauma center patients. *Journal of the American Medical Association, 277,* 1769–1774.

Solomon, R., & Corbit, J. (1974). An opponent-process theory of motivation: Temporal dynamics of affect. *Psychological Review, 81,* 119–145.

Solomon, L. J., Secker-Walker, R. H., Skelly, J. M., & Flynn, B. S. (1996). Stages of change in smoking during pregnancy in low-income women. *Journal of Behavioral Medicine, 19,* 333–344.

Sorensen, G., Thompson, B., Glanz, K., Feng, Z., Kinne, S., DiClemente, C. C., Emmons, K., Heimendinger, J., Probart, C., Lichtenstein, E., & Working Well Trial. (1996). Worksite-based cancer prevention: Primary results from the Working Well trial. *American Journal of Public Health. 86*(7), 939–947.

Southwick, L., Steele, C., Marlatt, A., & Lindell, M. (1981). Alcohol-related expectancies: Defined by phase of intoxication and drinking experience. *Journal of Consulting and Clinical Psychology, 49*, 713–721.

Speiglman, R. (1997). Mandated AA attendance for recidivist drivers: Policy issues. *Addiction, 92*, 1133–1136.

Stanton, M. D. (1980). A family theory of drug abuse. In U.S. Department of Health and Human Services, *Theories on drug abuse: Contemporary perspectives* (NIDA Research Monograph No. 30, pp. 147–156; DHHS Publication No. ADM 80-967). Washington, DC: U.S. Government Printing Office.

Stanton, M. D., Todd, T. C., & Associates. (1982). *The family therapy of drug abuse and addiction.* New York: Guilford Press.

Stanton, M. D. (1997). Role of family and significant others in the engagement and retention of drug-dependent individuals. In L. S. Onken, J. D. Blaine, & J. J. Boren (Eds.), *Beyond the therapeutic alliance: Keeping the drug-dependent individual in treatment* (NIDA Research Monograph No. 165, pp. 157–180). Rockville, MD: National Institute on Drug Abuse.

Steffenhagen, R. A. (1980). Self-esteem theory of drug abuse. In D. J. Lettieri, M. Sayers, & H. W. Pearson (Eds.), *Theories on drug abuse: Selected contemporary perspectives* (NIDA Research Monograph No. 30, pp. 157–163; DHHS Publication No. ADM 80-967). Rockville, MD: National Institute on Drug Abuse.

Steinglass, P. L., Bennett, L., Wolin, S., & Reiss, D. (1987). *The alcoholic family.* New York: Basic Books.

Stewart, M. A., & Brown, S. A. (1993). Family functioning following adolescent substance abuse treatment. *Journal of Substance Abuse, 5*(4), 327–339.

Stotts, A., DiClemente, C. C., Carbonari, J. P., & Mullen, P. (1996). Pregnancy smoking cessation: A case of mistaken identity. *Addictive Behaviors, 21*, 459–471.

Stotts, A. L., DiClemente, C. C., Carbonari, J. P., & Mullen, P. D. (2000). Postpartum return to smoking: Staging a "suspended" behavior. *Health Psychology, 19*(4), 324–332.

Sue, D. W., & Sue, D. (2002). *Counseling the culturally diverse: Theory and practice* (4th ed.). New York: Wiley.

Suris, A. M., Trapp, M. C., DiClemente, C. C., & Cousins, J. (1998). Application of the Transtheoretical Model of behavior change for obesity in Mexican American women. *Addictive Behaviors, 23*(4), 655–668.

Sutker, P. B., & Allain, A. N. (1988). Issues in personality conceptualizations of addictive behaviors. *Journal of Consulting and Clinical Psychology, 56*(2) 172–182.

Sutton, S. (1996). Can "stage of change" provide guidance in treatment of addiction? A critical examination of Prochaska and DiClemente's model. In G. Edwards & C. Dare (Eds.), *Psychotherapy, psychological treatments and the addictions*. New York: Cambridge University Press.

Sutton, S. (2001). Back to the drawing board? A review of applications of the Transtheoretical Model to substance abuse. *Addiction, 96*(1), 175–186.

Tarter, R. E. (1988). Are there inherited behavioral traits that predispose to substance abuse? *Journal of Consulting and Clinical Psychology, 56*(2) 189–196.

Tarter, R. E., & Mezzich, A. C. (1992). Ontogeny of substance abuse: Perspectives and findings. In M. Glantz & R. Pickens (Eds.), *Vulnerability to drug abuse* (pp. 149–178). Washington, DC: American Psychological Association.

Tejero, A., Trujols, J., Hernandez, E., Perez de los Cobos, J., & Casas, M. (1997). Processes of change assessment in heroin addicts following the Prochaska and DiClemente Transtheoretical Model. *Drug and Alcohol Dependence, 47*(1), 31–37.

Tobler, N. (1986). Meta-analysis of 143 adolescent drug prevention programs: Quantitative outcome results of program participants compared to a control or comparison group. *Journal of Drug Issues, 16*, 537–567.

Trull, T. J., & Phares, E. J. (2001). *Clinical psychology* (6th ed.). Belmont, MA: Wadsworth/Thompson Learning.

Tucker, J. A., Donovan, D. M., & Marlatt, A. (Eds.). (1999). *Changing addictive behavior: Bridging clinical and public health strategies*. New York: Guilford Press.

Tucker, J. A., Vuchinich, R. E., & Pukish, M. M. (1995). Molar environmental contexts surrounding recovery from alcohol problems by treated and untreated problem drinkers. *Experimental and Clinical Psychopharmacology, 3*, 195–204.

U.S. Department of Health and Human Services. (1980). *Theories on drug abuse: Contemporary perspectives* (NIDA Research Monograph No. 30; DHHS Publication No. ADM 80-967). Washington, DC: U.S. Government Printing Office.

U.S. Department of Health and Human Services. (1990). *The health benefits of smoking cessation: A report of the Surgeon General* (DHHS Publication No. CDC 90–8416). Washington, DC: U. S. Government Printing Office.

U.S. Department of Health and Human Services. (1993, October). *National household survey on drug abuse: Population estimates 1992* (DHHS Publication No. 93–2053). Rockville, MD: Substance Abuse and Mental Health Services Administration, Office of Applied Studies.

U.S. Department of Health and Human Services. (1997). *Ninth special report to the U. S. Congress on alcohol and health*. Washington, DC: Public Health Service, National Institutes of Health, and National Institute on Alcohol Abuse and Alcoholism.

Vaillant, G. E. (1995). *The natural history of alcoholism revisited*. Cambridge, MA: Harvard University Press.

Velasquez, M. M., Carbonari, J. P., & DiClemente, C. C. (1999). Psychiatric severity and behavior change in alcoholism: The relation of Transtheoretical Model variables to psychiatric distress in dually diagnosed patients. *Addictive Behaviors, 24*(4), 481–496.

Velasquez, M. M., Maurer, G. G., Crouch, C., & DiClemente, C. C. (2001). *Group treatment for substance abuse: A stages-of-change therapy manual.* New York: Guilford Press.

Velasquez, M. M., Hecht, J., Quinn, V. P., Emmons, R. M., DiClemente, C. C., & Dolan-Mullen, P. (2000). Application of motivational interviewing to prenatal smoking cessation: Training and implementation issues. *Tobacco Control 2000, 9*(Suppl.), iii, 36–40.

Velicer, W. F., DiClemente, C. C., Prochaska, J. O., & Brandenburg, N. (1985) A decisional balance measure for assessing and predicting smoking status. *Journal of Personality and Social Psychology, 48*(5), 1279–1289.

Velicer, W. F., DiClemente, C. C., Rossi, J., & Prochaska, J. O. (1990). Relapse situations and self-efficacy: An integrative model. *Addictive Behaviors, 15*, 271–283.

Velicer, W. F., Fava, J. L., Prochaska, J. O., Abrams, D. B., Emmons, K. M., & Pierce, J. P. (1995). Distribution of smokers by stage in three representative samples. *Preventive Medicine, 24*, 401–411.

Velicer, W. F., Prochaska, J. O., Rossi, J. S., & Snow, M. (1992). Assessing outcome in smoking cessation studies. *Psychological Bulletin, 111*, 23–41.

Velicer, W. F., Prochaska, J. O., Bellis, J. M., DiClemente, C. C., Rossi, J. S., Fava, J. L., & Steiger, J. H. (1993). An expert system intervention for smoking cessation. *Addictive Behaviors, 18*, 269–290.

Volpicelli, J. R., Pettinati, H. M., McClellan, A. T., & O'Brien, C. P. (2001). *Combining medication and psychosocial treatments for addictions: The BRENDA approach.* New York: Guilford Press.

Vuchinich, R. E. (1999). Behavioral economics as a framework for organizing the expanded range of substance abuse interventions. In J. A. Tucker, D. M. Donovan, & G. A. Marlatt (Eds.), *Changing addictive behavior* (pp. 191–220). New York: Guilford Press.

Wagenaar, A. C., O'Malley, P. M., & LaFond, C. (2001). Lowered legal blood alcohol limits of young drivers: Effects on drinking driving and driving after drinking in 30 states. *American Journal of Public Health, 91*, 801–804.

Walker, R. D., Lambert, M. D., Walker, P. S., Kivlahal, D. R., Donovan, D. M., Howard, M. O., Mail, P. D., Beauvais, F., Westermeyer, J., Sack, W., Mitchell, C. M., Cohen, F., Kraus, R. F., Miller, T., Trimble, J. E., & Dinges, N. (1996). Alcohol abuse in urban Indian adolescents and women: A longitudinal study for assessment and risk evaluation. *American Indian and Alaska Native Mental Health Research, 7*(1), 1–97.

Walsh, D. C., Hingson, R. W., Merrigan, D. M., Levenson, S. M., Coffman, G. A., Heeren, T., & Cupples, L. A. (1992). The impact of a physician's warning on recovery after alcoholism treatment. *Journal of the American Medical Association, 267*(5) 663–667.

Weaver, M. F., & Schnoll, S. H. (1999). Stimulants: Amphetamines and cocaine. In B. S. McCrady & E. E. Epstein (Eds.), *Addictions: A comprehensive guidebook* (pp. 105–120). New York: Oxford University Press.

Weinstein, N. D., Rothman, A. J., & Sutton, S. R. (1998). Stage theories in health behavior: Conceptual and methodological issues. *Health Psychology, 17*(3), 290–299.

Weiss, R. D. (1992). The role of psychopathology in the transition from drug use to abuse and dependence. In M. Glantz & R. Pickens (Eds.), *Vulnerability to drug abuse* (pp. 137–148). Washington, DC: American Psychological Association.

Werch, C. E. (2001). Preventive alcohol interventions based on a stages of acquisition model. *American Journal of Health Behavior, 25*(3), 206–216.

Werch, C. E., Carlson, J. M., Owen, D. M., DiClemente, C. C., & Carbonari, J. P. (2001). Effects of a stage based alcohol prevention intervention for inner-city youth. *Journal of Drug Education, 31*(2), 123–138.

Werch, C. E., Carlson, J. M., Pappas, D. M., Dunn, M., & Williams, T. (1997). Risk factors related to urban youth stage of alcohol initiation. *American Journal of Health Behavior, 22*(5), 377–387.

Werch, C. E., & DiClemente, C. C. (1994). A multi-component stage model for matching drug prevention strategies and messages to youth stage of use. *Health Education Research: Theory and Practice, 9*(1), 37–46.

Werch, C. E., Pappas, D. M., Carlson, J. M., & DiClemente, C. C. (1998). Short and long term effects of a pilot prevention program to reduce alcohol consumption. *Substance Use and Misuse, 33*, 2303–2321.

Werch, C. E., Pappas, D. M., Carlson, J. M., DiClemente, C. C., Chally, P. S., & Sinder, J. A. (2000). Results of a social norm intervention to prevent binge drinking among first-year residential college students. *College Health, 49*, 85–92.

Whitehead, P. C., & Wechsler, H. (1980). Implications for future research and public policy. In H. Wechsler (Ed.), *Minimum-drinking-age laws.* Lexington, MA: Heath.

Wholey, D. (1984). *The courage to change.* New York: Warner Books.

Wickizer, T., Maynard, C., Artherly, A., Frederick, M., Koepsell, T., Krupski, A., & Stark, K. (1994, February). Completion rates of clients discharged from drug and alcohol treatment programs in Washington state. *American Journal of Public Health, 84*(2), 215–221.

Wierzbicki, M., & Pekarik, G. (1993). A meta-analysis of psychotherapy dropout. *Professional Psychology: Research and Practice, 29*, 190–195.

Wild, T. C., Newton-Taylor, B., & Alletto, R. (1998). Perceived coercion among clients entering substance abuse treatment: Structural determinants and psychological determinants. *Addictive Behaviors, 23*(1), 81–95.

Willoughby, R. W., & Edens, J. F. (1996). Construct validity and predictive utility of the stages of change scale for alcoholics. *Journal of Substance Abuse, 8*(3), 275–291.

Wills, T. A., McNamara, G., Vaccaro, D., & Hirky, A. E. (1996). Escalated substance use: A longititudinal grouping analysis from early to middle adolescence. *Journal of Abnormal Psychology, 105*, 166–180.

Wills, T. A., & Shiffman, S. (1985). Coping and substance use: A conceptual framework. In S. Shiffman & T. A. Wills (Eds.), *Coping and substance abuse.* Orlando, FL: Academic Press.

Windle, M., & Davies, P. T. (1999). Developmental theory and research. In K. E. Leonard & H. T. Blane (Eds.), *Psychological theories of drinking and alcoholism* (2nd ed., pp 164–202). New York: Guilford Press.

Windsor, R. A., Woodby, L. L., Miller, T. M., Hardin, J. M. Crawford, M. A., & DiClemente, C. C. (2000). Effectiveness of agency for health care policy and research clinical practice guideline and patient education methods for pregnant smokers in Medicaid maternity care. *American Journal of Obstetrics and Gynecology, 182*(1), 68–75.

Winters, J., Fals-Stewart, W., O'Farrell, T. J., Birchler, G. R., & Kelley, M. L. (2002). Behavioral couples therapy for female substance-abusing patients: Effects on substance abuse and relationship adjustment. *Journal of Consulting and Clinical Psychology, 70*(2), 344–355.

Wolpe, J. (1958). *Psychotherapy by reciprocal inhibition.* Stanford, CA: Stanford University Press.

Wonderlich, S. A. (1995). Personality and eating disorders. In K. D. Brownell & C. G. Fairburn (Eds.), *Eating disorders and obesity: A comprehensive handbook* (pp. 171–176). New York: Guilford Press.

Yahne, C. E., & Miller, W. R. (1999). Enhancing motivation for treatment and change. In B. S. McCrady & E. E. Epstein (Eds.), *Addictions: A comprehensive guidebook* (pp. 235–249). New York: Oxford University Press.

Ziedonis, D. M., & Trudeau, K. (1997). Motivation to quit using substances among individuals with schizophrenia: Implications for a motivation-based treatment model. *Schizophrenia Bulletin, 23,* 229–238.

Zimmerman, G. L., Olsen, C. G., & Bosworth, M. F. (2000). A "stages of change" approach to helping patients change behavior. *American Family Physician, 61*(5), 1406–1416.

Zucker, R. A., & Gomberg, E. S. L. (1986). Etiology of alcoholism reconsidered: The case for a biopsychosocial process. *American Psychologist, 41,* 783–793.

Index